THE HEALTHY HEART PROGRAM

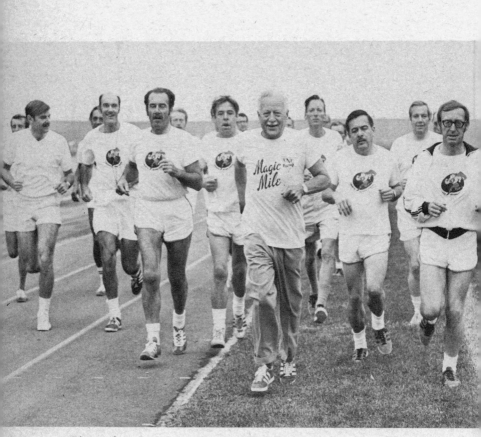

The author (extreme right) and cardiac patients jogging with former Governor General of Canada, Roland Michener (centre).

THE
HEALTHY
HEART
PROGRAM

Terence Kavanagh, M.D.

 Van Nostrand Reinhold Ltd., *Toronto*
New York, Cincinnati, London, Melbourne

For my mother
and
for Jo and "the guys"
who made it happen

Library of Congress Number 79-57601

Canadian Cataloguing in Publication Data

Kavanagh, Terence, 1927 —
    The Kavanagh program for a healthy heart

Expanded and up-dated version of the author's Heart attack? Counterattack! published 1976.

ISBN 0-442-29768-8

1. Heart — Diseases — Prevention. 2. Exercise therapy. I. Title. II. Title: Heart attack? Counterattack!

RC684.E9K38 1980   616.1′23062   *C80-094158-6*

Editorial consultant: Diane Mew
Graphs by Julian Cleva
Cover photograph by Paterson Photographic Works
Printed and bound in Canada by Webcom Limited

Photograph Credits

The Publisher is grateful for the assistance of those who have provided the photographs used in this book. Every care has been taken to acknowledge below the correct sources. The Publisher would welcome information that will permit the correction of any errors or omissions.

Rudy Crestle: 144 (top right, top left)
David Lee: 10
Rawlins Mohammed: 145 (bottom)
Noel Nequin, M.D.: 59, 107 (top)
G. Pinna: 128 (top)
Toronto Rehabilitation Centre (Chris Stutzman):106
Toronto Star Syndicate: ii
All other photographs have been provided by the author

80 81 82 83 84 85 86 10 9 8 7 6 5 4 3 2 1

Contents

Preface

Since the 1920s the incidence of heart disease has relentlessly increased, until today it has assumed the proportions of a pandemic. The now so familiar "heart attack" is the greatest single killer in the modern world.

This book is the outcome of eight years' work at the Toronto Rehabilitation Centre where I have directed the assessment and training of close to one thousand patients suffering from coronary artery disease. It attempts to provide an outline of the methods we have used at the Centre in the conditioning and training of patients who have sustained a heart attack. It also contains information which, I hope, will be of use not only to the person who has had a heart attack, but also to the coronary candidate — which in this day and age means any male over the age of forty.

The contents are intended primarily for the intelligent layman who would like to explore the fascinating fields of endurance exercise and rehabilitation medicine. Thus, there is enough elementary physiology as is needed to explain the changes which occur with physical fitness, enough medicine to help the layman understand the nature of heart disease and enough coaching technique to enable the exerciser to grasp the rationale behind an effective training regime. The specialist in any of these areas should look elsewhere if he expects to find erudition for erudition's sake. The approach is essentially pragmatic and the goal is quite clear-cut — to reduce the risk of heart attack by encouraging the development of a healthy, active lifestyle.

The first part of the book, therefore, deals with the various "risk factors" associated with the high incidence of heart disease.

You, the reader, should decide which of these may be applicable to you, and then try to modify your lifestyle accordingly. No matter where your susceptabilities may lie — whether it be a high level of blood fat, obesity, excessive cigarette smoking, or a bad family history of heart disease — I am confident that you will find a safer lifestyle more easily attainable if you adopt the cardiac training methods outlined in Part Two.

I am indebted to countless individuals for their help not only with the program, but also for their direct and indirect assistance with the manuscript itself. There are some, however, whom it would be churlish of me not to single out. Professor Roy Shephard, my very good friend and colleague, has been a constant source of help and reference. His good-natured response to my occasional cavalier descriptions of the more subtle intricacies of his speciality are an indication that despite his international reputation as a scientist, he retains to a high degree the pragmatism inherent in every good physician. My manuscript secretary Margaret Hepburn, has laboured long and hard in this past three years, enduring my erratic deadlines with incredible good humour, always ready with tactful suggestions both on content and the more mundane details of grammatical construction and spelling. Johanna Kennedy, track and field "expert", head of my Cardiac Rehabilitation Department, has provided invaluable advice and help, and her hand is evident throughout most of these pages. She and her team, including technicians, therapists, physical educators, and secretarial staff, deserve full credit not only for the success of the program, but also for the accumulation and preparation of much of the data upon which the book was based. Without such a team there would be no program to write about.

There are two other indispensable ingredients to the whole picture; the patients who are on the program and the physicians who referred them. May I go on record now with a sincere thanks for their trust and their confidence in the program and the people who operate it.

Needless to say, the ultimate responsibility for the content of these pages is mine, and I accept in advance full censure for any shortcomings, medical or otherwise.

Terry Kavanagh
Toronto
April 1976

Preface to the Second Edition

This year sees the second edition of *Heart Attack? Counterattack!* (now entitled *The Healthy Heart Program*), and the twelfth anniversary of the Toronto Rehabilitation Centre's Post-Coronary Exercise Program. The prime movers in the latter of these happy events, Johanna ("Jo") Kennedy, Professor "Robin" Campbell, and myself are still very much in the picture — even more so. In these times, when the emphasis seems to be on increased "mobility" and change, I like to think this is rather exceptional, and explains to a large extent why the exercise program is so phenomenally successful. Not only that, but of the eight men who ran that never-to-be-forgotten first Boston Marathon in 1973, all but Big John, who died in his sleep in 1975, are alive and well and running — five of them members of the TRC Joggers and each completing two or three marathons annually. And this year, 1980, our largest ever contingent of cardiac runners finished the Boston — an impressive total of sixteen.

As the years have gone by, increasing patient referrals to the program have led to the construction of a two-storey addition to the Centre. This is devoted solely to the rehabilitation of cardiac patients. It is fully equipped to deal, not only with the heart attack and post-aortocoronary bypass patient, but also the individual with the early symptoms of coronary artery disease, as well as those who fall into the "high risk" category. Jo Kennedy's staff has grown from its first humble beginnings of five part-timers in 1968 to twenty-five full-time professionals, including three physicians, and thirty-five part-time therapists. There seems little doubt that the concept of cardiac rehabilitation has achieved a high degree of acceptance with the medical profession and public alike. It is also gratifying to see the principles embodied in the first edition of this book play a major part in the formation of similar programs in places as far afield as Singapore and Cape Town, as well as some closer to home such as Chicago, Houston and Los Angeles.

This second edition updates where necessary. The section on cholesterol and diet has been rewritten and expanded, in line with newer thinking on the subject. An entire new section has been added in order to cater to the surge of newcomers to jogging and "fun marathoning," many of whom will welcome advice on training methods, precautions, recognition and treatment of injuries, et cetera. The aim, however, is the same: the presentation of important and useful physiological and medical information on exercise, fitness and coronary artery disease in a clear and comprehensible manner, without sacrificing accuracy for the sake of simplicity. To be perfectly frank, the degree to which I have been successful in attaining this goal is due in no small part to the efforts of my erstwhile manuscript typist, Margaret Hepburn, and my ever-patient, persuasive editor, Diane Mew (yes, same team as last time). Where I don't quite pull it off, I suspect I have insisted on having my own way!

T.K.
Toronto 1980

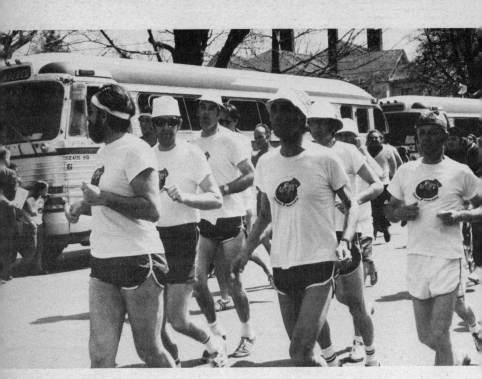

Starting out in the 1973 Boston Marathon; members of the T.R.C. *post-coronary program.*

Prologue

At twelve noon on April 15, 1973, a gun went off in the town square of the little town of Hopkinton, Massachusetts, marking the start of the seventy-seventh annual Boston Marathon. Before the echoes of the report had died, the cavalcade of over 1,500 runners had set out on the punishing 26-mile, 385-yard road course which would lead them from Hopkinton, through the town of Framingham, and on to the finish line in Prudential Square, downtown Boston. Lining the course would be the good citizens of Boston, ever ready to cheer the leaders, encourage the plodders, provide water and orange slices to the thirsty, and generally give succour to the limping, footsore and exhausted rearguard — the valiant losers who were determined to finish, no matter how long it took.

The seventy-seventh Boston was tough; the temperatures during the run were the highest ever recorded, in the high 70's and low 80's. Heat is the curse of the sweating marathon runner; it depletes his body of its water and salt stores, leaving him susceptible to heat stroke and all its attendant dangers, including kidney failure. It was not surprising, then, that in the 1973 race ten runners were admitted to hospital suffering from heat exhaustion. Many others dropped out, their initial high spirits changing to silent grim resolve and finally to grunting despair as their pace fell from a high-stepping stride to a monotonous jog and finally to a reeling walk. But, as usual, hundreds of determined runners did finish; and among them was a group of seven middle-aged men from Toronto, Canada. As, one by one, each of the seven crossed the finish line, they were embraced, congratulated and fussed over by a physician, a nurse and a medical technician who had accompanied them by car throughout the run; their body weights and blood pressures were measured, their electrocardiograms recorded, and samples of their blood and urine taken.

Why all this special care? The crowds of spectators still gathered in Prudential Square to cheer the latecomers little realized that these seven men had just achieved a milestone in the history of rehabilitation medicine. Incredibly, they were all heart attack victims; each had sustained a fully documented myocardial infarction (heart attack) one to four years previously; three of them had, in fact, suffered two attacks. Protégés of the Toronto Rehabilitation Centre's post-coronary rehabilitation program instituted by the author, their feat was the outcome of five years of experience and research into the effects of medically supervised exercise in the survivors of mankind's greatest scourge — coronary heart disease.

By the time you read this book, I hope it will be commonplace for the individual who has had a heart attack to be rehabilitated not only back to his former job, but also to the vigorous sports and activities of his choice. If so, it should be realized that this is a recent development. I can clearly recall that as a young, recently qualified intern (and that was only twenty years ago!), I was taught to maintain the heart attack patient on strict bed rest for four weeks, and then allow only gradual mobilization for a further two weeks. Very little activity was permitted for three months, and thereafter the watchword was "take it easy" — often for life. Small wonder the patient's morale was so low. Frightened to work, frightened to exert himself, frightened to have sex, he frequently became a rehabilitation nightmare. We now know that his enforced period of prolonged rest not only sapped his confidence, it also weakened his muscles, softened his bones and reduced even further the pumping efficiency of the very organ we were trying to strengthen — his heart.

However, we are ahead of ourselves. At the time when our seven men set out to jog the Boston Marathon, no other post-coronary had, to our knowledge, ever successfully attempted it. They were truly stepping into the unknown. After all, no amount of performance on the laboratory treadmill or the training track can equal the combined mental and physical stress of the real thing. The degree to which such attempts have become relatively commonplace is a tribute to them. A less likely looking group of heroes you will never see, but I view them as just that. The methods used in their physical restoration will be described in later chapters but I would like to begin with the story of their personal Everest and how they conquered it. I hope it will be an inspiration to you who have had a heart attack, or for whom (unless you take steps to avoid it) such an event lies in the future.

The Boston Marathon, 1973

Actually, eight post-coronary patients made the trip to Boston. The eighth man, 42-year-old Hal L., had decided from the outset that he would attempt only the "demi-marathon," or $13^1/2$ miles. This decision was not based on health reasons, but because his business commitments prevented him from putting in the extra hours of training necessary to ensure success. On the day of the race, he attained his goal comfortably, his only complaint being one of slight dizziness due to dehydration. Had he been able to train adequately, I have no doubt he would have been capable of jogging the whole distance. As it was, he followed medical directions implicitly, did not attempt more than his training program permitted, and deserves every bit as much credit as his seven colleagues.

The kernel of the Toronto Rehabilitation Centre's post-coronary program is exercise, the major activity being long distance jogging (that is, slow, relaxed running). In our experience, this is the best way to attain endurance fitness, which is the only form of fitness of benefit to the heart. But, as you will learn later, endurance fitness cannot be stored. You must work zealously to maintain it, otherwise it will deteriorate inexorably and become reduced by inactivity until finally it has all gone, and your ultimate state will be no better than your first — or maybe even worse, according to some studies. This means, for our cardiacs, staying on a jogging program for the rest of their lives — which we anticipate will be lengthy.

Man is by nature gregarious, and long-distance running is a lonely sport. Running in groups helps to alleviate the boredom (although personally, I find a two-hour solitary jog a stimulating experience), and tends to prevent "back-sliding" from the regular training routine. Thus it was that our most enthusiastic post-coronary joggers began to meet regularly at weekends for long easy runs through the pleasant park system which surrounds the Centre. Initially, these were made under medical surveillance with members of the staff accompanying the men on bicycles, and a truck containing resuscitation equipment cruising alongside. The accomplishment of the first five miles was a great achievement, only to recede into mediocrity as we managed seven miles, and then ten. Running with the men, I also gained confidence until ultimately I felt we could dispense with the medical cortege (although — and the men were never aware of it until this moment — for months, I continued to run with a hypodermic syringe, needle and three vials of heart medication strapped to my abdomen just in case!) Even I, an ex-sprinter and long-jumper, began to enjoy the long runs. We discussed the pros and cons of different routes through the park, the advantages and disadvantages of various brands of running shoes, the physiology of continuous as opposed to interval running, and so on. Heart disease was forgotten and gradually, over the weeks, my title changed from "Doctor" to "Doc" to "Coach." After our run one day, Ken S., a graphic designer and at 56 the senior member with two heart attacks to his credit, unveiled a crest for our running shirt — the figure of Superman proudly showing a large cracked heart on his chest! We were no longer a doctor/patient group. We had arrived; we were a running club.

For as long as I can remember, I have been involved in the sport of track and field, first as an indifferent performer, and then as an administrator, official and sports physician. I am as familiar with track clubs as I am with post-coronary exercise classes — and knew that there was a basic difference between a true track club and our new club. The driving force of any track club is competition, the desire to run faster, at your chosen distance, than any member of your own or any other club; in short, to knock the hell out of anyone rash enough to challenge you on the track, or die in the attempt. Obviously, I could allow no such choice of alternatives in our group; the men were running for their health. As the famous New Zealand coach, Arthur Lydiard, put it, their aim was "to train, not strain." Their ages varied widely, from Herman R. at 30 to Ken S. at 56. John N. had sustained his heart attack as recently as 15 months ago, whereas John R. was the first patient referred to our class after his second heart attack in 1968. John R., together with Harry B. and Ken S., had suffered more than one attack. For our group to indulge in racing one another would have been (and still is) not only imprudent, but pointless. Yet how to maintain club interest and motivation without the stimulus of competition? The answer was, of course, simple. Each man would compete against himself. There was no reason why each could not attain 15 or even 20 miles. Distance would be the goal. The variable would be the pace at which they accomplished it. The only limitations would be those imposed medically.

But, said the men, if distance was to be our aim, why not pick a distance which had the stamp of official recognition? Ever since the birth of the modern Olympic Games in 1896, the marathon run has been the pièce de résistance, the longest foot race in any official track and field contest. Commemorating the feat of Pheidippides who ran from the battlefield of Marathon to the city of Athens to announce the news of the Greek victory, it remains to this day one of the most gruelling tests of endurance an athlete can attempt.

One day, while we were changing after a five-mile run, someone half jokingly remarked how great an achievement it would be to finish a marathon. For a second or two there was complete silence, a few questioning glances, an uneasy grin, and finally one or two doubtful laughs. Then the moment was gone. But not for long. Gradually, week by week, the idea grew in our minds. What at first seemed to be a preposterous joke became a serious consideration and then a firm resolve. For me it was, in a way, the moment of truth. I had motivated these men to run; as far as I was concerned they were rehabilitated, and I had made no bones in telling them so. They had trusted me. To put it succinctly, the time had come to put up or shut up! I decided that we would make the attempt. Since that, for me, momentous decision, I have on two occasions heard my judgment publicly criticized. A prominent psychologist active in the field of coronary disease prevention, labelled the attempt as "silly." A well-known cardiologist, a pioneer in post-coronary exercise therapy referred to it as "showboating" — apparently forgetting how proud he was some years previously to announce that one of his rehabilitated heart patients was able to run five miles in 35 minutes. The difference between acceptable medical practice and ostentatious posturing would seem to be a question of mileage!

Our aim, then, would be to complete an official marathon

run. In that way, we would have the satisfaction of running over a road course which had been officially measured and certified. To come unscathed through such an ordeal without excessive strain or damage to the heart would not only be an achievement in itself, but it would have the added advantage of focusing attention on the value of exercise therapy in cardiac rehabilitation. Furthermore, it would restore confidence to other heart attack victims who felt that their active lives were over and that all they had to look forward to was a life of semi-invalidism.

As for the specific race, what better than the famous Boston Marathon. Held annually every Patriots' Day, and dating back to 1897, this event attracts runners from all over the world. Just four hundred miles or so down the highway from Toronto, we could drive there in a day. Official entry, however, was limited to those who had successfully completed a sanctioned marathon race in under $3^{1}/_{2}$ hours. Obviously, the men could not be official entrants — although at the time of writing, four of them could qualify. Fortunately for us, the Boston Marathon is renowned for its numerous "unofficial" entrants. On the day of the race, there are always hundreds of aspiring joggers from all over the United States and Canada at the starting line, minus official numbers but determined nevertheless to pit their endurance against the arduous Boston course. It was now August, and we had eight months of hard training before us if we were to join them.

If you want to run 26 miles non-stop, you have to attain an average weekly mileage of nearly twice that in training. The men were running 20 miles or so weekly at this stage, so they had a long way to go. The progression had to be slow and careful, otherwise their middle-aged muscles and tendons would injure, and they would miss valuable training sessions. Progress was checked by regular laboratory tests on the bicycle ergometer and treadmill. Their electrocardiograms were simultaneously recorded during these tests. From time to time, they were telemetered while running (a small radio-transmitter is attached to the runner's chest, and this transmits his electrocardiogram back to a receiver in the Centre as he runs around the track). It was agreed that at any time, the "coach" could revert to the role of the "doc" and imperiously forbid a man to take part in the run, even right up to the time of the gun. Lofty power indeed for a track coach, but one recognized to be essential under the circumstances. My responsibility was clearly to protect anyone who developed adverse signs or symptoms from allowing his enthusiasm and zeal to run away with his commonsense. The men saw it differently. "If anything happens to us," they said, "the Doc will be lucky to get a job in a remote jungle hospital so far away it will cost $10 to mail him a postcard!"

By Christmas, everyone was fitter than I would have believed possible, but the days were getting shorter and colder. Running in the dark became a necessity as the mileage increased. Luminous strips on shoes and sweat suits were adopted after Harry B. narrowly missed injury from an overtaking truck which decided to share the soft shoulder with him. We learned to run in temperatures as low as 10°F above zero (—12.2C), using suitable clothing and an "anti-angina" mask developed for the purpose. A visiting physician from a warmer clime was particularly disturbed by this and felt that such a practice was "suicide" for coronary patients. This has not been my experience, and the lessons we learned that winter have now been applied to the entire post-coronary class. With proper precautions, it is perfectly safe for such patients to walk and jog in temperatures down to 15°F above zero (—9.4C). As a matter of fact, I am much more concerned when the weather is hot and humid.

Throughout January, February and March we continued to train, and on only three occasions were we prevented by heavy snowfalls from using the roads. I can still recall vividly, however, the Sunday we decided to have our first trial attempt at 26 miles. An hour after the start, it started to rain — freezing rain! The men kept doggedly on, some managing the whole course, others having to quit after 18 to 20 miles because of the terrible conditions. Six-foot two-inch John R.'s sodden, frozen sweat suit weighed 10 lbs. at the finish. All of the wives must have thought their husbands insane on arrival home to report that they had run through one of the worst ice storms of the winter. Yet no one even caught a cold; if they could survive this, they could survive anything.

The weekend of the marathon fast approached. At first, it was decided that we would tell no one of the attempt until after the race was over. Then Don C., one of the runners who worked for CFRB, a Toronto radio station, intimated that Betty Kennedy, one of their leading interviewers, was interested in pre-taping an interview with some of us before leaving for Boston, and she would withhold the play-back until the day of the race. We agreed to this, and Mrs. Kennedy was as good as her word. She handled the whole interview in a most ethical manner, emphasizing throughout that this was a medically supervised endeavour and not a wildcat gamble. Furthermore, CFRB arranged for Charles Dearing, their news reporter, to cover the run, and he was able to send reports back to Toronto throughout. These were announced as they were received, thus alleviating some natural apprehension felt by the waiting wives.

We left Toronto to drive to Boston two days before the race. Accompanying the men were a medical team of three: myself, Johanna Kennedy, the nurse coordinator of the program, and Salah Qureshi, our chief medical technician. In addition to the usual resuscitation equipment, we carried instruments to measure body weight, blood pressure, electrocardiograms, as well as various substances in the blood, for we intended to learn as much as we could about the effect of such stress on the post-coronary patient. All sorts of people helped in varied and assorted ways, not the least of which were two of Canada's veteran marathon runners, Ron Wallingford and Bob Moore. Ron is now a professor of physical education at Laurentian University, Sudbury, and he gave us some valuable tips as to how to tackle the course; after all, he had completed it himself eight times. Bob Moore is a biochemist at the nearby University of Toronto, Sunnybrook Medical Centre, and he provided much of the technical advice regarding the biochemical tests. My colleague and friend, Roy Shephard, professor of applied physiology at the University of Toronto, is consultant physiologist to the Toronto Rehabilitation Centre, and his help on the testing procedures and later evaluation of the results was invaluable.

On the morning of the race, everyone was a little on edge. We had driven over the course the day before, and found that 26¼ miles seems even longer in a car than it does on foot. After all our winter training (the temperature when we left Toronto was in the 40's), we were mortified to discover a warm, balmy day. As the morning wore on, the temperature climbed. We occupied ourselves with last-minute measurements of weight, blood pressures and calculation of fluid intake. Finally, with five minutes to go, our eight stalwarts moved to the starting point, placing themselves well in the rear of the 1,500 or so packed runners.

If you've never witnessed the start of a large marathon, you may find it hard to understand what an emotional experience it can be. The tension mounts as the minutes tick off to the start. The officials bustle and shout instructions, the runners dance restlessly or stand morosely, as their personalities decree; some talk incessantly and laugh loudly, other cross themelves quietly, and the police motorcyclists who are to cover the whole route race their engines in an increasing crescendo of noise, as if anxious to be on their way. Finally, just as you think it will never come, there is the hoarse familiar command, "On your marks," the starting gun fires, the noise of the motorcycle engines increases to a deafening roar, and the whole pack is on its way, the top runners already fighting to get clear of the ruck and establish a strategic position.

On this occasion, I had little time to dwell on the scene. As our men left, Jo Kennedy and Salah Qureshi quickly gathered the discarded sweat suits, and the three of us ran to the waiting cars ready to drive to our first rendezvous a few miles down the course. We made the meeting place with minutes to spare and as each man passed, he seemed to be running easily and relaxed.

Throughout the remainder of the race, the medical team must have driven the course three times over. We knew that after the $13^1/2$-mile mark, provided all was going well, our runners would be strung out considerably. This meant that we could not accompany them as a group, but would have to "leapfrog" the cars, trying to check each man's condition every mile or so, while at the same time briefly meeting with each other to compare notes and decide who needed the most attention.

Hal L. made his half-way mark, and I quickly carried out my post-race examination — on the tailgate of our station wagon. He was in great shape and after he had hurriedly changed in the car, he acted as an extra driver for the medical team, and proved to be invaluable. As the miles wore on, Herman R., 32 years old, gradually pulled ahead of the rest; at the 24-mile mark he felt nauseated and developed stomach cramps and asked me if it was alright to continue. I checked him to assure that it was okay and gave him permission to carry on. He went on to cross the finish line, the first of our group to do so (and, as far as I know, the first post-coronary patient ever to complete the distance; if someone else can justly claim that honour, then Herman and I offer him our heartiest congratulations). Don C., age 40, was close behind and came in running strongly. Then one by one and so fast that I barely had time to get my measurements and Charlie Dearing to interview them, each appeared at the finish line.

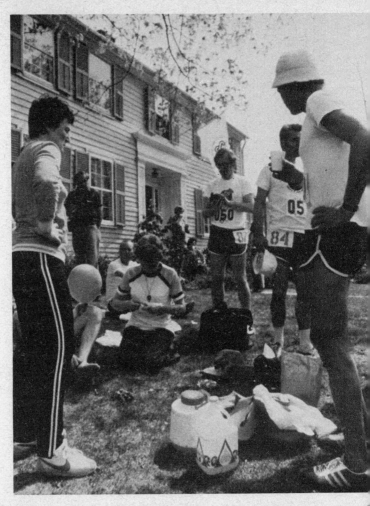

T.R.C. *marathoners: facing page, right, pride of achievement after t*
Honolulu Marathon, 1974; facing page, left, blood pressure check, Bost
Marathon, 1973; above, preparing to begin the 1976 Boston Marathon (
100 degree heat); lower right, a trophy presented to Supercoach, Dr. Ter
Kavanagh, by his patients, the world's "sickest" track club.

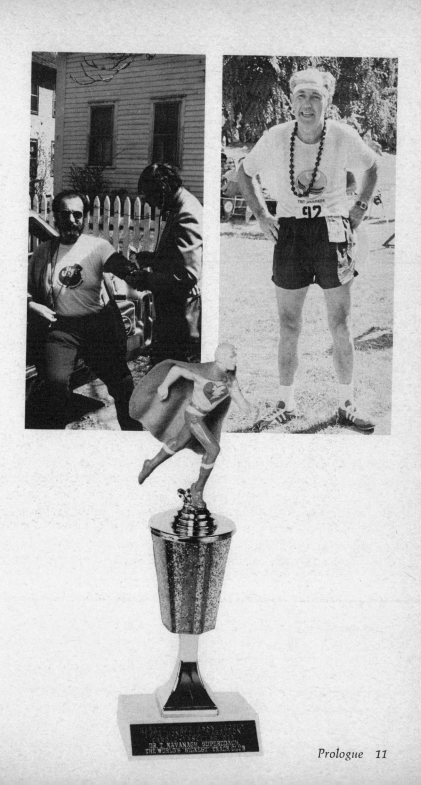

Dino V., followed by Harry B., then John N., John R. and finally Ken S. They were all tired, but happy and in excellent physical condition despite having lost an average of 8 lbs. body weight through dehydration. Each of them has his memories of the race: the girls' school at the 20-mile mark which raised a great shout of "Up Canada" as each one passed; the incredible experience of actually overtaking scores of other non-cardiac runners in the latter stages of the run; but, above all, the Boston crowds whose constant encouragement was a tonic. As Ken put it, "when I eventually got to Prudential Square, I thought everyone would have gone home. I couldn't believe it; here were hundreds of people clapping and cheering a 56-year-old s.o.b. who was so far back they'd lost count. I couldn't help it, as I crossed the line, for the first time since I was four years old, I broke down and cried."

That night, back in the motel, after all the post-race examinations and tests were completed, the eleven of us celebrated. The hard training had paid off, and we had proved our point. Hopefully, the days would be numbered when the heart attack victim is treated as a semi-invalid — automatically refused a private pilot's licence, cheated out of promotion because he would be "under too much pressure," and heavily rated by his insurance company. Old customs and attitudes die hard, but at least a crack might have been made in the wall of prejudice.

The publicity surrounding the run was extensive, and led Dr. Jack Scaff, a Honolulu cardiologist and long distance running enthusiast, to introduce a cardiac division into the First Honolulu Marathon held in December 1973. For the first time, post-coronary patients could enter a marathon officially. We were invited to participate, and I accompanied Herman R., Harry B. and Don C. to Honolulu. They finished a half hour faster than in Boston and in fine condition; we had learned from our previous experience and provided sufficient fluid before and during the race to reduce the weight loss to acceptable levels. Just as important, one of Dr. Scaff's post-coronary patients, Val N., a 42-year-old Hawaiian, also finished. He ran in Boston the following year as well, and became the first post-coronary American citizen to successfully complete the course.

Meanwhile, in Toronto, our club is now officially registered with the Canadian Track and Field Association and thus becomes the first track club in the world which requires that its president be a physician, its secretary a nurse, and all of its members to 'ave had a heart attack. Its members are recruited from the ranks of the Centre's post-coronary class. The club colours are funereal black, its constitution simple (see appendix), and its aim to promote long distance running as a means of combatting coronary artery disease. We refer to ourselves as the "sickest track club in the world." Within recent months, we have had four more of the group accomplish the marathon distance, including one who has had heart surgery. Herman's latest official time for the marathon is 3 hours, 11 minutes; Dino has a 3 hours, 22 minutes to his credit; Don, 3 hours, 28 minutes; and Harry, 3 hours, 29 minutes, while Ken is now down to 4 hours 20 minutes.

Now a personal note. Rehabilitation medicine is the poor cousin of the medical specialties. While lip service is paid to it by all governments and governing medical bodies, little has been done to elevate the status of the specialty. Many hospitals do not have a rehabilitation department; if they do, it usually occupies space in the basement (often next to the laundry), where it functions as a physiotherapy department providing heat and limited exercise to patients with musculo-skeletal disease.

But rehabilitation medicine is more than that — how much more would take me a whole new book to explain. Let's just say for now that it is encouraging the motivation that enabled the cerebral palsy victim, Christie Brown, to give the world his beautiful book *All Down the Days;* or teaching a paraplegic to become independent; or seeing a group of heart attack victims tackle and succeed in a task they never in all their lives thought they were capable of. Such events are what medicine, and life, is all about; they are basic to our survival as a species. Which is why all of the foregoing is written as if it really mattered to all of us; I happen to think it does.

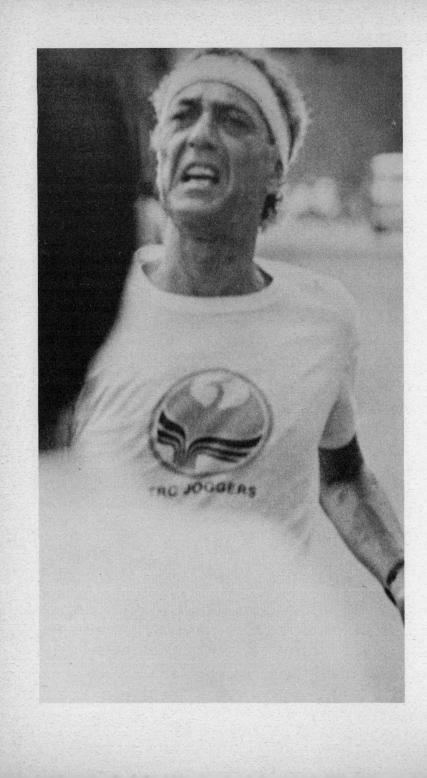

Part One

Courage was mine, and I had mystery
Wisdom was mine, and I had mastery.

Wilfred Owen

CHAPTER ONE

The Modern Plague

THE ancient Greeks believed in gods who could be both spiteful and capricious, from time to time playing cruel tricks not only on one another but also upon that vulnerable creature, man. Certainly the study of human history cannot help but leave one with the impression that whoever or whatever controls our fate possesses a malevolent sense of humour — with the joke inevitably being on us. If the current vogue in sick jokes is an updated version of this idea, then surely the sickest one-liner in history is that simple three-word title, "coronary care unit."

For those of you who have had a heart attack, a detailed description of a coronary care unit is likely both unnecessary and depressing. For those of you who have bought this book because you wish to avoid finding yourself in such a situation in the future, suffice to say that the ccu is one of the ultimate expressions of man's achievements in the field of medical electronics: a private observation ward where no privacy exists, where the patient's blood pressure, respiratory rate, heart action and other vital signs are constantly monitored, 24 hours a day, by automatic instruments which not only record every breath and every heart beat, but also alert the watching nurse by audio and visual signalling devices of any irregularity.

Only within recent years has such a unit become possible. Until the 1960's, we possessed only two of the three essential ingredients for a ccu — the nurse and the patient. The third ingredient, the highly sophisticated electronic instrumentation, is the product of our technological age. And herein lies the joke, for it now seems likely that this same era of science and the computer which gave us mastery of the air, journeys to the moon, and machines which think, has also imposed upon the human being a lifestyle incompatible with survival. An exaggeration? The World Health Organization has recognized the increased incidence of heart disease in modern times to be "of the utmost urgency." Dr. W. Kannel, medical director of a large-scale investigation of cardiovascular disease in the United States, goes further and refers to it as "the greatest sustained epidemic confronting mankind."

The plain facts are that heart attacks kill and disable more people in the western world today than any other single disease, and that includes cancer, chest disease, alcoholism and motor vehicle accidents. As the affluent life spreads to the non-western countries, so their incidence of heart disease begins to climb. Ironically, society seems to have developed the ability to furnish the ccu with both equipment and patients in the same era. Whether or not this curious relationship is coincidental or causal is a matter which we will explore later but, in the meantime, we will take a closer look at the villain of the piece, M.I.1 — as good a code name as any for today's number one killer, myocardial infarction, or the "heart attack" of popular parlance.

Profile of a Heart Attack Victim

John S. was entitled to feel pleased with himself. A professional engineer, at 41 he possessed all the contemporary hallmarks of success: a happy marriage, two teenage boys who were doing well at school, a comfortable house (almost paid for) in a desirable neighbourhood, and the imminent prospect of promotion to company vice-president. Mind you, he hadn't had too much time of late to count his blessings; a year previously the company plant started moving to a new location and, as production manager, he had found himself involved in a hectic work schedule. Even Mary, his usually so-patient wife, began to express concern as six- and seven-day work weeks became routine. Still, the job had to be done and "goodness only knows what a mess things would get into if I wasn't there to keep tabs on everything." Besides, when the move was completed, he could ease off a bit, maybe "play a little golf, or take a week's vacation and get in a little fishing." Maybe he would cut back on his smoking too; with all his stress and strain he was up to a pack and a half a day now . . . wouldn't do any harm to lose a little weight also, but that was difficult when one's meals consisted of an endless succession of hurried sandwiches interspersed with "two-martini luncheon meetings" and expense-account dinners.

Yes, he probably was a little out of shape — which no doubt accounted for the heartburn and indigestion pain he had begun to experience in recent months whenever he got up-tight at work or tried to lift anything heavy. He was "probably developing a a peptic ulcer," the almost prestigious occupational disease of all successful executives.

In due course, John's plant completed its move to the new location. But the transition phase brought with it teething problems which, naturally, only John could solve. Admittedly, weekends at the office were no longer routine (although they did occur from time to time), but the twelve- and thirteen-hour workday became commonplace. Always a hard driver, he was now hotly in pursuit of the presidency, and he dedicated himself to the task with all the energy and determination which had characterized his performance as one of the best linemen of his university football team. Unfortunately, he wasn't in his early twenties any more and while he still possessed the spirit and motivation of bygone years, his body was no longer fit enough to endure the tasks he placed upon it. His "indigestion" pain was bothering him more frequently now, and not only after eating. From time to time he experienced severe discomfort in his upper abdomen and chest when he ran up a flight of stairs, or walked quickly up an incline (not that he did too much walking nowadays). Usually, the pain would go away if he belched or rested for a minute or so.

He began to feel chronically tired. Never at any time, however, did he feel that he had any serious health problem. After all, he had always come through the annual company medical examination with flying colours; blood pressure, electrocardiogram, blood and urine checks always normal — which was, after all, only to be expected in a strong, 6'2" ex-college football player.

Then one day, while sitting dozing in front of the television set, he got a fright; the stomach pain came on quite suddenly. Only on this occasion, it was more severe, and seemed to have moved up into his chest. For a moment or two, he had difficulty breathing, as the pain radiated first into his neck and jaw, and then down both arms to his hands. He found he was sweating profusely. He didn't know what to do. When he tried to lie down, the pain seemed to get worse; moving around didn't do any good, and neither did belching gas. Mary, noticing his agitation and pale, sweating features, learned for the first time of his recurrent bouts of "indigestion." She wanted to call a doctor, but John persuaded her to wait and see if his condition improved. Fortunately (or unfortunately as it turned out), the pain subsided after about thirty minutes, although for the next day or two his chest felt very sore. In deference to Mary's wishes, he called in to see his family physician the following week, and told him that he had been getting the "occasional niggling stomach pain when I am over-tired or tense." A combination of John's natural tendency to downplay any evidence of physical weakness, together with what may have been a too-easy acceptance of his tale by the physician, led to a diagnosis of "nerves." An electrocardiogram was not carried out. Still, as John himself says, "hindsight is always 20/20."

During the following weeks, John continued his heavy work schedule, suffering only occasional and relatively mild "nerve" pains in his chest — until the week the plant workers went on strike. If the job was hectic before, it was frenetic now. Extra duties, extra hours, unpleasantness on the picket lines, all contributed to bring about a desperate situation. There seemed to be no solution. As a matter of fact, there was, and in John's case, it was almost the final one.

At four o'clock one morning, he was awakened by the most severe pain in his chest he had ever experienced. It was as if a terrible weight was pressing on his chest bone, squeezing and squeezing until he felt he could no longer breathe. He thought he was going to die. He put up no argument when Mary called the ambulance and, within half an hour, an electrocardiogram was carried out in the emergency department and the young, serious-looking doctor quietly gave him the news; he had sustained a severe heart attack and was to be admitted to the coronary care unit immediately.

John was six weeks in hospital, during which time he experienced a series of emotional reactions to his predicament. At first, he was stunned by the doctor's diagnosis. It was impossible for him to have had a heart attack; his heart wasn't weak, he had never had a day's illness in his life — there must be some mistake.

This period of "denial" lasted about 48 hours. Some patients never lose it even after discharge from hospital, persisting in their belief that the doctors have "made a mistake." In John's case, it was replaced by a sullen anger. What right had fate to treat him in this unfair fashion? Hadn't he worked hard to make his mark in life, to provide for his wife and family, to get on? What reward was this for living according to the rules?

After he came out of intensive care, his cardiologist told him he would probably be able to go home "in a couple of weeks." Always a stickler for accuracy, John interpreted "a couple" as being exactly two. When these two weeks were up, he was told he might be in hospital for another "few weeks." He now became dreadfully depressed. He felt the doctors were keeping something from him: he was going to die, or at best be an invalid for the rest of his life. He would never see his children again.

At the end of six weeks, he went home still in a depressed mood. The first day back in familiar surroundings was almost too much for him. He felt so fatigued he had to go to bed after only a few hours. He had lost his old aggressive self-confidence and was fearful of responsibility. Even after his return to work, ostensibly fully recovered, Mary was at first surprised and then perturbed to find that he continued to lean on her, reluctant to take the initiative in financial or domestic matters requiring a decision.

This state of affairs continued until his doctor, sensing a deterioration in the family relationship, had a talk with him and asked him if he would like to attend a new exercise rehabilitation class which had recently been instituted at the Toronto Rehabilitation Centre. John agreed. Later, he commented that the rehabilitation program was "like a lifebelt to a drowning man. It's the best thing since sliced bread."

The General Pattern

Of course, there is no such thing as a typical heart attack victim, patients coming in all shapes, sizes and types. John's story is a composite case history, drawn from the files of patients referred to me for post-coronary rehabilitation. But interestingly enough, an analysis of a hundred of these patients carried out in conjunction with Professor Roy Shephard of the Department of Preventive Medicine and Biostatistics, University of Toronto, in 1973 and published the following year in the *Canadian Medical Journal*, revealed a surprising similarity in the patterns of life prior to their heart attacks. Comparison with a matched group of healthy individuals showed that the patients who had sustained a heart attack also experienced a greater than average degree of business, financial and domestic stress in the year prior to their illness. In many cases, the stress factor was extreme.

In the last few weeks before the attack, a significant proportion had experienced vague pains in the chest, neck, jaw or arms, but had ignored these symptoms, ascribing them to "indigestion" or "nerves." Most described a feeling of incredible fatigue, one man actually falling asleep while dining with a business client, and another instinctively reacting to the news of his heart attack with the thought, "at least I'll be able to get a good sleep in hospital." Overweight, heavy smoking and lack of regular physical activity were all too common.

Often the attack itself occurred within 24 hours of a severe emotional experience or unaccustomed physical stress: for example, a violent row with the boss, or half an hour of trying to start a recalcitrant outboard motor. In at least one case, the emotional and physical were combined, when a patient undertook a long and exhausting journey to see a boyhood house full of bittersweet memories of early struggle.

Another study I carried out at the Centre, also published in the *Canadian Medical Journal*, showed that many of these patients go through a phase of denial after the infarction, but then all too frequently become depressed, lacking in confidence, and fearful for the future. They feel they have lost their masculinity, and they worry about their future ability to perform the role of husband and father with the same success as previously. They hide their depression very well, even from their wives, and it requires careful questioning by the physician and the psychologist to uncover it. Where depression exists, however, it is always profound. Oddly enough, the depressed post-coronary patient invariably feels that he is the only one in the whole group who feels this way. His fellow sufferers are as convincing in their show of false bonhomie and cheerfulness as he is.

By now, you should be getting a picture of the manner in which coronary artery disease can strike its victim, often nowadays an apparently healthy, busy man in his forties. Women are much less affected, and we will see the reason for this later.

But what exactly is coronary artery disease, and what causes it? In order to answer these questions, we must take a brief look at the anatomy and physiology of the heart and blood vessels, and then make a short excursion into the field of epidemiology.

What is Coronary Artery Disease?

The heart functions just like a mechanical pump. Its sole function is to supply the force by which blood is driven through the blood vessels to all parts of the body. Its walls consist of muscle tissue which possesses the unique property of contracting involuntarily; it works day and night, irrespective of whether its owner is awake or asleep. But, like all of the body's tissues, the heart muscle needs to be supplied with oxygen-rich blood. This it receives from two small arteries which branch off from the base of that major artery, the aorta, through which the rest of the body's blood supply needs are met (Figure 1). These small arteries are known as coronary arteries, and they are the heart's private blood supply system, operated by the heart and for the heart.

Each cycle of the heart's pumping action is divided into an active contracting stage when the various chambers are ejecting blood into the general circulation, and an inactive resting stage when blood is being sucked from the great veins into the non-contracting, almost empty heart. The active stage is referred to as systole, the inactive stage as diastole. If you place the palm of your hand over your left breast, you may be able to feel the impulse of your heart beating regularly against your chest wall (provided, of course, that you are not covered by a too generous layer of fat); this impulse is due to the heart contracting in its stage of systole. A unique feature of the coronary circulation is that blood flows through it most actively when the heart is in the phase of diastole. This is in direct contrast to the blood flow to the rest of the body which occurs, of course, in the stage of systole. It will be seen later when we come to consider the effect of exercise training on the heart, that this fact is of considerable significance.

What happens when someone has a heart attack? What causes the "attack"? The disease responsible is called atherosclerosis, a medical term for fatty thickening which occurs in the walls of blood vessels. The condition, when it develops, may affect any of the arteries in the body, but the consequences are

Figure 1

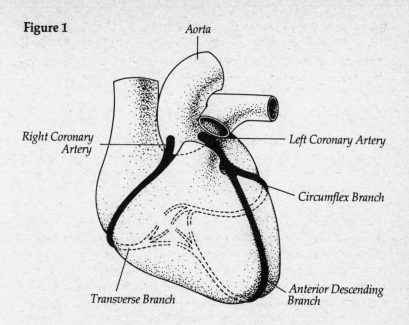

Aorta

Right Coronary Artery

Left Coronary Artery

Circumflex Branch

Transverse Branch

Anterior Descending Branch

The Coronary Arteries , Your Heart's Blood Supply

most serious in the coronary vessels. These are often not much thicker than a drinking straw. The fatty infiltration of their walls leads to a gradual narrowing of their inner diameter, with the result that they are unable to supply sufficient blood to the heart during times of high demand. When a hard-working muscle is partially deprived of its blood supply, it develops a cramp-like pain; put a tourniquet around your upper arm so as to cut off the blood supply, and then clench and unclench your fist for a few minutes, and you will quickly see what I mean. The heart muscle is no exception. Thus a patient who is suffering from atherosclerosis of the coronary arteries may find that emotional tension or physical exercise induces a form of cramp in his heart which he feels as an acute pain in the chest or, to use the medical term, angina pectoris — which is Latin for the same thing.

Walking up stairs or uphill, hurrying on the level, or suffering a severe shock, are notorious examples of daily incidents which bring on angina pectoris. A common situation in which both emotional and physical factors occur together is the all-too-familiar struggle through one of our modern overcrowded airports carrying a heavy suitcase. As soon as our atheromatous victim slows down or stands still, the workload on his heart is reduced; the narrowed coronary arteries can now cope with the blood requirements of the heart, and the cramp-like pain subsides.

Is angina pectoris, then, the same thing as a heart attack? Not really. The heart attack represents a further stage in the progress of the disease, and it should be noted that this may occur in a patient who has never experienced anginal pain. The narrow bore of the coronary artery may be plugged by the fatty substance which is accumulating in the walls; or a piece of the fatty substance may break off and be carried downstream by the blood flow until it reaches a portion of the artery which is too narrow to penetrate. Sometimes the cause of the blockage may be a piece of blood clot (a thrombus) which has previously formed on the surface of the fatty patch (referred to medically as a "plaque") and then breaks loose.

Sometimes no blockage can be demonstrated at post-mortem examination, and we then must assume that a sudden increase in the workload of the heart has created a situation where the blood supply simply could not keep pace with the demand. Whatever the mechanism, the end result is the same. A portion of the heart muscle is deprived of its blood supply to the point where it dies. Our patient classically complains of severe and continuous chest pain which, unlike angina pectoris, refuses to go away despite resting, taking indigestion pills, or belching gas. He shows all the signs of shock, such as sweating, pallor, slow pulse rate, and falling blood pressure. Within a few hours, his electrocardiogram tracing will show changes from the normal because the electrical potentials from the heart muscle are being modified by the presence of dead tissue. There is also a rise in the blood level of various substances released by the breakdown of heart muscle tissue. These substances are known as enzymes; their importance lies in the fact that they can be detected in the blood by laboratory tests and so are of diagnostic value in those patients who have all the signs and symptoms of a heart attack but whose electrocardiogram tracing is equivocal.

If the area of damage to the heart is great, then death is likely. There may be an electrical failure of the entire heart ("cardiac arrest" or "ventricular fibrillation") immediately, or it may occur up to 48 hours after the attack. If it does, then we may be able to restore the normal electrical activity of the heart quickly by applying an external "defibrillating" electrical current to the chest wall, in which case the subject may live. This is one of the values of having the patient in the coronary care unit, for here his heart can be monitored continuously and if electrical failure develops, he can be resuscitated within seconds.

Unfortunately, cardiac arrest is most likely in the first few hours of the attack when decisions are still being made to call a doctor or arrange admission to hospital.

Provided the patient survives the immediate emergency of the attack, his outlook rapidly improves. The dead heart muscle is replaced by fibrous scar tissue, and in about six weeks the process of repair is complete. Patients often ask if the repaired area is as strong as before. It depends on what you mean by "strong." If the damage is not too extensive, then the fibrous patch will stand the strain of the heart's pumping action without difficulty. Occasionally, when the area of damage is large, or if the patient remains too active during the acute stage of the attack, the patch may weaken, thin and bulge outwards; this bulge is known as an aneurysm, and its presence can be a contraindication to intensive exercise therapy. However, this a rare occurrence, and the physician can easily detect it by electrocardiograms and specialized x-ray techniques.

Obviously, while fibrous repair tissue may be strong, it does not contain specialized heart muscle cells and so does not possess the ability to contract rhythmically and regularly so as to produce the "heart beat." To this extent, therefore, the more replacement fibrous tissue present, the less flexible will be the heart wall and so the less efficiently will it stretch during the resting phase (diastole) or shorten during the pumping phase (systole). Essentially then, a heart attack is death of heart muscle due to blockage of blood supply; or, to put it medically, myocardial infarction (heart muscle death) due to coronary occlusion (blockage).

A Look at the Epidemiology of Coronary Artery Disease

Epidemiology is the study of diseases occurring in groups of people. One of its many uses is to help answer the questions related to the cause, incidence and prevention of a specific disease in the community. Because of the high incidence of coronary heart disease, a solution to the problem becomes urgent. It is no longer enough to study each case on an individual clinical basis; we must also examine large numbers of persons suffering from the disease, hoping to find some common denominator.

While there has been some indication recently that the number of heart attacks is decreasing slightly in the United States, nevertheless it is still responsible for approximately 50 per cent of all middle-aged male deaths in North America, the United Kingdom, and most western countries.

The alarming rise in coronary artery disease dates back only to the 1920's. Prior to that, physicians were familiar with the disease, but came across it infrequently in practice. Angina pectoris was first described by Heberden, an English physician, in a paper presented to the Royal College of Physicians in London in 1768. By that time, he had observed about twenty cases; eighteen years later he wrote, "I have seen nearly a hundred people with this disorder." Not a great number for a lifetime of practice. The famous physician, Sir William Osler, in 1892 described coronary heart disease as being "very rare." What was it, then, about the early decades of the twentieth century that spawned this modern plague? Since we don't know the cause of the disease, we can only attempt educated guesses in answer to the question.

To discover the causes of a disease is no small task. It may take years, even generations, of observation and research. The Black Death, a grimly accurate description of bubonic plague, ravaged the known world throughout recorded history, and still occurs sporadically to this day in certain parts of the globe. Yet it was only in 1894 that the causative agent, the deadly plague bacillus, was jointly discovered by the Japanese Shibasbauro Kitasato and the Frenchman, Alexandre Yersin. Even that knowledge was not as valuable as it might have appeared, as we still had no idea how the bacillus actually infected man. It was not until 1914 that the true culprit was discovered — the rat flea. Sucking blood from the stricken rat, it ingests hordes of the plague bacilli into its gut, and then transmits them into the blood stream of its healthy, human host. It took over two thousand years to find the answer, following a myriad of false clues, dead ends and spurious leads. Hopefully, we will be more speedy with coronary heart disease; but no matter how we telescope it, the process remains the same: observation, experimentation and more observation — together with that stroke of luck, or genius, that is the brilliant deduction.

But perhaps we don't need to actually know the cause of a disease in order to deal effectively with it. Let me draw another example of what I mean, again from the fascinating pages of medical history. John Snow, a nineteenth-century English physician, was concerned about the recurrent epidemics of Asiatic cholera which ravaged London in 1831 and again in 1848 and 1853. Considered by earlier healers to be a visitation from God upon the evil-doer, the condition was a deadly killer, with no known cure. Once contracted, it was invariably fatal in a matter of days. From his epidemiological observations, Snow inferred that the disease was caught by healthy individuals from persons who were already afflicted. He furthermore theorized that, whatever the actual causative agent, it was in some way eliminated in the patient's excreta, which was then accidentally swallowed by the next victim in whom it multiplied and reproduced cholera. Since all of the cases occurred in a district of London which obtained its drinking water from the River Thames, he blamed the spread upon the pollution of the river by infected human waste. Accordingly, he advised the then up-to-date measures of improved sewage disposal, as well as purification of the water supply by filtration through sand and gravel.

In 1854, Snow had the opportunity to test his theory. In a small area of central London a particularly virulent outbreak of cholera resulted in five hundred deaths in a two-week period. Following a painstaking house-to-house survey of each case, he established that all had a common source of drinking water, a pump in nearby Broad Street. He advised the removal of the pump handle, and immediately the number of new cases diminished to zero — a dramatic vindication of his theories!

These cases illustrate why the epidemiological approach is sometimes the only one open to us, and how at times it can be of immense practical value in helping us to control or even eliminate a disease — even if it may sometimes lead us to do the right thing for the wrong reason.

Risk Factors

We have seen that atherosclerosis consists of an infiltration of the blood vessel wall by a fatty substance which, in time, calcifies in the form of plaques, narrowing and possibly even blocking the artery channel. A process such as this takes time, and there is now ample evidence to suggest that it commences in childhood.

An English research worker called Osborn has carried out some excellent studies showing that early signs of the disease can be detected in the coronary arteries of children as young as 5 years of age; by the time they are 15, dangerous lesions are relatively frequent. Between the ages of 16 and 20, over half the population shows evidence of atherosclerosis of the coronary arteries. This is the quiescent stage of the disease. The patient is not aware of any abnormality; in fact, he often feels in excellent health. Routine check-ups, including electrocardiograms, are often negative. Occasionally, a laboratory test may show a higher than normal amount of fat in the blood, but more frequently this reading will be normal. The newer and more sophisticated methods of measuring coronary blood flow such as exercise stress testing, coronary angiography (x-ray of the coronary arteries using a radio-opaque dye), radio-isotope studies, may be of value in early detection, but as yet are not available routinely. Eventually, with the passing years, the process of artery-narrowing matures until it leads to alteration in blood flow of sufficient magnitude to affect the function of the heart. When this occurs, the subject for the first time experiences symptoms, usually chest pain or breathlessness on exertion. The overall process may occupy a span of forty years.

Nowadays, we are used to seeing the acute episode, myocardial infarction, at an earlier and earlier age. The youngest patient who came to my attention was a 27-year-old doctor who was training as a cardiologist. He first noticed chest pain when he ran up a flight of stairs to attend a cardiac arrest! Three days later, he sustained a heart attack. Herman R., the first post-coronary patient to finish the Boston Marathon in 1973, suffered his attack when he was 29. While atherosclerotic changes of one sort or another are present in practically all of us from infancy, there is individual variation in their degree of severity. Slight fatty infiltration of the coronary vessel wall may never progress to the stage where it causes symptoms. But heavy involvement at an early age will invariably lead to a full-blown clinical picture of coronary heart disease. Since we do not as yet understand the mechanism by which the fatty invasion of the vessel wall occurs, we are unable to say why some of us seem more susceptible than others. However, epidemiological studies can give us clues to the answer mainly by identifying the so-called risk factors. These are traits or common denominators shared by individuals or groups of individuals in whom the disease has a high incidence. If you possess a large number of these risk factors, you are "coronary-prone," and the likelihood of your developing the disease is high. Obviously, it is of great practical importance to know what these risk factors are since, as we will learn later, a significant number of them are subject to change or at least control.

One of the most famous epidemiological investigations is the Framingham Study. Sponsored by the United States Public Health Service and started in 1948, it studied the pattern of coronary heart disease developing over twenty years in a group of 5,000 residents (2,336 males and 2,873 females) in the small town of Framingham, Massachusetts. Each subject was medically examined every two years; body weight, blood pressure, chest x-ray, electrocardiogram, blood fat levels, smoking habits, and other details were carefully noted. The findings demonstrated that males who had elevated levels of fat in their blood, suffered from high blood pressure or diabetes, and smoked, had ten times the standard risk of developing coronary heart disease; if those factors were absent, the likelihood was reduced to one-third the standard risk.

Other studies elsewhere emphasize additional risk factors, including race, family history, emotional stress, and physical inactivity. This book is mainly concerned with the effects of physical training but, for a complete understanding of the problem, each of the factors will be dealt with under a separate heading.

Sex, Race Young women are relatively free from coronary heart disease, provided they do not suffer from diabetes, high blood pressure or very elevated blood fats. After they reach the menopause, however, their immunity is partly lost, and the incidence climbs until it is the same as males of comparable age. The reason for this is unknown, but it may be connected with the possible protective effect of female hormone. One study in the United States attempted to establish this by administering female hormone to coronary-prone males; unfortunately, the incidence of annoying and harmful side-effects caused the experiment to be abandoned.

One of the highest incidences of coronary heart disease is reported from Finland, particularly the eastern part of the country. There is no valid single explanation for this, although dietary habits and smoking have been variously incriminated, and it has been reported that blood cholesterol levels as well as blood pressures are higher than average.

The black population of the United States has an even higher death rate from heart disease than the white, possibly the result of being more susceptible to hypertension. Yet the Bantu people in South Africa have a very low incidence of heart disease, as does the black population of Haiti. Post-mortem examinations on young American soldiers killed in battle in Korea, average age 22, showed that a high proportion of these young men had atherosclerotic narrowing of one or more coronary arteries in excess of 50 per cent; similar evidence of advanced coronary atherosclerosis has been shown in young soldiers killed in Vietnam, and also in young accidental death victims in Great Britain and in Israel. Chinese soldiers, on the other hand, did not have these changes to anything like the same extent. Similarly, the death rate from heart disease in Japan is only one-sixth of that in the United States. One might be tempted to say that the Asiatic has a racial immunity to the disease, were there not now evidence to suggest that Japanese who emigrate to the United States and who adopt the western way of life lose their apparent immunity and succumb to the same extent as the Caucasian.

I am inclined to reject the influence of race in favour of environment and cultural factors. It seems to me that the low mortality rate from heart disease in the Scandinavian countries is less likely to be due to the inhabitants' Teutonic origin than it is to their lifestyle — just as the Finns must surely owe their coronary-proneness to some factor other than their supposed Mongolian antecedents. After all, the Eskimos of Canada's far north are pure Mongolian, and yet have very little heart disease.

And yet, there is the intriguing paradox of the Ashkenazy (European) and Yemenite (Asian) Israeli. The former is reported as having many times the incidence of heart disease as the latter. This seems to correlate with studies which show that Ashkenazy children between the ages of one to ten have a greater degree of early atherosclerotic changes in their coronary arteries than Yemenite children. Would the presence of such changes at this early age be the result of an unfavourable lifestyle? A different infant diet, maybe? But then, is it fair to say that the presence of these early tissue changes in the coronary arteries are connected with adult myocardial infarction?

High Blood Pressure   The association of high blood pressure, or hypertension as the condition is referred to medically, and coronary heart disease has been known for some time. The Framingham Study showed that hypertensives have about four times the likelihood of developing severe coronary atherosclerosis as the normotensive subjects. Electrocardiogram changes indicative of diminished coronary blood flow are seen more frequently during exercise tests in subjects with high blood pressure. Unfortunately, we still don't know the cause of 90 per cent of cases of hypertension encountered in practice. Nevertheless, there are now a series of prescription medications which can be used to reduce high blood pressure and keep it within normal limits. This obviously is a risk factor which can be detected during the regular physical check-up and then controlled by medical treatment, although to date there is no experimental evidence to suggest that controlling hypertension results in a reduction in the incidence of myocardial infarction.

The Cholesterol Connection   If there is one word that has made the scene in North America in the past twenty years, it's cholesterol. The paradox is that while everyone has heard of cholesterol, few know precisely what it is. There seems to be a number of misconceptions. For instance, most people think that cholesterol is some kind of dangerous fat that is present in certain foods, that it causes heart attacks by "furring" the inside of the blood vessels, and consequently should be eliminated entirely from our diet. At best, this picture is too simplistic, at worst, it's just plain nonsense. Let us try to clarify the situation. What exactly is cholesterol and how did it gain its bad reputation? Before we answer that question and so that we can understand the various terms used, we must take a brief look at the chemistry of fatty foods.

When we eat fat, it is broken down into what we call *fatty acids*. These are substances which are mostly made up of carbon atoms and hydrogen atoms. The carbon atoms are arranged in long chains, and the hydrogen atoms are attached to the carbon atoms at intervals along the chain (Fig. A). Each carbon atom has four grappling hooks, or bonds as the chemist calls them, which allow it to link up with any four other atoms. As you can see from the illustration, one bond is attached to each of two hydrogen atoms, and the remaining two to two adjoining carbon atoms. When all four bonds of the carbon atoms are occupied in this way, we refer to the fatty acid as being *saturated*. Where the hydrogen atoms are sparsely scattered along the carbon chain, however, many of the carbon atoms have bonds to spare. The spare bond usually "doubles up" with another carbon-to-carbon bond where it is readily available for use if needed (Fig. B). This type of fatty acid is known as a *polyunsaturated* fatty acid.

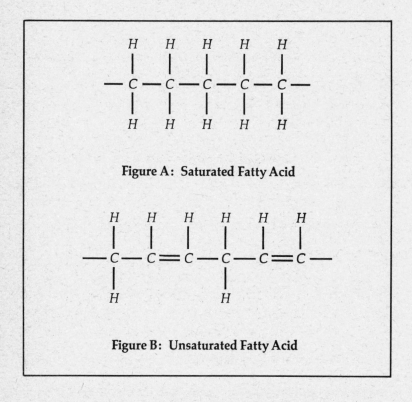

Figure A: Saturated Fatty Acid

Figure B: Unsaturated Fatty Acid

When not being used as fuel for the various metabolic processes of the body, fatty acids join up with an alcohol called *glycerol*, three fatty acid molecules to one glycerol molecule, and the resultant package is known as a *triglyceride* (Fig. C). This is the form in which fat is stored in your body. When a muscle or organ remote from the fat storage site wants to burn fatty acids for energy, triglycerides have to be transported to the scene of action. As we have seen, the blood stream is the body's only transportation system, and herein lies a snag. Since blood is 80 per cent water, substances using it as a freeway must be water soluble. As any schoolboy knows, fat is not soluble in water. The problem is solved by combining the triglyceride with two other substances, both of which can dissolve in water, in a package called a *lipoprotein* (Fig. D). The two other substances are blood protein and cholesterol.

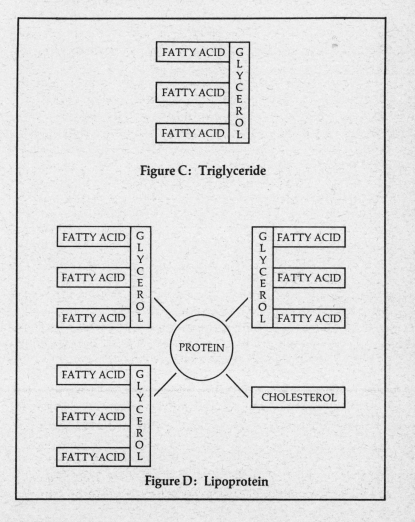

Figure C: Triglyceride

Figure D: Lipoprotein

Cholesterol, although it has some of the physical properties of a fat, is really not a fat at all. It resembles more closely an alcohol. It is in fact a sterol and is an essential constituent of all the cells in the body; in particular, those which go to make up the tissues of our brain, spinal cord and nerves. It is a major ingredient of bile juice and helps to manufacture our body's supply of natural cortisone and sex hormones. Its presence in the deeper layers of the skin prevents us from being poisoned every time we handle or touch potentially dangerous acids or solvents which would otherwise penetrate the skin barrier and enter the blood stream. It also saves us from dying from dehydration by helping to prevent excessive evaporation of body water from the skin. As you can see, without cholesterol, the human body could not survive. Thus it is widely distributed in nature and can be found in many of our foods, being particularly abundant in egg yolk and "organ" meats such as liver, kidney and brain. However, just in case we don't get enough cholesterol in our diet, our bodies have the ability to manufacture their own cholesterol. This process takes place principally in the liver, which is capable of synthesizing up to six times more daily than is found in the average diet!

But if cholesterol is so vital to our continued health, how did it become the villain in the piece? To answer that, you have to go back to 1911 when a Russian, Dr. Nikolai Anitschkov, carried out an experiment in which he demonstrated that he could cause atherosclerosis in rabbits by feeding them on a diet of egg yolk. Since the atherosclerotic plaques which developed in the linings of the rabbits' blood vessels contained quantities of cholesterol, he concluded that the cholesterol in the egg yolk diet had been absorbed into the blood stream and then, because of its high concentration, had eventually clogged the arteries by forming a deposit along their inner walls. At that time it seemed reasonable to assume that atherosclerosis in humans as well as rabbits was due to a diet too rich in cholesterol-containing foods. Taking the argument one step further, it was thought possible to prevent the development of atherosclerosis by restricting our cholesterol intake. In practice, however, this didn't work too well. Only in a minority of cases was it possible to alter blood levels of cholesterol by varying the amount of cholesterol eaten. We now know, of course, the reason for this: the body has another source — itself.

In any event, it isn't the amount of cholesterol per se in our blood that matters; more important is the total quantity of circulating fat, or lipoprotein. It so happens that it is easier to identify and measure the cholesterol part of the lipoprotein molecule and use this as an indicator of blood fat levels. Nowadays, we can also use the triglyceride portion of the fat packet in the same way, but cholesterol still remains the most convenient index of blood fat levels.

Why do we think that blood fat levels might be important? Well, for some time scientists have noticed that in countries like Japan, where the population derives much of its source of dietary fat from vegetable fats rather than animal fats, the average blood fat levels are lower than in, say, North America and the incidence of atherosclerosis is very low indeed. You will recall that some fatty acids are heavily saturated with hydrogen atoms, whereas others are relatively unsaturated. The saturated fatty acid is almost invariably found in animal fat, has a relatively high melting point and so, at room temperature, is solid in consistency. Typical examples of saturated fats are meat fat, dripping, lard, butter. Unsaturated fatty acids have a low melting point, and constitute the vegetable and fish oils — for example, corn oil, peanut oil, cod liver oil. As a result of these observations, it was recommended that in countries where there was a high level of coronary atherosclerosis, the diet be changed so as to reduce the amount of animal fat and increase the amount of vegetable oil used.

This is pretty well the state of the art today. The majority of physicians would recommend that those of us who live in the more affluent countries reduce our intake of animal fats and dairy products and, where possible, substitute vegetable oils. The results of such an approach are, unfortunately, not as clear-cut as we would like. The all-important experiment of altering the dietary habits of infants and children in order to assess the effect on heart disease incidence in adult life has not yet been undertaken. We are still uncertain as to whether reducing blood levels of fat is synonymous with reducing the likelihood of having a heart attack.

Furthermore, while it is relatively straightforward to demonstrate the association between a low animal fat diet, low blood fat levels and low incidence of heart attack in a whole population such as the Japanese, it is much more difficult to explain discrepancies within a given population. For instance, why is it some North Americans have extremely high blood cholesterol levels and others have very low ones despite the fact that their overall dietary habits may be similar? To make the situation even more complex, a number of studies purporting to show the beneficial relationship between a low fat diet, low blood fat levels and protection from heart disease have given conflicting results.

At the time of writing, the most recent large-scale study comes from Europe and has involved some 15,745 men living in Edinburgh, Budapest and Prague. After measuring blood cholesterol levels and noting those in whom the reading was high, medication was used to bring it down. Treatment was continued for an average of five years. During this time, the average decrease in cholesterol levels was only 9 per cent. Even more puzzling is the fact that while this was accompanied by a definite reduction in the occurrence of primary *non-fatal* heart attacks, there was no reduction whatsoever in the incidence of angina or the development of *fatal* primary heart attacks. In the United States, the Coronary Drug Project, a study involving 53 centres and some 8,000 heart attack patients, failed to show with any degree of certainty that the reduction in blood cholesterol brought about by diet and medication had any effect on subsequent mortality from recurrent attacks.

Yet, despite all this, few sensible physicians would deny that there does seem to be some association between excessive ingestion of fats and the development of atherosclerosis. For instance, we now know that a high intake of animal fat stimulates the liver to produce more cholesterol, while a high intake of unsaturated fat has the opposite effect. The tantalizing thing is that most of the pieces of the puzzle seem to be available to us; they just don't fit together to form a clear picture.

What's new on the horizon? While it seems reasonable to dismiss both cholesterol and triglycerides as the "cause" of heart disease, there is growing interest in the third and final component of the lipoprotein molecule — the blood protein to which both cholesterol and triglyceride are attached. Investigation of this substance is a recent development, and since it looks like being the most productive of all, we should take a few minutes to discuss it.

There are actually two forms of protein which can be involved in the lipoprotein molecule. One is large and light, like a soccer ball; the other is smaller and heavier, like a billiard ball. The larger type is referred to as the low density lipoprotein (LDL), the smaller type as the high density lipoprotein (HDL). It has been known for some time that individuals with abnormally high levels of LDL are prone to heart attacks. Recently, it has been observed that there is an equally striking but *inverse* relationship between the amount of HDL in the blood and the incidence of atherosclerosis. In other words, the higher the proportion of HDL fat you possess, the lower your chances of heart attack. This inverse relationship has been demonstrated in population studies carried out in Hawaii and also in Framingham, Massachusetts, which might explain why some individuals with high total (i.e., HDL, and LDL cholesterol) blood cholesterols do not suffer heart attacks. Females, for reasons as yet unknown, tend to have higher average levels of HDL than males, and this may be the reason why they are less likely to suffer from coronary artery disease. It is possible that LDL fat cannot pass through the blood vessel wall, becomes trapped, and over the years forms the familiar fatty plaques of atherosclerosis. On the other hand, HDL fat apparently encounters no such difficulty.

Assuming that such a theory is found to be true, the next step would be to find a method of changing our LDL fat into HDL fat, at least in those individuals in whom LDL levels are high. So far, no drug has been found that will accomplish this. A very strict low-fat diet is useful, but it takes considerable time to work and is not successful in everyone. Exercise, on the other hand, has been consistently shown to be associated with high HDL levels.

In 1974 Dr. A. Lopez, Associate Professor of Medicine at the Louisiana State University Medical School, published a report describing the effects of a seven-week training program (30-minute sessions, four times weekly) on thirteen young medical students. There was a significant fall in LDL and a concomitant increase in HDL. Two years later, Dr. Peter Wood, an English biochemist now working in the Stanford University School of Medicine, reported his investigation of forty-one joggers, average age 47, who had been jogging in excess of 15 miles a week for a year. When compared with a group of sedentary men of similar age, all the joggers had considerably higher levels of HDL. He remarks in his article that "these very active men exhibited a plasma lipoprotein profile resembling that of younger women rather than of sedentary middle-aged men. This characteristic, and apparently advantageous, pattern could be only partially accounted for by differences in adiposity [amount of body fat] between runners and control subjects."

Since then, several reports have appeared in medical journals.

Recently, I have started to measure HDL levels in my post-coronary patients on entry, after six months, and after one year on the jogging program. HDL levels are low at the outset and rise significantly with the walking/jogging regime; the highest readings of all are found in the post-coronary marathoners. Admittedly, it may not be jogging or exercise per se which is the potent factor, although some very recent studies suggest it is. However, it could be because the joggers are leaner, or smoke less. Only time and further investigation will tell.

These findings might also explain the apparent paradoxes which have dogged the experimental work associated with blood cholesterol in the past. It could, for instance, explain why individuals with blood cholesterols in the 400s and 500s still avoid heart attacks while others with blood cholesterols in the high 200s succumb. If those with the high cholesterol counts had most of their lipoprotein in the form of HDL, or alternatively, those with the low cholesterol counts had most of their lipoprotein in the form of LDL, this would explain the apparent discrepancy.

There is yet another area of controversy. I have already said that the present dietary trend is to substitute animal fats with vegetable oils — that is, to replace saturated with unsaturated fats. This, however, poses a problem for the food industry. One can use liquid corn oil as a substitute for cooking lard, but what about a liquid substitute for butter? How would you like to pour margarine onto your toast in the morning? The solution is something of a compromise. Food chemists have devised a method of partially saturating the unsaturated vegetable oils. They place the oil in a large tank and bubble hydrogen gas through it. This adds hydrogen atoms to the carbon chain. The process is known as hydrogenation or hardening, and the result is a vegetable oil which has a higher melting point and is closer in consistency to an animal fat. Consequently, it is easier to package and use. In the words of the ad, your margarine is now as "spreadable as butter."

Hydrogenation is also used for another purpose. The empty spaces in the unsaturated fatty acid chain are just a little bit too available to any passing molecule that happes to be homeless at the time. The most commonly available molecule is oxygen; so, over a period of time, the inclusion of oxygen in the carbon chain causes the fatty acid to change its properties. It develops a rather unpleasant odour and taste. In other words, it has become rancid. Obviously, if you attach hydrogen atoms to the spaces along the chain, you reduce the likelihood of rancidity. In short, if you want to prolong the shelf-life of any foodstuff which contains an unsaturated fat, you merely hydrogenate that fat.

Herein lies the controversy. Some experts say that hydrogenation defeats the whole purpose of eating unsaturated fats; since you have now turned the unsaturated fatty acid into a saturated fatty acid by hydrogenating it, you might as well have stuck with eating animal fat. Some scientists go even further, maintaining that you are actually worse off because instead of eating the natural fat, you are ingesting an artificial material which, for all we know, might be dangerous. How could that be so? Well, the molecules of the unsaturated fatty acid can present chemically in two forms, each a partial mirror image of the other. One form, known clinically as the *cis* form, looks like this:

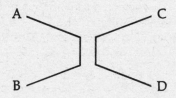

The other, the *trans* form, looks like this:

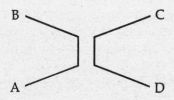

It so happens that the cis configuration is the one most frequently found in naturally occurring unsaturated fatty acids. However, the process of hydrogenation converts the cis into the trans form and it is this type, therefore, that is found in certain brands of margarine, peanut butter, etc. When we eat these substances, the fatty acids are incorporated into the cells in our body and while the evidence to date suggests that they do not produce any ill effects, there are some food scientists and physicians, among them the eminent Dr. Mann of Vanderbilt University in Nashville, who feel that the ingestion of abnormal trans fatty acids is injurious to health. At the present time the whole matter remains unresolved.

There is one vegetable oil used extensively in the food industry which is probably more dangerous in terms of causing atherosclerotic heart disease than any animal fat. That is coconut oil which, despite the fact that it is an oil, is the most saturated of all the saturated fats. Why is it used? Largely because it is relatively cheap, but also because when added to a variety of food stuffs, it gives them a creamy consistency and a pleasant taste. Today it is used widely, and is found in cookies, salad dressings, bread, margarine, coffee creamers, even certain infant formulas. The amounts used are probably small, but remember that the highest incidence of coronary artery disease in the world has been found in primitive tribes which, lacking both meat and dairy products, have relied on a combination of fish and coconuts as the two main staples in their diet.

Having read all this, you are bound to be perplexed. Accordingly, I have attempted to summarize in point form the dietary policies which are most generally accepted by the medical profession at this time. I have avoided the more extreme and bizarre recommendations — of which there is no shortage in this day and age — confining myself to suggestions which are founded on a legitimate body of data.

1. The most important rule is to maintain your ideal body weight (see page 295). If you can achieve this, it means that there is a perfect balance between food intake and energy expenditure. It really doesn't matter what you eat, it's all fuel to drive the body machine. I have often thought that if I were in a remote area, miles from any laboratory service and with no means of measuring blood fat levels, I could probably estimate fairly accurately those individuals with a low cholesterol count merely by putting them on a scale and pinching the skin folds of their abdomen, chest and waist. The light, lean, skinny individual with minimal subcutaneous fat is usually free from atherosclerosis. If you eat more than you need, then you will invariably store it in the form of fat. The 30-mile-a-week jogger can eat a great deal more than the sedentary office worker and still stay slim and trim.

2. Reduce your intake of fat so that it accounts for about 30 per cent of your daily caloric intake. These days, the average

Western diet contains far too much fat — about 50 to 60 per cent of the calories eaten each day. The trouble is that not all of the fat you eat looks like fat. It's easy to see the fat on a piece of pork or a slice of bacon. But you also have to be aware that many hot dogs contain anywhere from 60 to 80 per cent fat, that a hamburger is considered lean if it contains only 20 per cent fat, and that there is often beef fat or lard in white bread, cookies, packaged pastries, prepared salad dressings, fried chicken and a whole host of packaged edibles.

So if you want to reduce the amount of fat in your diet, you not only have to cut down on fatty meats, you must also read the contents label carefully before you buy. In general, you might try to eat more veal, poultry and fish. Approximately one-third of the fat you consume should be animal fat (saturated), and the remaining two-thirds vegetable fat (unsaturated). One way to achieve this is to cook in vegetable oil rather than lard or butter. When you buy packaged or canned foods, read the label to see whether the fat or "shortening" which has been included is saturated or unsaturated. But again a warning: the more hydrogenated the vegetable fat, the more it will resemble animal fat. Needless to say, it is almost impossible to avoid some degree of hydrogenation in modern foodstuffs, but settle for partial rather than full hydrogenation. Also, where the ingredients are listed something like this: vegetable oil and/or beef fat and/or lard — assume the worst. If you buy margarine, choose the soft type that comes in a plastic tub; if it's wrapped in parchment, you know that the vegetable oil in it has been heavily hydrogenated, in which case you might as well buy butter.

3. Butter, along with other dairy products such as whole milk and whole milk cheese, are classed as animal fats. Although I would not advocate their complete exclusion from your diet (unless you have a major problem with high blood fat levels), they should be used in moderation.

4. We have seen that reduction of cholesterol in the diet usually results in only modest changes in blood cholesterol levels. We also know that the absorption of cholesterol is enhanced by your intake of animal fat. Nevertheless, most authorities agree that we should hedge our bets and cut back on those foodstuffs which contain cholesterol in particularly high

concentrations. These are egg yolk (use the whites of the egg, or limit yourself to three whole eggs a week, and remember this includes whole eggs or egg powder used in cooking), organ meats (liver, kidney, brains), and certain shellfish (oysters, shrimp, lobster, crab).

5. Finally, don't forget the Golden Rule: All things in moderation. Only if you have grossly elevated blood fat levels and have been given strict instructions from your physician to follow a rigid diet should you become too meticulous. The above guidelines represent the middle-of-the-road thinking. But then, the middle of the road isn't a bad place to be — especially when the traffic starts to reverse! In the present state of our knowledge, you can't afford to pin all your hopes on diet. Regular exercise, stopping smoking, regular check-ups to detect the presence of high blood pressure or diabetes are all part of a well-balanced attack on the disease. The emphasis you place on each is an individual matter and will depend on your own particular weaknesses. It's not much use smoking fifty cigarettes a day and then bragging that you have trained your wife to buy skim milk and trim the fat off your meat!

Smoker's Heart   The link between cigarette smoking and coronary heart disease has been verified in several large epidemiological studies carried out in the United States, Canada, Great Britain and elsewhere. Male smokers under the age of 65 have twice as high an incidence of heart disease as non-smokers, and a similar, though smaller, risk exists in female smokers. Furthermore, smokers seem to suffer from a more severe form of the disease; crippling angina is more frequently encountered, and the incidence of sudden death is four times as great. It's as though smoking decreases the heart muscle's threshold for electrical failure, or fibrillation. The heavier one smokes, the higher the risk. Cigar and pipe smokers resemble non-smokers in incidence — provided they are not ex-cigarette smokers; this is possibly because of the cigarette smoker's inability to forsake the habit of inhaling.

Recently, the ill effects of smoking have been demonstrated in a very concrete way. Post-mortem examination of the hearts of smokers has found a marked thickening of the walls of the coronary arteries and also a thickening of the small arteries which course through the substance of the heart muscle. These appearances are so distinctive and so characteristic of smokers that the investigator, Dr. Auerbach, has labelled them "smoker's heart."

A word of consolation to the long-term cigarette smoker who would like to quit but is discouraged by the thought that it is probably too late to gain any benefit. I can assure you that stopping smoking promptly reduces the liability of coronary artery disease to the level of that for non-smokers — provided, that is, the ex-smoker does not have a plethora of other risk factors. In reality, he often has a high blood cholesterol, is hypertensive, and out of shape physically. Misery loves company!

Diabetes   Atherosclerosis takes a more severe form in diabetic patients, involving a greater number of the smaller blood vessels than usual. The clinical course of coronary heart disease, therefore, is likely to be more severe and the progression more rapid. Both the young and middle-aged diabetic male have a high mortality rate from myocardial infarction, four times higher than the non-diabetic, and the female diabetic loses her immunity and becomes six times more prone to heart attack.

It is imperative, then, that diabetics, especially young diabetics, adhere strictly to their treatment regimen, striving to keep their disease under control at all times.

Heredity   A study by Gertler and his co-workers showed that twice as many fathers of coronary patients had died of a heart attack as had the fathers of an equal size non-coronary group; 10 per cent of mothers had succumbed to a myocardial infarction as opposed to 7.7 per cent in the control group, and 9 per cent of the brothers and sisters compared with 1 per cent in the controls. Thomas, in another study, demonstrated that when both parents have heart disease, their sons have a five times greater chance of developing the same disease than if both parents were healthy. When only one parent has the condition the risk is only two-fold.

It seems doubtful that there is a specific genetic factor for coronary disease. The familial tendency is more likely explained by the predisposition for other risk factors to run in families — for example, hypertension, diabetes, high blood lipids, smoking — and some of these are probably the result of environmental background and training rather than genetic traits.

Obesity   This factor above all others has been considered the major villain of the piece. A series of studies in the past has associated overweight directly with an increased incidence of heart disease, which goes to show how carefully you must interpret the epidemiological "evidence." Recent researchers have demonstrated that, in the majority of cases, obesity is associated with other well-proven risk factors such as diabetes, hypertension and physical inactivity; consequently, obesity has been blamed for the ill-deeds of the company it keeps. On its own (a rare enough occurrence, admittedly), it appears to be blameless. On the other hand, obesity may be the cause of high blood pressure and high blood cholesterol.

Stress and Personality   Of all the factors considered to be associated with the increased incidence of heart disease, emotional stress is the hardest to evaluate. Workers such as Buell and Russek in the United States have found a correlation between stressful work habits and coronary artery disease. The mechanism is not explained, although it may be due to the excessive release of stress hormones (adrenaline and noradrenaline) into the blood stream, with a consequent rise in blood pressure. Prolonged stress is also said to raise blood fat levels.

Against these findings is the study of Hinkle, who followed 270,000 employees of Bell Telephone Company over five years, and found a lower incidence of heart disease in senior executives with heavy responsibility. Theorell, in Sweden, studied a group of heart attack victims in Stockholm and compared them with a matched control group who were free from coronary disease. The control group actually carried greater responsibility at work, were more involved in supervision, and spent more of their free time in committee work of various types. The patients differed from the control group mainly in that they took less time to relax at home and took less physical exercise.

Recently, Friedman and Rosenman have described a "Type A" behavioural type who is, they say, particularly susceptible to heart disease. This individual is characterized by competitiveness, excessive ambition, impatience with delay, and irritability. He is very time-conscious and has a compulsion about punctuality. He is constantly setting goals just beyond his reach, is never satisfied with any achievement. "Type B" behaviour is the opposite; low ambition, no desire to compete, and has a phlegmatic approach to problems. According to Friedman, the Type B individual rarely, if ever, sustains a myocardial infarction.

Apart from the fact that a Type A is associated with other

risk factors, such as smoking, it seems difficult to accept that such a clear-cut definition can distinguish the coronary-prone. I am constantly impressed by the wide spectrum of personalities attending for post-coronary rehabilitation and, in my experience, the coronary disease population is not at all homogeneous.

While it would not seem conclusive that emotional stress can cause atherosclerosis, our own studies have shown that it may be a factor in triggering a myocardial infarction. Dr. Peter Nixon, Chief of Cardiology at the Charing Cross Hospital, London, holds similar views. He believes that the heart attack represents a breakdown in the body's equilibrium, due to the effects of prolonged and excessive fatigue. The warning signs of irrational outbursts of temper, inability to cope and steadily decreasing productivity, all obvious to the onlooker, go unrecognized by the victim and are accompanied by such physical changes as increases in blood pressure, blood fats, blood stickiness and ultimately disruption of heart function. An intriguing and unique aspect of Nixon's approach is his use of the French mathematician René Thom's Catastrophe Theory and his own Human Function Curve to help his patients to chart and recognize dangerous levels of environmental stress. Examples of such stress cited by other workers include intense disappointment, failure or lack of appreciation after intense effort, dissatisfaction with achievement, and recent bereavement. The stress of external factors, then, seems to be a greater hazard than the possession of a coronary-type personality — if, indeed, such a thing exists.

CHAPTER TWO

Exercise and Heart Disease

THE early years of this century saw the development of an invention which was destined to have a profound effect on the lifestyle of all of us. I refer, of course, to the internal combustion engine. Cheap, efficient and effortless transportation became the order of the day. For those of us who could not afford an automobile, there was always the bus, motor-driven by sixteen horse-power instead of hauled by two. And if Henry Ford's Model T symbolized the height of personal driving luxury, England's unique double-decker bus became equally famous as the modern city's answer to the now-universal demand for mass transportation.

Herein lies a most interesting paradox, for that same double-decker bus was to figure prominently in an article written by Professor Jeremy Morris of the British Medical Research Council, which appeared in the medical journal, *The Lancet*, in 1953. The title was "Coronary Heart Disease and Physical Activity of Work." It compared the occurrence of heart disease in two groups of workers in the London Transport Department: the bus drivers and the bus conductors. The conductors were found to have one-third less heart disease than the drivers, and they sustained only one-half the number of fatal and non-fatal heart attacks.

The likeliest explanation of this seemed to lie in the different nature of their jobs. Driving is a sedentary activity requiring a low expenditure of energy; the conductor, on the other hand, has to collect fares, and in a double-decker this necessitates making an average of up to twenty-four trips an hour up and down the winding staircase of the moving vehicle, in addition to walking back and forth along the aisles of the upper and lower compartments. Over an eight-hour shift, the energy expenditure is considerable, equal to walking from the basement to the top floor of a sixty-storey skyscraper twice a day.

Morris and his colleagues were quick to point out that this very significant association between physical activity and immunity from heart disease was precisely that — an association; there was no proof of cause and effect. For instance, it might be that a process of self-selection was at work; the coronary-prone individual might be more likely to seek employment as a driver than as a conductor. Nevertheless, despite this very legitimate caution, Morris' pioneer work was quickly recognized as being of the utmost importance, and soon other researchers in the field set about trying to duplicate his findings.

The results almost invariably were the same. In the United States, Zukel showed that sedentary workers had six times the incidence of heart disease as did individuals who engaged in heavy work. Taylor compared active U.S. railroad switchmen and sedentary ticket clerks; he found the latter had one-third higher death rates from heart attacks. Kahn, also in the United States, as well as Morris in England, looked at postal workers, comparing mail carriers and sorting clerks; the active carriers had one-third to one-half less heart disease than the sedentary clerks and even greater protection against rapidly fatal heart attacks.

Israel has a high prevalence of heart disease, which is likely why its doctors have carried out so much excellent research on the subject. Probably the best known to physicians is the work of Dr. Daniel Brunner. In pursuing Morris' findings, Dr. Brunner made use of a unique feature of Israeli life, the existence of the kibbutzim. In these communities, people live in a uniform environment, eating the same food, experiencing the same climate, and largely subject to the same stresses. Their standard of living is not influenced by their occupations. Obviously a study carried out in such a setting eliminates many sources of error. In analyzing the causes of death of ten thousand residents of a kibbutzim over a period of fifteen years, Brunner ascertained that "the incidence of anginal syndrome, myocardial infarction and fatalities due to ischaemic heart disease was found to be 2.5 to 4 times greater in sedentary workers than in non-sedentary workers." That same study contributed a further significant piece of information: no difference could be found in the serum cholesterol values of sedentary and non-sedentary workers. An argument against the confirmed "cholesterol watchers"?

In talking to Dr. Brunner a few years ago, I found that he ranked physical inactivity much higher on the list of risk factors for a heart attack than either blood fat levels or racial origin. We discussed the incidence of coronary heart disease in Jews of European and Oriental origin, and he was forthright in stating that this was much more likely due to their level of daily physical activity than to any racial or psychological characteristics.

Closer to home, Dr. Curtis Hames, a family physician practising some sixty miles from Savannah, Georgia, was intrigued by the apparent selective manner in which heart disease attacked his patients. Whites seemed to suffer more heart attacks than blacks; yet the black population not only had a higher incidence of hypertension, but also consumed a high animal fat diet. Determined to seek the answer to this anomaly, Dr. Hames instigated a series of epidemiological studies which commenced in 1960 and continued throughout most of the decade. The Evans County Study, as it came to be known, confirmed Dr. Hames' clinical impression; heart disease was found to be four times more prevalent in whites than in blacks.

And yet this difference could not be explained on the basis of any known risk factors such as hypertension, smoking, obesity, or high blood fat levels. However, it was noted that the incidence of heart disease varied inversely with the nature of the job. The harder a man laboured, the less heart disease he suffered, irrespective of his race or colour. Since the majority of the black people were manual labourers and field workers, they showed an immunity to coronary disease. As if to underline this point, it was further found that the white of lower socio-economic status who shared the toil of his black brother, also shared that immunity. During the 1960's, Evans County became more industrialized, and this brought with it an upward mobility for the poor white. At the end of the decade, less and less whites could be found resistant to heart disease; the only ones remaining immune were those who, for various reasons, had not made it in the race for affluence — in other words, the sharecroppers, who still worked hard and long in the fields.

These are only some examples of the studies which have been carried out since Morris' article first appeared in 1953. With a few exceptions, they have all demonstrated that those who are physically active have a significantly reduced incidence of morbidity and mortality from heart disease. As for studies which have not shown the protective benefit of heavy physical work, the answer is to be found in modern technocracy which has reduced the energy cost of so-called "heavy" jobs to very modest levels. As one European expert in the field has said: "The discrepancy can be explained by the fact that nowadays work labelled as 'heavy' is not heavy at all, so that the study population was not divided into appropriately different categories of physical activity, but rather into different categories of physical *inactivity*."

This is borne out by the work of the American epidemiologist and physician, Dr. Ralph Paffenbarger of Berkeley, California, who over a period of twenty-two years has studied the incidence of heart disease in some 6,351 longshoremen living in the San Francisco Bay area. Paffenbarger's work is noteworthy in showing the encroachment of modern methods on this traditionally heavy labouring field. He has been able to stratify his subjects into light, moderate and heavy workers. He found that the light workers had two and one half times the incidence of fatal heart attacks and three times the incidence of sudden death from cardiac causes as did the heavy or moderate physical workers. Interestingly, this benefit persisted even when the ill effects of high blood pressure, obesity, previous heart disease and cigarette smoking were taken into account. According to Paffenbarger, analysis of the figures showed that the effect of heavy work was to reduce the chance of a fatal heart attack by 54 per cent; he estimated that stopping smoking or reducing high blood pressure would cut the risk by 27 and 29 per cent respectively.

Another approach has been to use insurance company statistics. The Health Insurance Plan of New York was able to categorize its members into those who had a high level of both on- and off-the-job physical activity and those who had a low level. The low-level individuals had twice the number of heart attacks as the high-level members; there was also a striking difference in the two groups with regard to death within the first 48 hours after the attack — 48 per cent death rate in the sedentary as compared with 22 per cent in the active.

In recent years, there has been increasing interest in off-the-job physical activity, since heavy physical work has become increasingly rare. Once again, the pioneer Jeremy Morris was first to look at this aspect of the problem. In February 1973 he published a preliminary report in *The Lancet* which dealt with the beneficial effect of leisure-time exercise in a group of 17,000 British civil servants. He found that those who reported carrying out vigorous recreational activities in their leisure time such as brisk walking, swimming, digging in the garden, and other similar vigorous activities in excess of thirty minutes, had about one-third the incidence of coronary disease as those whose behaviour was similar, except that their recreational activities were of a more sedentary nature. The more vigorous the exercise, the lower the incidence of coronary disease. Light exercisers, on the other hand, had no greater immunity than non-exercisers. In this particular report, the vigorous exercisers did not seem to differ significantly from the rest of the group with regard to other coronary risk factors (e.g., family history of heart disease, high blood pressure, high cholesterol levels or Type A/B personality). This suggests that one of the ways exercise exerts its beneficial effect is by blocking the other risk factors. A further source of comfort for those of us who are past our prime is Morris' finding with this group that the beneficial effect of exercise did not fade with advancing age. Morris concludes: "Habitual vigorous exercise during leisure time reduces the incidence of coronary heart disease in middle age among male sedentary workers."

In addition to looking at heart disease in longshoremen, Paffenbarger has also studied the effect of vigorous physical activity in leisure time. In following 17,000 Harvard University male alumni aged 35 to 74 for a ten-year period, he recorded a 64 per cent greater incidence of heart attacks in those with sedentary recreational habits as compared with vigorous exercisers. The difference applied at all age levels (35-44, 76 per cent; 45-54, 32 per cent; 55-64, 47 per cent; 65-74, 31 per cent). The charge of "pre-selection" (that is, that individuals who are genetically endowed with healthy hearts automatically tend to choose vigorous pursuits while those prone to atherosclerosis are more sedentary in nature), is largely forestalled by the fact that college athletes who became sedentary in adult life showed no protective effect, while academicians who had taken up vigorous sports after leaving school did. A further refinement of this particular experiment was the emergence of a "threshold" of exercise at which the maximal degree of protection pertains. This worked out to be 2,000 kilocalories a week — or 20 miles of jogging a week.

It must be realized that the perfect epidemiological observation is impossible; all the investigations which associate inactivity with heart disease can be faulted on some score or other, as Morris himself was the first to point out. Nevertheless, it has been estimated that to provide even minimal statistical proof of the exercise theory, you would have to set up a prospective study involving some 8,000 individuals randomly allocated to an exercise and a non-exercise group and followed for a minimum of five years to see how many in each group suffered a heart attack. The project would be a major undertaking, and a costly one. For argument's sake, let's say that the organization of the whole scheme, including recruitment, follow-up, provision of exercise facility, etc., amounted to $1,000 per annum per subject. You are looking at a $40 million bill. When you consider that attempts to measure the effects of differing lifestyles on mortality and morbidity are fraught with innumerable intangibles, all of which can affect your result, it's understandable that there have been no takers. Nevertheless, I think it is fair to say that the evidence in favour of exercise is increasingly compelling. As more people begin to exercise in their spare time, more data will become available. For myself, I am satisfied at this stage that there is ample justification to advocate habitual physical activity as a major health measure.

Lessons from Primitive People

Would you like to live to be one hundred? For years, we have heard tales of communities where centenarians are commonplace; not only that, but are healthy and alert enough to work until they are past 80. Lately, scientists and gerontologists (physicians who specialize in the treatment of the aged) have become particularly interested in these reports. The three regions of the world most renowned for longevity are the Ecuadorian Andes, the Karakoram mountains in Kashmir, and the Abkhazia region of the southern Soviet Union. On-the-spot research in these areas verified that ages of one hundred years and up are not unusual. Heart attacks are extremely rare. Why is this so?

The inhabitants of high Ecuador and Kashmir eat sparingly of a diet low in animal fat; conversely, the Abkhazians eat well, with meat and dairy products as regular items. Smoking is common in all three areas, and many of the old people enjoy their wine, vodka and local spirit. Researchers have remarked that in all three areas, the lifestyle is characterized by lack of stress, contentment with one's station in life, and heavy involvement of the aged in both family and civic affairs. People expect to live to a ripe old age, and assume they will work for as long as they are capable. Any or all of these factors may be important contributions to their longevity. A more objective finding, however, is their high degree of cardiovascular fitness. This is due to the nature of their work: heavy physical labour interspersed with a great deal of walking, not infrequently over hilly terrain. Dr. David Kakiashvili, a Russian cardiologist who is intensely interested in this subject, is convinced that it is this active lifestyle, commencing in early childhood and continuing for eighty years or more, which confers the high degree of cardiac health and results in such lengthy lifespans. In other words, if you have a fit cardiovascular system, then the odds are that you will live for a long time.

Two features always considered to be an inevitable consequence of aging are a deterioration in the blood flow to the brain, and a reduction in the body's ability to utilize oxygen. The former results in apathy, forgetfulness, depression, and many of the other mental hallmarks of senility; the latter in a decline in physical vigour. A United States Department of Health study cast a new light on the matter. A large number of elderly males from an Old Age Home were medically examined and from these were selected twenty-seven men aged 65 and over who were completely free from atherosclerosis. Further comprehensive tests revealed that these favoured individuals had the same cerebral blood-flow and oxygen consumption as a group of 21-year-olds. It is not chronological aging *per se*, then, which is responsible for many of the stigmata of aging, but rather the presence of diseased arteries. Which is probably why some Abkhazians are able to work efficiently into their nineties and older, and reportedly sire children while in their late eighties! In a recent television program dealing with this subject and shot on location, one of the attractive female directors commented that a resident in his late eighties made a very determined pass at her. So, if we can keep atherosclerosis at bay, we may have more to look forward to than just the old age pension!

However, to return to the question of physical activity. Dr. Alexander Leaf, an American cardiologist who has made a study of these people in their own environment, repeatedly found a high level of endurance fitness in the aged and was obviously impressed with their capacity for heavy work. He wrote of "Markhti Tarkil, who walks half a mile downhill to his daily bath in the river and then climbs uphill again. Surely any day a man can do this he must be too fit to die. The next day he repeats this physical activity and so on, day after day while the years roll by, and at 104, Tarkil is still much too fit to die!" On one occasion, Dr. Leaf toiled up a steep mountain side to interview a 106-year-old shepherd. The journey took him six hours, and the going was so rough that two of the four-man party, including the interpreter, had to turn back. The cardiologist's pride on making it to the top was, however, short-lived; it turned out that the ancient shepherd did the journey regularly in three hours!

Dr. Leaf truly took the lesson to heart, for on his return home, he commenced jogging as a hobby. At a recent meeting of the American Medical Joggers Association (a group of physicians dedicated to jogging, which I shall talk about later), it was reported that he continues to jog regularly and still feels very enthusiastic about the beneficial effects of regular endurance-type exercise.

Man has become domesticated only within the last ten thousand years; for one million years before the discovery that we could grow and eat grain (provided we stayed around long enough to reap it), man was a nomad, a hunter. He moved with the game, walking, running, stalking, and constantly setting up and breaking camp. Is ten thousand years long enough to extinguish the needs of his body for activity and motion? If it were, why is the child still afraid of the dark? Why does our hair stand on end and our pupils dilate in preparation for fight or flight when we are startled? We are closer to our stone age ancestors than we sometimes choose to admit.

Wherever pockets of primitive peoples are still to be found, they are relatively free from heart attacks (recognizing the fact that some may not survive to the age at which heart attacks become common). The Australian aborigine, the Kenyan Masai tribesman, the Mexican Tarahumara Indian, the peoples discussed previously in this chapter, all rely mainly on their legs for loco-motion. The Tarahumara call themselves the Raramuri, which literally means runner, and part of their culture rites consists of a one-hundred-mile foot race over rugged terrain at 7- to 8-minute mile pace, at the same time kicking a small hand-carved wooden ball! Their freedom from cardiovascular disease is well documented.

To sum up, there is a substantial volume of evidence indicating that regular physical activity carried out over many years protects against a heart attack. The degree of protection is considerable, with about one-third the incidence of fatal and non-fatal myocardial infarctions among active as opposed to non-active workers. Furthermore, evidence is now accumulating that sedentary workers who indulge in vigorous physical pastimes of an endurance type have a similar degree of immunity.

But if regular exercise, either as part of work or play, protects us from heart disease, do we know how it accomplishes this? Not precisely. Exercise physiology, or the study of the effects of short- and long-term physical activity on bodily mechanisms, is a relatively new subject. It has made great advances in the past twenty years or so, but it still hasn't got all the answers. Nevertheless, there is sufficient known for us to be able to consider a number of the beneficial effects of physical fitness, and from this, choose the likeliest contenders for the honour of "heart disease antagonists."

To follow the discussion fully, however, we must understand something about the mechanism of physical activity itself; we must know how our lungs, heart, blood stream, and muscles work to counteract gravity and move our skeletal form around.

The Physiology of Exercise

We all know that man is an aerobic creature; that is, he requires a constant supply of oxygen to survive. A few short minutes without oxygen, and the cells of his body begin to die, starting with the most sensitive in the brain. The environment of this planet is, as far as we can tell to date, unique within our own solar system in that its atmosphere consists of a mixture of gases containing 21 per cent oxygen. Our bodies are designed to utilize that fact, and the specific mechanism concerned is referred to as the "oxygen transport system." This provides a steady supply of oxygen to the muscles, and is obviously heavily taxed when we exercise vigorously. It works as follows. A series of "feedback" systems throughout the body keep the brain constantly supplied with information as to the level of oxygen in the blood stream and the tissues. When the oxygen content falls below a critical level, the brain, acting through a relay of nerves, causes the diaphragm and other chest muscles to contract. The chest cavity expands, the lungs follow suit, and air passes down through a sequence of ever-smaller air passages — the bronchi and then the bronchioles, finally reaching the myriad of tiny terminal air sacs known as the alveoli. The walls of the alveoli contain fine hair-like capillary blood vessels which are part of the lung's blood circulation. In accordance with the laws of physics, oxygen passes from the region in which it is in the highest concentration to that where it is in the lowest, that is, from the alveoli to the capillary blood vessels. Here, the major part of the oxygen combines with red cells in the blood stream: more specifically, with a protein substance in the red cells known as hemoglobin. In this form, it is carried away from the lungs to the left side of the heart. From here, it is pumped through the arterial system. The arteries branch and subdivide, becoming smaller and smaller, until eventually they form capillaries again, this time in the muscles. Thus, oxygen-rich blood is carried to active muscles. Once in the muscle tissue, the oxygen separates from hemoglobin, under the influence of various environmental conditions such as the heat of muscle contraction, acidity, and the presence of myoglobin, a protein substance in the muscle fibre, which has a greater affinity for oxygen than hemoglobin. The net result is that the oxygen-poor muscle receives a fresh supply of oxygen from the capillaries. The de-oxygenated blood is then returned to the right side of the heart through the great veins, from where it is pumped once more to the pulmonary capillaries, and the whole cycle starts again (Figure 2).

Muscle Contraction   We must now take a closer look at what happens in a muscle when it contracts, and the precise manner in which it uses oxygen. As recently as thirty years ago, what follows would have been largely conjecture, but the invention of the electron microscope has enabled us to examine the minute cells which make up the various tissues of the body, with the result that we now know that our muscles consist of bundles of partially interlocking strands of protein. These strands, or filaments, are two in type; one is composed of the protein actin, and the other, the protein myosin (Figure 3). When a muscle contracts, it shortens in length and, by an interlocking action, the actin fibrils slide over the myosin fibrils to produce an overall reduction in length; expressed chemically, the two proteins combine to form actinomyosin (Figure 3). Energy is required to start and continue this process. The immediate source of energy is a chemical substance known as adenosine triphosphate or, more commonly, ATP. Each muscle fibre contains small quantities of ATP which are ready for use when a message from the brain calls for muscle action. The message passes down the spinal cord, and then along a nerve to the muscle. When it arrives at the muscle, it releases minute particles of calcium. The calcium triggers off the breakdown of ATP to a lesser substance known as

Figure 2

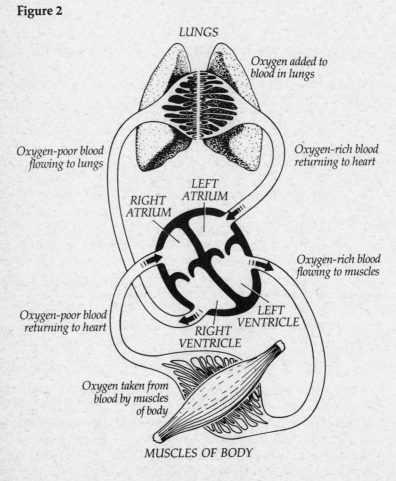

LUNGS

Oxygen added to
blood in lungs

Oxygen-poor blood
flowing to lungs

Oxygen-rich blood
returning to heart

LEFT
ATRIUM

RIGHT
ATRIUM

Oxygen-rich blood
flowing to muscles

Oxygen-poor blood
returning to heart

LEFT
VENTRICLE

RIGHT
VENTRICLE

Oxygen taken from
blood by muscles
of body

MUSCLES OF BODY

Your Heart is a Pump

adenosine diphosphate (ADP), with the simultaneous release of energy — energy to initiate the sliding movement of actin and myosin. Hence the muscle shortens, or contracts.

It should be noted that ATP is the *only* immediate source of energy acceptable to the muscle. Therefore, the body must be able to replace the muscle's local store of ATP quickly, and for as long as the muscle contraction requires it. The ultimate source of all our energy is the food we eat. In terms of ATP formation, the major short-term energy resource is the breakdown of a substance known as glycogen — the principal form in which carbohydrate-type foods are stored in the muscles and the liver. So you see, it's what you eat that makes you go!

Figure 3

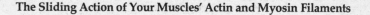

The Sliding Action of Your Muscles' Actin and Myosin Filaments

By a process known as glycolysis, glycogen is broken down to glucose and then oxydized into simpler compounds, i.e., carbon dioxide and water. But — and this is a big but — a plentiful supply of oxygen is needed if the process is to continue to its ultimate end, which is the formation of carbon dioxide and water. In the absence of sufficient oxygen, breakdown of glycogen halts part-way and less ATP is synthesized. Furthermore, an undesirable substance known as lactic acid accumulates both in the muscles and in the bloodstream. High lactic acid levels block the formation of more ATP, are associated with the sensation of fatigue, and eventually lead to cessation of muscle contraction. The exercising subject is forced to rest. Depending upon the intensity of effort, this point may be reached in anywhere from 20 seconds to a minute. The type of exercise which leads to this state of affairs is known as *anaerobic* activity — that is, an effort that deliberately outstrips the rate of oxygen supply. It occurs when we swim underwater, or if we run for a bus at our maximum pace.

Work which is carried out anaerobically gives rise to an oxygen debt, and like all debts, this must be paid back after the spending spree is over. The accumulated lactic acid must be removed from the system; some is burned by the heart and inactive muscles, but the majority is changed to glucose. This takes place in the liver, by a process which also requires oxygen. Thus, we can appreciate why the sprinter is breathless for some time after he has stopped running — he needs additional oxygen to rid him of his excess lactic acid. For the same reason, the heart continues to beat at a faster rate than normal following a race, for, as we have seen, the heart has a major part to play in supplying oxygen to the muscles.

Some individuals have a greater ability than others to sustain a high level of anaerobic work. World champions, whether sprinters or distance performers, are born rather than made. Training can improve both speed and the ability to incur large oxygen debts, but this acquired improvement is not sufficient to make the difference between an indifferent performer and a record-holder. The potential record-holder in the anaerobic events such as sprinting probably possesses not only larger muscles but also muscle chemical systems and/or a type of muscle fibre which adapt easily to the process of operating efficiently in oxygen debt.

Let us return to the mechanism of muscle contraction. If the rate of muscle contraction (that is, the intensity of exercise) is such that it does not outstrip the supply of oxygen, then the breakdown of glycogen proceeds without interruption to the production of carbon dioxide and water. This *aerobic*, or "with oxygen," process is altogether more efficient than the anaerobic route; twice as much energy is obtained from a given amount of carbohydrate, and thirteen times more ATP is produced. If the

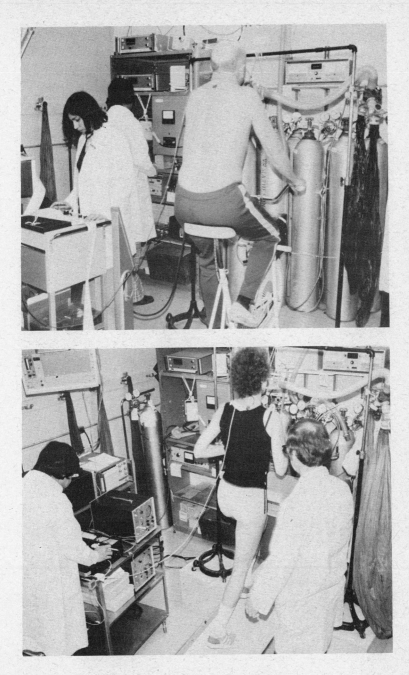

Exercise stress testing: bicycle ergometer and treadmill.

degree of muscle activity is moderate, then a fine balance is achieved between the rate with which the muscle uses oxygen, and the speed with which it is supplied to the muscle: thus there is little tendency for lactic acid to accumulate.

Endurance Fitness From what has been said, it is apparent that the ability to sustain muscle contractions of moderate force is dependent upon a steady supply of oxygen to the muscle tissue: in other words, an efficient oxygen transport system. A good long distance runner or swimmer possesses such a system. Exercise physiologists usually measure this in terms of the maximum volume of oxygen an individual can utilize per minute (litres of oxygen per minute or, to take into account the factor of body weight, millilitres of oxygen per kilogram of body weight per minute). The more oxygen one can use per minute, the higher is one's oxygen consumption, and the higher is one's ability to perform aerobic-type or endurance-type work. We shall be particularly interested in this measurement when we come to discuss the details of exercise training in post-coronary rehabilitation.

Thus, other factors being equal, the individual with a maximum oxygen consumption (vo_2 max.) of 80 ml/kg/min (that is, 80 millilitres per kilogram per minute), will also perform better in a 5,000 metre race than a competitor with a vo_2 max of 70 ml/kg/min. This does not tell us precisely how the two individuals differ. By definition, the oxygen transport system of one is superior to that of the other, but this is merely a label which leaves us no wiser as to the true basis for that superiority. We must look at each of the links in the oxygen transport system and see which is the most important in terms of increased or decreased fitness.

Provided there is no evidence of chest disease such as chronic bronchitis or emphysema, the ability to get air into the lungs is not a critical factor in oxygen transport. While the first-class athlete may have a large lung capacity, this is often a reflection of body build and muscle strength. Lung capacity in itself should not account for any great difference in performance since it does not limit the healthy individual's capacity to exercise. The same applies to the rate of breathing. The ability to breathe quickly and deeply is not a fundamental index of high-level performance. Blood leaving the lungs is almost always fully saturated with oxygen, and no additional quantity of oxygen can be carried as a result of more vigorous breathing.

However, when there is a reduction in the content of blood hemoglobin, fully saturated arterial blood has a relatively low oxygen content. Hemoglobin molecules contain iron, and their formation requires adequate body stores of that metal. Chronic blood loss (from say, excessive menstrual bleeding or a bleeding ulcer), leads to a depletion of body reserves of iron and unless this is compensated for by an increased dietary intake, the subject becomes anemic and, therefore, less efficient in transporting oxygen to the tissues. There is some evidence that athletes occasionally suffer from anemia, but this is not a limiting factor in the average healthy individual, male or female.

At the other end of the oxygen transport chain, we have to consider the process by which oxygen is given up to the active muscles by the blood. The delivery of oxygen depends both upon the speed of local blood flow and the amount of oxygen extracted from the bloodstream by the muscle (the arteriovenous oxygen difference or avO_2). Exercise usually increases local muscle blood flow and also avO_2 difference by causing a rise in muscle acidity, temperature and waste products. There is some evidence that a trained and physically fit individual has a greater ability to extract oxygen from the blood in his muscle capillaries. This is probably due to the development of a more efficient muscle chemical system of oxygen extraction which can be a definite factor in characterizing the individual with an efficient oxygen transport system. However, it does not play a fundamental role in determining oxygen supply.

Which leaves us with our remaining link, the heart pump. It is here that an individual's ability to transport oxygen is ultimately decided. The quantity of blood pumped by the heart each minute is known as the cardiac output. It is the product of the amount pumped per beat (stroke volume) and the number of beats per minute (heart rate). Each individual has a characteristic maximum heart rate, and this maximum rate decreases with age. Similarly, there is an upper limit to an individual's stroke volume. From a practical point of view, therefore, we can say that one's maximum oxygen consumption is mainly a measure of one's maximum cardiac output. We can also conclude that fitness is determined very largely by the body's ability to transport and utilize oxygen.

Finally, an efficient oxygen transport system implies efficient lungs, an adequate hemoglobin level and blood volume, an efficient distribution of cardiac output and an efficient chemical system within the muscles, but above all, an efficient heart.

The Benefits of Regular Physical Activity in Coronary Heart Disease

After that brief physiological excursion, we can now return to our original theme. There is a good deal of data available on the effects of exercise on the heart. Unfortunately, until recently, most of the studies in this field have involved young men and women in their teens and early twenties, many of them competing athletes. Since the highest incidence of myocardial infarction occurs in the middle-aged, some allowance has to be made in interpretation of the results. However, the emergence of physical inactivity as a possible cause in heart disease has led to greater interest in studying the middle-aged exerciser, and a considerable amount of scientifically valid information is accumulating.

The Heart Rate   The most obvious result of regular exercise, repeated over weeks, months and years, is a drop in the heart rate. This is referred to medically as a bradycardia, and in the fit person it is present both at rest and at exercise. It is so characteristic of fitness, that if it does not occur in the individual who is on a training program, then you can be sure that the subject is either not adhering faithfully to the program or the training regime is badly designed. At the same time as the heart rate is dropping, the stroke volume is increasing. The cardiac output, therefore, remains the same at rest or at any given effort short of maximum. In effect, the heart is pumping the same amount of blood, but with less strokes. In general, this is accomplished by the heart muscle contracting more strongly for the same time period per beat — an arrangement which reduces the workload of the heart. Each stroke is, therefore, more powerful and efficient.

The reason for the bradycardia is still unknown. The resting heart rate is regulated by a specialized portion of the heart muscle tissue which acts as a pacemaker and is known as the sino-atrial node. This basic rate is subject to modification by a specialized set of nerves known as the autonomic system. The autonomic nerves are distributed throughout the body and are concerned with the function of those organs and structures which operate independently of the will, such as the digestive tract, various internal glands, the heart and blood vessels. Two groups of fibres are recognized, the parasympathetic and the sympathetic; these tend to have opposing actions. Thus the parasympathetic nerve (the vagus nerve) slows the heart down, while the sympathetic nerve speeds it up. The entire system controls basic primitive functions such as digestion of food, or removing one's self from danger. At times of fear or anxiety, it is the sympathetic nerves which prepare the body for "fight or flight" by increasing the heart rate and blood pressure, redistributing the blood flow from skin and viscera to muscle, quickening the rate of breathing.

Modern inactive man responds to the constant mental stresses of daily living in much the same way as his primitive ancestor reacted to physical danger; he increases the activity of his sympathetic nerves, or "sympathetic drive." But since he rarely fights or takes flight in the literal sense, the acceleration of heart rate, rise of blood pressure and other signs of increased sympathetic activity are superfluous. When constantly repeated, these exaggerated responses may be damaging to the organs involved. For instance, we know that sympathetic stimulation increases the irritability of the heart, and thus the risk of ventricular fibrillation. The rise of blood pressure increases the work load on the heart, and may also lead to greater deposition of fat in the blood vessel walls, thus aggravating the condition of atherosclerosis. Regular physical exercise would appear to have a two-fold effect on the autonomic nerve supply to the heart. Parasympathetic effect is enhanced at rest, while sympathetic drive is decreased during exercise. The end result is to slow the heart rate both at rest and during exercise. Not only that, but the cardiovascular system is less susceptible to the harmful effects of sudden shocks or stresses.

The stimulus for this alteration in autonomic nerve control probably operates as follows. Muscular activity massages the limb veins, thus increasing the volume of blood returned to the heart. This immediately results in a greater stroke volume, and the brain, realizing that it can now achieve the same cardiac output with fewer heart beats, takes steps to reduce the heart rate. This increased "priming" of the heart pump is maintained by another effect of regular exercise — an increase in the volume of the blood.

Increase in Heart Size   In a young subject, the more powerful
contractions of the heart which are necessary to attain the increased stroke volume result in an increase in the size of the
heart. The so-called "big-heart" of the trained endurance athlete
has long been recognized. The work of Dr. Joel Morganroth
of Philadelphia has now identified the nature of that enlargement.
Using a specialized ultrasound x-ray technique, he has shown it
to be due to a lengthening of cardiac muscle fibres, resulting in
an increase in the volume and capacity of the ventricles or pumping chambers. Such volume enlargement does not occur in weight-
lifters, wrestlers, sprinters, shot-putters and the like. These
explosive-type performers develop hypertrophy, or thickening of
the walls of the heart, but no particular change in overall cardiac
dimensions. In fact, their hearts resemble more closely those of
the "normal," sedentary, population.

The healthy enlargement of the heart of the long distance
runner, swimmer, or cyclist must be distinguished from the
enlargement due to the dilatation of a failing heart. They may
look the same on a routine chest x-ray, but the athlete's heart
never exceeds a critical weight of 500 grams, whereas the dilated
diseased heart will frequently attain much greater weights. The
distinction is, of course, an academic one. Weighing a heart is
hardly a routine clinical procedure! And yet, differentiation is
important, otherwise the ultra-fit young endurance athlete may
find himself labelled as "abnormal" and ordered to abstain from
any exertion (or even put to bed), for months, by which time his
fitness has gone, his heart has shrunk to sedentary size, and he is
"normal" again. Nowadays, such an error is less likely to occur,
since various methods exist to ascertain that the big heart is
actually functioning normally.

But the main safeguard against such unnecessary invalidism
is an awareness on the part of the physician. Sad to say, I still
come across cases of athlete's heart labelled by the well-meaning
radiologist as "abnormal enlargement."

Can the middle-aged jogger develop a beneficial increase in
cardiac volume? As yet this has not been recorded. However, we
cannot say firmly that it does not occur. It may be that the middle-
aged exerciser is to date unaccustomed to carrying out the very
heavy training regimes of the young athlete. Now that the 40-
year-olds and over are becoming more fitness conscious, studies
may begin to show that the trained older heart may be capable

of obtaining a healthy and beneficial increase in size.

The Blood Supply   As the heart increases in size, there is a proportional increase in the diameter and number of branches of the coronary vessels, together with an increase in the tiny capillary blood vessels which course through the substance of the heart muscle. In this way, blood supply keeps pace with demand. Clarence de Mar, a famous American long distance running champion, died of cancer in his seventies; an autopsy of his heart revealed that his coronary arteries were unusually large. While this may have been the result of natural endowment, it seems more likely to have been brought about by his many years of intensive training. Large coronary arteries are of distinct advantage in that they are extremely unlikely to be blocked by even a lifetime's deposit by fatty atheromatous material. Maybe this is why myocardial infarction is a rare occurrence in active marathon runners, even though a significant number of these men are middle-aged.

In the previous chapter, we noted that oxygen-rich blood flowed through the coronary arteries to supply the heart muscle *between* beats (that is, during the resting phase, or diastole). Thus, the higher the heart rate, the shorter the time between beats. Conversely, the slower the heart rate, the greater the proportion of time spent in diastole. Fitness bradycardia, therefore, is synonymous with a lengthening of diastole and an increase in coronary blood flow.

As if an improved blood supply to the heart were not enough, the fit exerciser has further advantage over his sedentary counterpart. Fitness brings with it a reduction in the blood supply requirements of the heart. The slowly beating heart muscle uses oxygen more sparingly, and so the blood flow does not need to be so vigorous. It is a case of living well within one's cardiac budget. The oxygen income is potentially high, while at the same time, the expenditure is low. Obviously, this affords a high measure of safety, with adequate protection from the vicissitudes of modern life, including disease.

Blood Pressure   Heavy physical labour, or athletic training, is associated with a low, or normal, blood pressure. While this is often evident at rest, it is most striking during effort. Since in a significant proportion of cases a link can be found between the heart attack and a bout of unaccustomed severe effort, this may be another important factor in the reduced tendency for heavy workers to sustain an attack. An unusual heavy exertion on the sedentary heart will lead to a precipitant rise in blood pressure, and if there is pre-existing disease of the coronary arteries, this sudden increase in cardiac workload may be sufficient to trigger a myocardial infarction. Isometric muscle contractions, such as straining to lift a heavy weight or moving a heavy piece of furniture, are particularly dangerous since the rise in blood pressure is disproportionately high. Fit individuals, however, can accomplish heavy physical tasks with relatively low increments of pressure. A number of investigations indicate that people who regularly indulge in heavy exercise have less increase in their blood pressures with advancing years. Indeed, Kraus and Raab have included several forms of hypertension in their list of so-called "hypokinetic diseases" — diseases caused by too little movement.

Other Advantages of Physical Activity

In addition to the benefits accruing to the heart itself, the active have certain other advantages over the inactive in areas which are pertinent to our topic. We have seen that heart attack is often precipitated by a blood clot forming over the fatty plaque, thus increasing the size of the obstruction to blood flow. It has been shown that increase in fitness may be parallelled by a lengthening of clotting times; the blood becomes less "sticky," and thrombosis is less likely to occur. High levels of blood fat can be reduced by prolonged exercise, and one study on Finnish soldiers showed that, following a high-fat meal, there was a significantly greater reduction in the blood fats of those who shortly after went on a ten-mile march than in those who rested. Dr. Peter Wood of Stanford University, California, has demonstrated that middle-aged men, following a jogging program, had much higher than average levels of "protective" HDL cholesterol (see page 36) in their blood. In terms of experimentation, animal studies have shown that an atherosclerotic-producing diet was highly successful in developing the disease in inactive subjects, but not in those which were kept physically active. Other animal studies demonstrated how muscular activity was effective in increasing the breakdown of radio-actively labelled cholesterol.

Finally, some studies show that physical training improves sugar tolerance in the mild diabetic. Interestingly enough, exercise was a main form of therapy for diabetes before insulin was discovered, but it seems to have been neglected by physicians since then. The active diabetic requires less insulin, and it is well known clinically that the sedentary diabetic requires to increase his insulin dosage. The precise mechanism by which this comes about is uncertain, but it seems to be connected with the development of a more efficient carbohydrate metabolism. There may also be an indirect connection between certain high blood fats and a tendency to diabetes, and so reduction in the former could be of benefit to the latent diabetic. Weight control is an important feature in the management of diabetes and so a reduction in weight due to physical activity may be yet another aspect of the problem.

Few would deny that the above is an impressive list of potential benefits, any or all of which could protect the fit individual from a heart attack. We now need to consider the implications. Heavy work is becoming a thing of the past, and so we must pursue fitness in our leisure time. Since most of the physiological changes described have been demonstrated in amateur athletes rather than heavy workers, this seems a feasible proposition. However, we still have certain questions to answer pertaining to our particular need. What type of exercise produces the most cardiovascular fitness? How intensive need the exercise be? How frequently should it be carried out, and for what duration? Finally, and most important, can a training program benefit the individual who has had a heart attack and devoutly wishes to avoid another? These topics, and others besides, will be the subject of our discussions in the next chapter.

CHAPTER THREE

The Beneficial Effects of Exercise

WE have seen how regular physical activity protects against a heart attack. However, most of the studies quoted dealt with occupational exertion — with people who work as bus conductors, farmers, mailmen. The mechanism by which such work could have protected the heart was deduced from the results of scientific investigations carried out on trained athletes. Are we justified in concluding that the effects of heavy work and heavy sports training are comparable? The answer is yes.

One way to measure the amount of effort expended on a physical task is to estimate the amount of calories the body burns to accomplish it. The active and heavy workers in the studies mentioned averaged between 400 and 900 calories per day over and above the sedentary worker; this was the effort required to evoke the mechanism which gave them a high degree of protection from heart disease. An international endurance athlete trains seven days a week, often twice a day, burning around 1,000 calories in each session. Small wonder that long distance runners and cyclists and the like, provided they remain active, have almost total immunity from heart attacks. However, such dedication may not be necessary. Even the 170 lb. "hobby" runner expends 700 calories if he goes for a one-hour jog. You will note that the physical worker's effort is more likely to be spread over an eight-hour day, so that his work costs him an extra two calories per minute. The jogger, on the other hand, concentrates his effort into 60 minutes, burning about 10 calories per minute. This seems to make little difference although, as we shall see later, there is a critical intensity of exertion below which cardiac benefits fail to occur.

For practical purposes, we can divide all exercise into two types — aerobic and anaerobic (see Chapter 2, page 58). The latter consists of short, sharp bursts of activity lasting only a matter of minutes, and leaving us gasping for breath in order to pay back the oxygen we "borrowed" to accomplish the task. Sprint runners and cyclists, weight-lifters, hockey players, are typical examples of anaerobic performers. Aerobic exercise, on the other hand, is less intense, more prolonged, and is carried out without any, or only slight, breathlessness. There is no need for the muscles to function without oxygen because the task required of them is well within the capacity of the oxygen transport system. It is this type of long, steady endurance exercise which is associated with benefits to the cardiovascular system and which will, therefore, be of primary interest to us. Running, cycling and swimming for long distances, cross-country skiing, canoeing and rowing are all sports in which a high degree of aerobic effort is needed. Active participants in these activities, if they are to be successful, must be capable of using large quantities of oxygen. By definition, this is synonymous with a highly efficient oxygen transport system — in other words, a healthy and effective heart pump.

We have now progressed to the crux of the whole situation. If all successful aerobic performers possess such superior cardiovascular systems, can the bulk of the sedentary population attain equal benefits by the regular practice of similar activities? Exercise physiologists and physical educators now think that this is so. Neither the physical labourer nor the long distance runner chooses these activities *because* he has a healthy cardiovascular system; he is healthy *as a result* of the activity. Admittedly, individuals such as Roger Bannister, the Englishman who first broke the four-minute mile, and mythical figures such as John Henry of American railroad fame, likely have to thank their forebears for a proportion of their legendary ability. But that does not alter the fact that the bulk of their greatness came from regular practice and training.

Thus, if we wish to see our children grow up with healthy cardiovascular systems, we will ensure that they are introduced to endurance type sports in their early school days, and we will provide the facilities and motivation for them to continue with these activities into adult life. Unfortunately, many schools in North America devote little or no time to sports, or if they do, only to those which are professional, spectator, and anaerobic in type, such as football, ice hockey and basketball. The adult of today is the product of this short-sighted system and is currently paying the penalty for it. But is it too late for the middle-aged citizen to catch up? The answer is no — with reservations. All the evidence suggests that the beneficial exercise-induced cardiorespiratory changes which occur in the young also take place in the individual who starts to train for the first time in his (or her) middle years. However, there are some differences in the reaction of the middle-aged heart to effort, and these are more evident when the heart is the site of coronary artery disease. Thus, if we are going to advocate exercise for the 30-year-old and over, we must examine these differences more closely. Exercise can help us beat heart disease, but if we are to employ it, we must use it like any other medication. We must be familiar with its indications and contra-indications, its optimal dosages, its side affects, and its adverse reactions. We must also be able to measure its effects in an objective manner so as to be able to adjust the dosage accordingly. Like any potent medicine, exercise does wonders when used wisely but can be useless or even dangerous when dispensed with ignorance.

Exercise and the Normal Middle-Aged Heart

We must distinguish between the physiological changes caused by acute and by chronic exercise. The former refers to an isolated bout of activity; its effects on the heart are clear-cut and have been referred to briefly in Chapter 2 when describing the oxygen transport system. In essence, acute exertion stresses the whole body in a specific manner. Constant repetition of that stress at regular intervals, on the other hand, constitutes chronic exercise, and here again, the long-term bodily effects are specific.

An increase in physical activity requires an increase in the supply of oxygen-carrying blood to the muscles. The heart responds with a higher output. As we have seen, it can achieve this in three ways: either by an increase in the number of strokes per minute, in the amount of blood ejected with each stroke, or by a combination of both. In the untrained, the oxygen require-

Figure 4

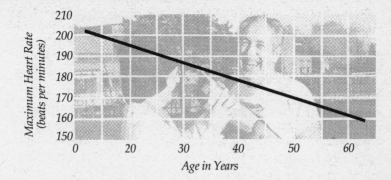

The Older You Are the Lower Your Maximum Heart Rate

ments of casual exertion are largely met by a speed-up in heart rate. This accounts for the extremely rapid heart beat which accompanies even mild exertion in the sedentary. The trained heart increases its output largely by stepping up the stroke volume.

Our blood pressure depends upon three factors: the force with which the blood is pumped into the general circulation by the heart; the elasticity or "give" of the arterial walls; and the resistance to flow experienced by the blood as it courses through the vessels in the muscles, skin and internal organs. During endurance-type exercise there is a rise in blood pressure, probably because the vigorously contracting muscles squeeze the blood vessels in the legs and arms, thus necessitating an increase in the force required to move the blood around the body. The more intensive the exercise becomes, the more the blood pressure rises.

The middle-aged heart suffers to some extent in terms of these adaptations. It is a physiological fact that each of us possesses a maximum heart rate. This maximum varies slightly from person to person, but once reached, it cannot be exceeded no matter how much the intensity or duration of the exercise is increased. Furthermore, the maximum heart rate declines with age (Figure 4). Thus, whereas an individual of 25 might have a maximum heart rate of 190 beats per minute, this declines to 160 heart beats per minute at age 65. The net result is that the older exerciser has a smaller potential increase of heart rate. Also, the middle-aged heart contracts more slowly, and this has the effect of lengthening the phase of systole at the expense of the phase of diastole. A shortening of diastole means less time for coronary blood flow. Finally, middle-aged muscles are often flabby from disuse, and so have to work closer to all-out effort in order to achieve a given workload; thus, for any given effort, the rise of blood pressure is much more marked.

Despite these differences, the normal middle-aged heart is perfectly capable of sharing in the benefits of an exercise program, provided that these differences are borne in mind when the exercise regime is designed.

Exercise and the Atherosclerotic Heart

So far, we have been considering the response of the healthy heart to activity, with some allowance made for age. We will now look at the effects of acute exercise in coronary artery disease. This is of supreme importance to the heart attack patient who becomes involved in an exercise rehabilitation program. It also has value for the middle-aged exercise neophyte who, without knowing it, may already have significant atherosclerosis of his coronary arteries — which probably includes most of us over 40!

Severe coronary disease may be complicated by an irregular heart rhythm, weakening or stiffening of the wall of the heart from previous scarring or, if an actual heart attack has taken place, weakness and debility as a result of a period of sustained bed rest following the attack. For this reason, a great deal more caution must be used when prescribing exercise in these individuals.

In the normal individual, there is a close relationship between the increase of heart rate and the increase of intensity of effort. However, occasionally the heart rate of the atherosclerotic patient may not rise in such a linear manner. This may be due to a narrowing of the artery which supplies blood to the heart's primary rhythm regulator, the sino-atrial node. Thus, there is a sluggish response to the body's demand for an acceleration of heart rate. In extreme cases, this can be dangerous, and Dr. Ernst Jokl of the University of Kentucky has ascribed some unexplained sudden "exercise" deaths in apparently healthy individuals to a deficient blood supply to the sino-atrial node.

The condition may reveal itself during an exercise stress test when it is found that an increase in workload does not bring about the anticipated increase in pulse rate. Vigorous exercise is contra-indicated in such individuals.

Atherosclerosis may equally affect the blood supply to other parts of the electrical conducting system of the heart. This may cause different portions of the heart to beat out of phase, giving rise to so-called "dropped" or "skipped" beats. These are readily recognized on the electrocardiogram, which will also indicate to the physician which part of the heart is contracting irregularly. Irregular beats, unless they occur very frequently, are usually not a contra-indication to exercise, although most physicians would like to control their frequency with medication before permitting training.

In the absence of damage to the pacemaker or the rhythm-conducting system, the heart rate and stroke volume will usually increase normally in response to exercise, despite disease of the coronary arteries. On the other hand, subsequent to a heart attack, pumping may be sustained with the scarred part of the muscle wall contributing nothing to the squeezing action, or even bulging outwards and thus absorbing part of the force developed by the healthy muscle. This may affect the stroke volume, which in some cases may actually decrease in response to demand for higher output. Pressures inside the heart may rise excessively, with a consequent abnormal increase in "back-pressure" both in the general circulation and also in the lung capillaries. In such cases, exercise will cause swelling of the legs and feet, or excessive breathlessness. Blood pressure may rise excessively, and this will increase the cardiac workload and possibly induce angina pectoris. The patient becomes anxious, his blood pressure rises further, the pain increases, and a vicious circle is established.

The heart's ability to function as a pump may also be adversely affected by "ectopic" or "skipped" beats. There seems to be an innocent form of this irregularity which is present at rest and clears up during exercise. Such cases are often discovered in youth and are probably due to excessive sympathetic drive in a highly strung individual. In the absence of other signs of heart disease, they are not considered by physicians to be harmful. When irregular beats first appear, or become more frequent with exercise, they are more serious in import, and since they interrupt the regular rhythm of the heart, they can reduce the quantity of blood being pumped around the body per minute.

"Asynergy" of cardiac muscle, or inability of all parts of the wall to contract together as one, may result from either an electrical conduction defect or fibrous scarring. It also gives rise to a less effective pumping force. The valves of the heart may be involved in the atherosclerotic process, and may not function efficiently when the heart is beating rapidly, thus decreasing the amount of blood being delivered around the body.

Finally, there is the emotional aspect of exercise. The average post-coronary patient may see a bout of exercise as a threat to his health. Excessive stress hormones (adrenalin and noradrenalin) are secreted, the heart muscle becomes more irritable and liable to "skipped beats," the heart rate and blood pressure increase, and the workload of the heart rises. Thus, while many patients with coronary artery disease apparently respond to exercise in the same manner as normal, healthy middle-aged individuals, some will react in an abnormal and potentially dangerous manner. The more serious and extensive the disease, the greater the likelihood that the heart will respond abnormally. Therefore, the post-coronary patient should approach exercise with due caution. Neither exercise stress tests nor post-coronary exercise classes should be undertaken lightly. Why then, you may ask, take the risk at all? Do the benefits of training outweigh the possible hazards?

A study carried out in conjunction with Dr. Roy Shephard showed that of 203 consecutive cases referred for post-coronary rehabilitation, 60 were engaged in vigorous physical activity at or shortly before the time of their heart attack. The breakdown was as follows:

Heavy domestic chores	14	Baseball	1
Walking	13	Soccer	1
Snow-shovelling	9	Basketball	1
Running	8	Hockey	1
Curling	4	Squash	1
Tennis	2	Gymnastics	1
Sexual intercourse	2	Dancing	1
Ice-breaking	1		

If acute exercise can cause a heart attack, how can chronic exercise be a suitable form of therapy? The answer is that an acute bout of unaccustomed physical activity merely reveals the presence of a diseased coronary artery system which is already highly susceptible to physical and mental stress. This is largely unavoidable; most of us face excessive activity at some time or another. Training prepares us for such emergencies and reduces the danger of such episodes.

Training and its Benefits in Coronary Artery Disease

We have previously looked at the beneficial effects of training on the normal middle-aged heart and have described the conditions which occur in training post-coronary patients: bradycardia and prolongation of diastole, increased stroke volume, reduced blood pressure, increased extraction of blood by the muscles, reduction in clotting time, and decrease in blood fats. Of more obvious value, a training program frequently reduces or eliminates the occurrence of exertional angina pectoris. Why is this so?

In 1957, Eckstein carried out a most interesting study in which he took a group of dogs and tied off a branch of their coronary artery tree so as to induce a non-fatal myocardial infarction. He then divided them into two groups, one of which was exercised regularly, the other restricted to their cages and forced to be sedentary. As time went by, it was found that the exercised dogs developed new coronary blood vessels which grew around the blocked vessels and eventually made up for the lack of blood supply; these new blood vessels are referred to by the medical term "collaterals." The sedentary dogs, on the other hand, showed no such beneficial effect. The implication was obvious. However, the use of coronary angiograms (an x-ray technique by which a radio-opaque dye is introduced into the coronary arteries to show their number and calibre) has only occasionally demonstrated such changes in human post-coronary patients who are involved in exercise programs.

This does not mean, of course, that collaterals do not develop in humans. It may be that the vessels are so fine that they exist only in the micro-circulation, and so our present rather crude angiograms cannot detect them; or it may be that we haven't studied enough cases as yet. After all, post-coronary patients who are doing well on an exercise program are understandably reluctant to submit to angiography. Finally, it may be that more arduous training might be necessary to obtain the desired results; many post-coronary training regimes are rather light in intensity.

However, assuming for argument's sake that training does not increase coronary collateralization in the atherosclerotic heart, there is an additional mechanism by which improvement can occur. The coronary blood flow answers the requirements of the heart muscle for oxygen. There are three major factors determining the amount of oxygen consumed by the contracting heart — the heart rate, the blood pressure, and the velocity of heart wall contraction. For practical purposes, the third factor may be ignored, and we can obtain an adequate approximation of the heart's oxygen requirements from the first two components. We merely multipy the heart rate and the blood pressure together. The resultant figure is known as the Rate Pressure Product (RPP). The clinical value of this product as an index of myocardial oxygen consumption is suggested by the fact that patients with angina pectoris frequently have a constant Rate Pressure Product at which pain first appears.

Let us suppose that an individual develops angina at a RPP of 18,000. Such a figure could be attained arithmetically by various combinations of heart rate and blood pressure: for instance, a heart rate of 120 per minute and a systolic blood pressure reading of 150; or a rate of 106 beats per minute and a blood pressure of 180. This explains why a patient's angina may be triggered by different levels of activity, or indeed can result from excitement or anxiety even while at rest. For instance, hot and humid weather may give a disproportionate rise in heart rate during physical activity, while in cold weather weight-lifting may accentuate the rise in blood pressure. An argument with the boss may increase both heart rate and blood pressure, even while sitting at a desk.

A carefully designed training regime can reduce or eliminate angina pectoris at increasing workloads. Even if this were not due to increased collateralization, it could be explained on the basis that training results in a slower heart rate and a lower blood pressure, and this gives rise to a lower RPP.

As the angina improves, we often see changes in the exercise electrocardiogram. Again, this can be explained either on the basis of increased coronary blood flow, or reduced RPP at that workload. We have shown that post-coronary patients can be brought to a high level of fitness through an intensive training program. Evidence to date suggests that these fortunate individuals not only get relief from chest discomfort at a given workload, but also push their critical RPP threshold higher and higher, until they can perform large muscle exercises such as treadmill running to their maximum without developing subjective or objective evidence of cardiac ischemia. These are the men who have attained jogging distances of four miles and up, averaging 25 or more miles a week over two years or more.

But why is it that some post-coronary exercisers are unable to attain such intensity of training? Is it a question of being less motivated? Or is it that they are physiologically incapable of meeting the demands of the program, either because of age, or because of the severity of their disease? These are questions which we cannot as yet answer, but hopefully we will be able to as our research progresses.

If we consider the benefits discussed above, it seems fair to argue that the task of training post-coronary patients is no mere academic exercise. In particular, the reduction of the RPP at a given intensity of work is unquestionable. There is no shortage of evidence that training is physiologically beneficial. But can it increase the lifespan of the heart attack victim by reducing the frequency and severity of recurrent attacks? And if it can, what is the optimum intensity, duration and frequency of exercise sessions required? Are men who devote themselves to the demanding program of 20 or 30 miles of jogging each week going to gain a more decisive advantage over those who remain content with one or two weekly sessions of calisthenics?

These and similar problems will be discussed more fully in the second part of this book which deals with the inception and operation of a post-coronary exercise rehabilitation program over the past seven years. However, before closing this section, we must examine the method by which response to training is measured. This is a vital part of any exercise program, providing feed-back not only for the exerciser, but also for the trainer, be he coach or physician.

Exercise Testing and Fitness

In recent years, exercise physiologists and physical educators have become increasingly interested in the measurement of endurance fitness, leading them to invade areas long regarded as the province of the physician. Laboratory testing of high-performance endurance athletes has shown that the most valid measurement of superiority is maximum oxygen consumption — which is another way of saying efficiency of the oxygen transport system. The most vital link in this system, of course, is the heart, which pumps the oxygen-rich blood to the muscles.

In principle, measurement of the amount of oxygen an individual can utilize is easy. The air we breathe in contains 21 per cent oxygen. Analysis of the air we breathe out (the technical term is "expired gas") will show a reduction in this figure; the difference represents the amount of oxygen consumed by our muscles. The more vigorously the muscles contract, the more oxygen they require. Ultimately, however, the point will be reached where the oxygen transport system is no longer effective and cannot satisfy the increasing demand of the muscles for oxygen. Heart rate and stroke volume have reached their zenith. So far, and no further, they say; or to use a modern analogy, the engine has run out of gas.

Testing for Maximum Oxygen Consumption   Posed with the task of measuring someone's maximum oxygen consumption, you would need to estimate the oxygen consumed in carrying out increasingly vigorous physical tasks until exhaustion supervenes, taking the final figures as the vo_2 max. Expressed in scientific jargon, what you have done is progressed the subject through multi-stage standardized workloads while continuously measuring oxygen intake; the end point is reached when the subject cannot continue because of exhaustion.

A discerning reader may detect a weakness in this description. What if the subject voluntarily quits before his muscles have reached the limit of their performance, before they are totally exhausted? It may be that his threshold for physical discomfort is low and that he is not prepared to push himself to this limit. There is no doubt that motivation plays a large part in the successful accomplishment of a maximum test, and this is one of its drawbacks. It is, however, possible to tell in retrospect if the maximum level has been reached, for analysis of expired gas samples will show that the amount of oxygen consumed has plateaued, despite an increase in the final workload. For example, increasing the speed of walking will increase the amount of oxygen used in a linear fashion until eventually an increment in speed will outstrip the muscle's ability to function aerobically. At this point, anaerobic muscle contraction will take over; but, as we have seen, this is a wasteful and self-limiting process, building up lactic acid and forcing matters to a halt within sixty seconds or so. Measurement of the oxygen content of the expired gas will now show that it is the same or only fractionally more than that for the speed immediately preceding it. Professor Roy Shephard has recommended that an increase in oxygen consumption of less than 2 ml/kg.min for a 10 per cent increase in workload intensity can be accepted as proof that the subject has attained maximum effort; this is the standard used in our laboratory. Another indication of supreme effort is the high level of lactic acid in the blood as a result of the final few seconds of anaerobic activity. Of course, there will also be the more usual signs of acute exhaustion, such as leg fatigue, staggering gait, facial pallor, nausea, gasping for breath and extremely high heart rate.

It will now be obvious that measurement of endurance fitness by maximum testing is a somewhat arduous procedure. It is usually carried out in the exercise laboratory on a treadmill, a piece of equipment which consists essentially of a moving belt, approximately three feet wide, on which the subject walks or runs. The speed and/or elevation of the belt is increased in a step-like manner every two or three minutes. The treadmill is bulky, noisy and frightening to subjects who have never been on one before. At high speeds, it is potentially dangerous, especially when the subject has become unco-ordinated as a result of maximum effort. In general, then, the sedentary middle-aged and the elderly are unsuitable candidates for maximal testing. How then can we assess the cardiovascular fitness of these individuals?

Sub-maximal Testing Fortunately, there is a method which is based on two very convenient facts. One is that oxygen consumption increases in a straight line in response to augmentation of effort (Figure 5). The second is that heart rate and oxygen consumption are related in the same fashion (Figure 6). And since everyone has a maximum heart rate which decreases with age, this has led to the construction of tables containing average values for the population at large. A little reflection will enable

Figure 5

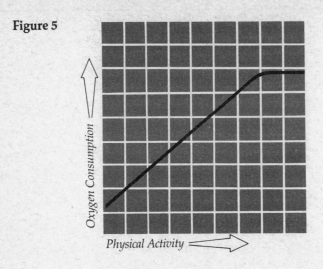

The More Vigorous Your Physical Activity, the More Oxygen Your Body Uses.

us to put these three pieces of information together and come up with a method of predicting an individual's maximum oxygen consumption from the measurement at a sub-maximal level of exertion.

Simply, the procedure is to bring the heart rate up to 50 and 75 per cent of the maximum as read from the tables, measure the oxygen utilized at each of these levels, join these two points and extend the line to the estimated maximum heart rate; the point of intersection is then dropped to the baseline, where it is read off as the predicted vo_2 max (Figure 7). Formulas have been developed which obviate the necessity for plotting a graph, and enable a prediction to be made from oxygen analysis at one workload only, usually the one which results in a heart rate of about 75 or 80 per cent maximum.

It usually takes a few minutes for the heart rate and oxygen consumption to stabilize at any given workload, and the test protocol calls for the subject to work a minimum of three minutes at each load to ensure the so-called "steady state" as being reached. A further simplification of the sub-maximal test is the use of tables which relate heart rate and oxygen consumption. Thus one can plot heart rate against workload and obtain the

Figure 6

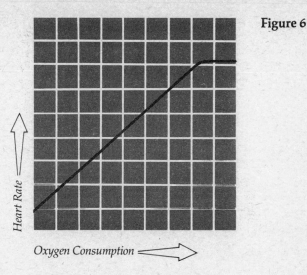

Heart Rate

Oxygen Consumption

As You Use More Oxygen in Physical Activity, Your Heart Rate Increases Accordingly

predicted vo₂ max from a table of average equivalents, removing the necessity to collect and analyze expired gas.

The validity of sub-maximal testing is dependent upon the accuracy of the maximum heart rate tables, and while purists will prefer to establish the actual figure by maximum testing, by and large the tables are correct to within a range of 10 per cent. For practical purposes, this is quite adequate, and is a reasonable trade-off for the inherent difficulties and dangers of maximum testing. When measuring the fitness level of patients who are suffering from coronary heart disease, one has to be particularly careful, and sub-maximal testing has obvious advantages. However, some physicians argue that the maximum heart rate is frequently reduced in such cases and the use of heart rate maximum tables is not justified. In a recent study in which I compared the results of maximum and sub-maximum tests in a group of heart attack patients, the results indicate that maximum heart rates are frequently within normal limits, and that the predicted values for vo₂ max are acceptably close to actual measurement.

Sub-maximal testing can be performed on a treadmill, a set of steps, or a stationary bicycle. Steps are awkward if the subject is expected to breathe into a gas collection bag. The stationary

Figure 7

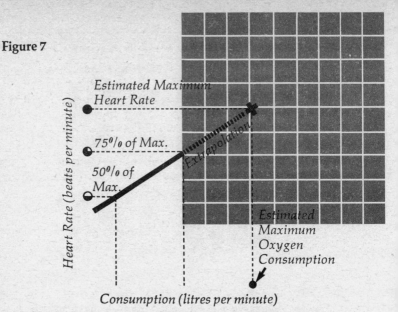

How to Estimate Your Maximum Oxygen Consumption

bicycle is the most convenient, provided the thigh muscles are not so weak that they give out before the heart rate has achieved the desired level — an occasional occurrence in North Americans who are unaccustomed to cycling (actually, this is one of the major reasons for choosing the treadmill over the bicycle in maximal testing). The type of bicycle used delivers a measured workload by applying resistance to the drive-wheel either mechanically by means of a friction belt, or electrically by a variable magnetic field. The resistance must be constant, and accurately reproducible from test to test. Incidentally, the home exercise bicycle which uses a crude screw and tension spring arrangement to adjust workload is useless for this purpose. The great advantage of the stationary bicycle is its cost ($400 to $500 as opposed to $3,000 and up for a motor-driven treadmill), and the fact that it allows the upper portion of the body to remain relatively free from movement during the test. This makes for greater convenience in collecting expired gas and obtaining blood pressure readings and good quality electrocardiograph tracings.

Use of the Electrocardiogram in Testing   So far, we have only considered the application of exercise testing to the measurement of maximum oxygen consumption. This requires the recording of heart rate and, in most cases, the collection of expired air in large rubber balloons for later analysis. A heart rate may be counted manually by feeling the pulse at the wrist or in the neck, or it may be obtained by the use of a cardiotachometer, an instrument which picks up the heart beat from an electrode applied to the chest and transmits it by a solid wire lead to the dial of a counter. The more normal method, however, is to connect the subject to an electrocardiogram so that a simultaneous ECG tracing is obtained throughout the test. This has two advantages: it allows the physician to count the number of electrical complexes every few seconds, thus obtaining a very accurate heart rate count; it also permits detection of irregularities in the rhythm and shape of the electrical signals indicative of cardiac stress.

As a matter of fact, it is this simultaneous recording of the ECG tracing during exercise which has interested the cardiologists most in the past ten years, ever since it was discovered that latent coronary heart disease could frequently be detected in this manner. A patient with advanced atherosclerosis of his coronary arteries and consequent impairment of blood supply to his heart will often show evidence of this in his resting (or static) ECG. But what if the atherosclerotic narrowing is not so severe, and the myocardial blood supply only becomes inadequate when the heart has to work hard? In such cases, the static ECG might well be normal. Only an ECG recorded during exercise (a dynamic ECG) will demonstrate the abnormality. The milder the degree of disease, the higher the intensity of exercise needed for its detection.

In the final analysis, sub-maximal or maximal exercise testing can be used to diagnose hitherto unsuspected heart disease in an individual who has no apparent evidence of any abnormality. By the same token, the completion of a maximum exercise test without the development of ECG irregularities is highly indicative of freedom from coronary disease.

The work of Robb and Blackburn has indicated that such testing may be able to predict whether or not the subject will have a heart attack in the future. Over a twelve-year period, they subjected a group of 1,659 life insurance applicants to an exercise test which involved stair-stepping followed by immediate post-exercise electrocardiograms. All of the applicants were free from impairment which would call for rejection of their applications. The cardiac response to exercise testing was abnormal in 269 individuals (16.2 per cent), and when followed over the years, these subjects had a death rate from heart attacks two and a half to thirteen times higher than those with normal exercise tests, the frequency increasing with the abnormality of the exercise response. Furthermore, even in those subjects who were considered on the basis of pre-test medical evidence to have probable or definite coronary heart disease, the dynamic electrocardiogram proved to be a significant forecaster of mortality; a positive exercise response in these people was followed by a five-fold increase in coronary death rate; a negative response meant a more benign outlook despite the previous poor history.

While underlining the diagnostic value of the step-exercise test, the authors in their report went on to postulate that there may have been some cases of heart disease undetected "because they were not exercised enough to make it manifest." Hence, the increasing interest by cardiologists in maximal and high sub-maximal treadmill and bicycle tests, with simultaneous dynamic electrocardiogram recordings.

Warning Signs in Testing

In recent years, a number of objective criteria for labelling an exercise test "abnormal" or predictive of ischemic heart disease have emerged. They are: (1) ST segment depression, (2) irregular heart action, (3) inappropriate blood pressure response to exercise, and (4) inappropriate heart rate response to exercise. Since this requires some explanation, we will deal with each separately.

ST Segment Depression or "Silent Angina" The beating heart muscle produces minute amounts of electricity which, when amplified, can be recorded on a piece of moving graph paper (figure 8). Each spike on the tracing is labelled by a letter for convenience of reference, and represents electrical activity in a different portion of the heart. The P wave is caused by the upper chamber of the heart, the atrium, contracting. The QRS complex is caused by the ventricles "discharging" as they squeeze blood out of the chambers. The T wave marks the recovery phase when the ventricles "recharge" their electrical energy. The portion of the tracing between the s and the start of the T wave is known as the ST segment.

Figure 8

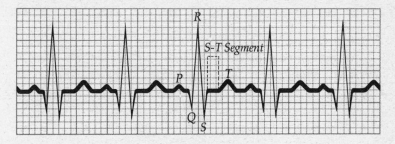

Normal Electrocardiogram

You will notice that in the normal heart each labelled deflection of the tracing returns directly to the mid-line, or "iso-electric" line, as soon as it has reached its peak. The iso-electric line represents electrical neutrality. When the ventricle has completed its contraction (the s point of the QRS complex), it has discharged its electricity, and so the trace returns quickly to neutral before commencing to recharge again (T wave). In other words, the ST segment ascends vertically and without delay to the iso-electric line. In cases of ischemic heart disease, however, this prompt ascent may be delayed, in which case, the moving graph paper will show a "depression" of the ST segment (figure 9).

Figure 9

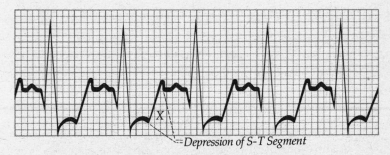

Depression of S-T Segment

**Electrocardiogram Showing Depression of the S-T Segment
Indicating Reduced Blood Flow Through the Coronary Arteries**

The greater the degree of depression (measured as x in the diagram), the more severe the degree of ischemia. Actually, this change in the sᴛ segment merely tells us that the heart muscle is short of oxygen; it does not tell us why. For instance, the patient may be anemic, or may be suffering from a form of thyroid disease, or may be taking a type of medication which results in a similar picture. However, since coronary heart disease is by far the most common cause of heart muscle ischemia these days, depression of the sᴛ segment has become characteristic of that condition. Obviously, the physician will know if the patient is on the sort of medication which gives a "false" sᴛ segment depression.

In practice, the electrocardiogram tracing at the beginning of the test may well be normal. Only as the level of work increases does the sᴛ segment begin to sag. Sometimes this may not occur until the patient is exerting himself to 85 per cent or more of his maximum. Not infrequently the depression will revert to normal almost immediately on stopping the exercise — hence the insistence of some physicians on obtaining concurrent tracings during the test rather than relying on immediate post-exercise electrocardiograms. By international agreement, a depression of the sᴛ segment measuring more than 2 mm is considered abnormal. It is highly likely that such a response is evidence of coronary heart disease, and the greater the depression, the higher the likelihood of a heart attack in the future. That is not to say that a positive test is an irrevocable portent of tragedy. No test is one hundred per cent certain. Nevertheless, the evidence favours acceptance of a high degree of predictability — enough to make the individual with a positive exercise test take steps to avoid future trouble by altering his lifestyle in such a way as to reduce his risk factors. Similarly, while a negative test carried out to maximum intensity does not absolutely guarantee freedom from myocardial infarction in the future, it makes such an event unlikely.

In some subjects with clearly established atherosclerosis, exercise-induced sᴛ segmental depression is not accompanied by typical anginal pain. We know that the sᴛ changes are an indication of shortage of blood to the heart muscle, but unfortunately the patient cannot feel anything wrong. In discussing this type of situation with a patient, I usually tell him that his exercise electrocardiogram has shown evidence of "silent angina"; in other words, we know from his electrocardiogram that at a given level of exertion he develops myocardial ischemia, but for a number of reasons this does not give rise to the usual cramp-like pain. We therefore prescribe a level of exertion below that at which the electrocardiogram changes appear. This helps him to understand why we are asking him to walk or jog at a slower pace than he feels capable of.

Finally, sᴛ segment response to exercise may change, some individuals regressing from a negative test to a positive test, others progressing from positive to negative; in my experience, the latter is a fairly common result of an exercise rehabilitation course.

Irregular Heart Rate　In a healthy heart, the electrical events follow a relatively fixed time sequence. The ᴘ wave, representing atrial contraction, rarely lasts more than 0.08 seconds; the ǫᴙs complex, representing the ventricular contraction, also takes 0.08 seconds; from the beginning of the ᴘ wave to the start of the ǫ wave is never more than 0.2 seconds. These intervals, together with many others, can be quickly read off the electro-cardiogram paper by the physician, using the standard graph paper (1 mm squares) and standard paper speed (25 mm per second), so that each of the squares corresponds to 0.04 seconds. Not only are the events within the cardiac cycle on a time and sequence basis, but the intervals between each cycle, or heart beat, are also regular. Obviously, as the heart beats quicker or slower, these inter-beat intervals will change, but the alterations will occur evenly in the same manner as a well-tuned automobile engine accelerates and decelerates. However, if the heart is starved of blood, then an increase in tempo will result in a short-age of oxygen to the myocardium, with resultant "misfiring" which gets worse as the rate accelerates. These irregular beats are known as "ectopics" or "extrasystoles" and we have referred to them earlier as "skipped beats" (figure 10).

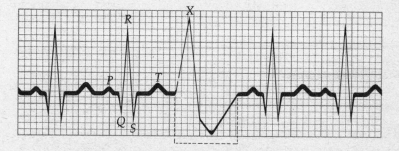

**Electrocardiogram Showing an Irregular Beat, Normal Heart Rhythm
Interrupted by One Irregular Beat**

Note that the extra complex is followed by a prolonged pause; the heart is recovering from the unexpected interpolated effort, and the recharging process takes a little longer. The shape of the ectopic beat is abnormal, as is the sequence and timing of each event, so that the P wave is missing altogether, and the QRS complex lasts longer than 0.08 seconds.

The development of such ectopic beats during exercise and their increasing frequency as the intensity of the exercise is raised, is considered to be an adverse sign. Very frequent irregularities can be dangerous and, by general agreement, the exercise test is terminated when they exceed 3 in every 10 normal beats.

It should be pointed out that there is an innocent form of irregular heart beat which occurs at rest, is often present from childhood, and which disappears as the heart rate increases with exercise. There is no evidence that these types of extra beats are due to, or are even a forerunner of, heart disease.

Another variant of benign ectopic beats is sometimes found in very fit individuals whose resting heart rates, as a result of training, have fallen to low levels, such as the 50's or the high 40's. Here, the gap between beats is so long that the muscle of the ventricles becomes impatient for the electrical impulse to arrive from the sino-atrial node, and so they "escape" from the influence of the vagus nerve and initiate an early contraction on their own.

Inappropriate Blood Pressure Response to Exercise   The increased demand imposed by exercise on the pumping ability of the heart is evidenced by a rise in blood pressure. If for some reason the ventricles are unable to pump vigorously, then the blood pressure will fail to rise concomitantly with the workload. Even worse, it may fall, signifying a serious state of affairs in which the heart is the seat of so much damage that it gives up the struggle to keep pace with the demand. This may be because previous heart attacks have caused so much scarring that healthy contraction is no longer possible.

So far, we are considering the systolic blood pressure, or pressure in the arteries during the heart's pumping phase. When the heart is resting between beats, or in its phase of diastole, the diastolic pressure obviously remains steady, being unaffected by exercise. If the diastolic pressure starts to rise, it means that the pressure within the chambers of the heart is rising abnormally due to increasing back pressure or damming up of blood from ineffectual onward pumping. A stationary or falling systolic pressure then, and/or a rising diastolic pressure during the exercise test, is a signal for the physician to halt the procedure. While not characteristic of coronary disease, it does denote pump failure, and in the context of today's high incidence of atherosclerosis, probably means ischemic heart disease.

Inappropriate Heart Rate Response to Exercise   In 1972, Hinkle and his associates noted that a sluggish heart rate response to an exercise test in middle-aged men was often the forerunner of a later heart attack. Dr. Myrvin Ellestad has observed a similar relationship. In a study published in 1975, he reported that of 2,700 patients with and without evidence of heart disease who were subjected to a maximum treadmill test, those with normal ST segments but with a low heart rate response to exercise went on to develop the same incidence of coronary events (sudden death, myocardial infarction, angina pectoris) as patients who had an ischemic ST segment depression. While there is no doubt that *failure* of the heart rate to increase with workload is a dangerous sign, and probably indicates damage to the pacemaker or electrical conduction system of the heart, *slowness* of response is more difficult to define. Dr. Ellestad has established standard heart acceleration rates for his particular test protocol. Sufficient data have not as yet been accumulated to permit their application in other test procedures. Various medications, as well as a high fitness level will affect rate of response. For the time being, then, although this sign has intriguing possibilities, it does not have the same degree of predictability as the previous three described.

Before leaving the matter of adverse criteria, mention should be made of maximum oxygen consumption. Dr. Robert Bruce of Seattle, using maximum treadmill testing, has ascertained that the maximum oxygen consumption is reduced in coronary artery disease; he believes that this is due to a drop in maximum heart rate. The amount by which maximum oxygen consumption is reduced represents, he believes, a measure of the disease's severity. He refers to the patient's "functional aerobic impairment," and has constructed tables to calculate this parameter from the results of his treadmill test.

We have now come full circle, tracing the use of exercise testing in the evaluation of fitness, the diagnosis of latent coronary heart disease, and the combination of both. In recent years, additional uses have developed. These include the guidance of normal individuals who wish to undertake an exercise program, the determination of suitability for entrance to rehabilitation exercise programs, and the prescribing of safe and suitable training activities based on individual requirements.

Needless to say, exercise testing carried to maximum or even sub-maximal levels can be hazardous in patients with heart disease and, for this reason, should never be carried out on such individuals by unqualified personnel, or without a physician being present. Furthermore, it is not enough for the physician to play a passive role in the proceedings, being prepared to act only if resuscitation is required. He or she should be thoroughly conversant with the testing protocol. In addition to observing the patient's reaction, reading the simultaneous electrocardiogram, and taking the blood pressure at regular intervals, he should designate successive increments in the workload and halt the test at the first evidence of untoward signs or symptoms. The experienced physician will rarely have to take emergency measures; his handling of the test will not infrequently prevent the need arising.

Physical educators and technicians have little or no training in the process and manifestation of disease and so cannot be expected to carry out testing on cardiac patients, except under medical supervision. To some extent, the same applies to the random testing of middle-aged normals. A proportion of these over the age of 40 will invariably be found to have latent heart disease, often to a severe degree, and accidents are inevitable unless this is borne in mind.

I am prompted to mention this because of the increasing popularity of "fitness testing." From time to time, one comes across physical educators or kinesiologists carrying out "field work" in shopping malls, sports stadia and the like. Armed with a bicycle ergometer, a blood pressure cuff, stethoscope and an electrocardiograph machine, and determined to satisfy the requirements of a "project," or promote the gospel of fitness, these individuals, often undergraduates, will encourage all and sundry to volunteer for testing. Without suitable medical screening, one cannot be sure that all of the volunteers are free from disease.

Under such circumstances, the possibility of an accident occurring is high. Such a happening would be doubly tragic, since the procedure which led to it was not essential. I am aware of the argument that if fitness testing is to await the availability of a physician, it will wait forever. But at the very least the presence of a suitably trained nurse should be mandatory when such testing is being carried out by individuals whose training should limit them to working with only healthy persons.

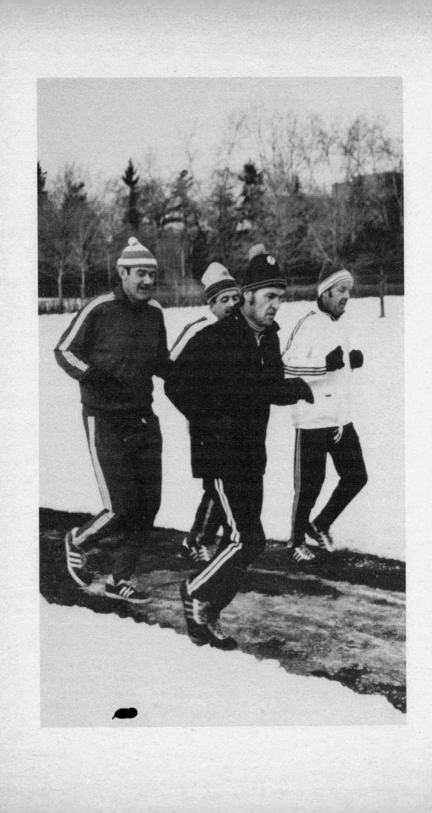

Part Two

Better to hunt in fields, for health unbought,
Than fee the doctor for a nauseous draught.
The wise, for cure, on exercise depend;
God never made his work for man to mend.

John Dryden

CHAPTER FOUR

The Rehabilitation Program

"**THERE** is no way you can go back to your old job," said the physician.

Bill H., a 39-year-old construction worker, stared across the desk in disbelief. "What can I do?" he said. "I don't know any other trade. How will I get by?"

Firmly, the doctor reminded him of the facts. Bill had just been discharged from hospital having sustained his second serious heart attack. The first was a year previous. Both attacks had been severe, and an additional factor to take into account was the family history. Bill's father had died at the age of 42 from a heart attack. One older brother had died, again in his 40's, from a heart attack, and another brother had sustained a heart attack at the age of 38.

It was essential, said the doctor, that Bill take all sensible precautions to see that he had recovered completely before exposing himself once more to the stress of heavy physical effort. His wife would have to go out to work, and he would have to stay at home to look after their two children, preparing their meals and carrying out the routine housework.

This "role reversal" is a familiar rehabilitation technique, used primarily when the male breadwinner is so incapacitated from disease or accident that he is no longer employable. To Bill, however, this approach was hard to take. His common sense told him that his doctor was right; he was not in fit shape to withstand the physical strain of his old job. On the other hand, it was difficult to see himself as disabled. He looked the picture of health, as do many convalescent heart attack patients. He felt that he was essentially a strong and healthy individual who had merely had a stroke of bad luck.

Thus, as the months went by, Bill became more and more morose. Never what you would call an abstainer, he began to drink heavily. His tenseness and anxiety increased, and instead of benefiting from the enforced rest from work, he became worse. He would wake up in the night restless and sweating. In the daytime, he began to notice chest pains, some of which he thought were angina and others he thought were "nerves." He was irritable with the children and downright ugly to his wife.

Fortunately, his doctor was astute enough to realize that things weren't working out the way he had hoped. He still felt that return to work was not the answer, and yet neither was sitting all day at home.

"The less I do, the flabbier I get," said Bill, plaintively. "At this rate, I'll never work again."

Doctor and patient gazed speculatively at one another, each trying to find a solution.

Then Bill had a thought. "Why not send me to one of the "Y's" fitness classes? Wouldn't that build up my strength again?" As he spoke, his voice became more enthusiastic. Already he was seeing himself active and vigorous again, participating in the games and sports he had enjoyed at school.

The physician was torn. There was no doubt of the morale-boosting effect of a fitness program, but what of the safety factor? How could he entrust Bill and his damaged heart to a fitness class geared to the needs of essentially healthy individuals? Then, a half-awakened thought stirred in his mind. Hadn't he read somewhere recently that a local rehabilitation centre had just started a post-coronary rehabilitation program? He promised Bill he would enquire further, and let him know the outcome the next day.

He was true to his word and the following week, Bill was waiting in the lobby of the Toronto Rehabilitation Centre. It was 1968, and he was one of the first patients to be referred to the new exercise rehabilitation program for heart attack patients.

Stuart K. was 54 years old. He had "had it with doctors." This was largely because his doctors had almost "had it" with him.

A highly successful executive, Stuart was a prime example of the unco-operative patient. He was also a magnificent example of a type of patient seen all too often in the coronary care unit.

He had just been discharged from hospital after recovery from his second heart attack. The first was only three months earlier, and his reaction at that time had been most businesslike — keep a stiff upper lip and stay in there fighting. In Stuart's terms, this meant denying that he was suffering from anything other than a minor setback, and dispensing with medical assistance as soon as possible. Accordingly, he took his own discharge from hospital one week earlier than his cardiologist advised, and then returned to work the following week. Shortly after this, he put himself on an exercise training program as outlined in a popular book on fitness. Naturally, he considered himself already a rather fit individual, and so quickly skipped through the precautionary chapters of the book, written for "old guys and crocks," and started half-way up the training table at a level suitable for those whose fitness rating was good.

In short, Stuart did all the wrong things. Small wonder that six weeks later, while on a business trip and shortly after attempting to run a seven-minute mile through Stanley Park in Vancouver, he experienced severe chest pain. On his return to Toronto, he was diagnosed has having sustained another and this time more extensive heart attack. He was lucky enough to survive, and one would have thought that after that experience, he would have adopted a more cautious approach. Obviously, this was not his nature; if nothing else, one has to give him A for persistence. He was still determined to work, worry and play at his customary pre-attack level.

He presented his hapless cardiologist with an ultimatum: "Tell me how to get fit and strong again, or send me to someone who can."

His physician, feeling that Stuart had had a great deal more luck than he deserved, and anxious to protect him from further excesses, recalled reading of an exercise rehabilitation program that was being carried on in the city. He recommended that Stuart attend this program.

"My God," said Stuart. "Rehabilitation! You mean basket weaving?"

"Not quite," said his doctor, but feeling that maybe he might have scored a point in that encounter!

Harold D. was thoroughly depressed when he came out of hospital. He had been taking part in a curling championship play-off five weeks earlier when he had felt intensely nauseated and sweaty. Within minutes, he developed intense, crushing pain in his chest, and an hour later found himself in the emergency department of the local hospital. A myocardial infarction was diagnosed, and he was admitted. Four weeks later, he was discharged. His progress had been uneventful and free from complications. On the day of his discharge, his wife came to help him pack and drive him home. He felt weak, and unsure of himself. Would he be able to go back to his old job? Would he be able to curl again? What restrictions and limitations would the doctors place upon him in the future?

Unwittingly, one of his wife's first actions as they left the hospital seemed to reinforce all his fears. "Don't carry that, dear," she said, lifting his suitcase. "It's too heavy for you."

As they walked across the lobby, he deliberately fell behind, ashamed of his weakness in not being able to carry his own case.

The following day, his doctor phoned him. He was going to be referred to a post-coronary exercise program which had been instituted in a nearby rehabilitation centre. His feelings were mixed. Such places were for the severely disabled, the handicapped. Well, if that is what he had become, he might as well accept it. But hadn't he read somewhere that a group of heart attack patients had recently taken part in a two-mile demonstration run? Maybe they were from the same program. Well, he'd have to see. There was no sense giving up now.

The rehabilitation program to which these men were referred was unique in that it stressed prolonged endurance exercise. If Stuart expected basket weaving, he was in for a shock. From the outset each participant would be asked, depending on his condition, to walk or jog for half an hour, five times a week. Within a matter of weeks, the time would be increased to one hour. His immediate goal would be to jog four miles in 48 minutes; ultimately, he could look forward to jogging six miles in 72 minutes (were he under 45, his prescription would amount to six miles in 60 minutes).

His starting level and rate of progression would depend upon the results of rigorous cardio-respiratory fitness testing. His exercise plan would be carefully tailored to accommodate his two-fold need: developing endurance fitness, and doing so with minimal risk to his already damaged heart. He would be given an individual prescription specifying duration, intensity and frequency of exercise: in short, the distance he would have to jog, the time it should take, and the number of times a week it should be carried out.

He would be expected to attend exercise classes regularly until he achieved his fitness potential. During these supervised sessions, he would be observed by physicians, therapists and physical educators to see how he performed. If he developed cardiac symptoms he would be examined again, or his electrocardiogram monitored while he exercised. He would be instructed in the art of taking his own pulse, reading a stop watch, pacing himself, and jogging in an easy and relaxed manner so as to avoid minor injuries to his muscles, tendons and joints.

Physician-led discussions would deal not only with the physiological and medical aspects of endurance training, but also the significance of exercise-induced symptoms associated with coronary heart disease. Individual advice as to whether or not he should participate in other sports such as squash, weight-lifting, tennis or curling, would be available to him. The value or otherwise of vitamins, low-fat diets, soft water versus hard water, would be some of the topics relevant to his disease which would be covered in the short pre-exercise discussions.

In point of fact, he was in for the experience of a lifetime. For the first time in his life, he was going to be subjected to a systematic, medically directed, scientifically designed onslaught on his deplorable and heinous state of unfitness. In the process, some of his long-cherished beliefs and prejudices about training were going to be exploded; he was going to discover that many of the sports he had taken part in, under the impression that they were good for his health, were actually of little value in attaining true worthwhile fitness; and that a set of singles tennis played on odd occasions throughout the year to a perspiring, gasping, knee-trembling finish did more harm than good. But most important, he was going to find that he was expected to work constantly and assiduously on his own, changing his lifestyle to accommodate to five one-hour sessions of exercise every week. His reward? Something that money cannot buy. The attainment of a quality of life far surpassing anything he had experienced before: the relaxed, confident satisfaction that only regular exercise can bring.

He would experience the sheer physical elation of being fit.

Not only that, there was an additional bonus. At the initial induction lecture it had been carefully pointed out that the outlook for an individual who had already had a heart attack was somewhat gloomy. This statement in itself had been a bit of revelation, in more ways than one. First, he had not fully realized this sombre fact; and secondly, he was accustomed to his physician wrapping unpalatable news in a more attractive package. To be told that the recurrence rate among heart attack survivors was high, that in fact some 25 to 30 per cent are dead from a second attack within five years of the primary one, had been quite a jolt. Yet the physician (who incidentally was clad in a track suit and seemed curiously jocular about such bad news) produced the results of a series of different studies to back his statement. He put the case bluntly:

All of you here listening to me have to face the fact that your life expectancy is less than normal. I tell you this for one reason only: so that you understand right from the outset that the task facing us in post-coronary rehabilitation is a formidable one. Our job is to try to increase your life expectancy, by reducing the incidence of fatal recurrences.

Can we do that? We offer no guarantees, but the evidence is highly suggestive that we can. Regular exercise has been found to be a powerful factor in the primary prevention of fatal heart attacks. Individuals who have been engaged in heavy work before their attacks have a higher survival rate (two to three times as high) both immediately and over a five-year follow-up. It is not unreasonable, therefore, to theorize that an exercise program instituted *after* your heart attack will have a similar protective effect. Furthermore, there is enough presumptive evidence around now to say that it does. Of course, if you want more definitive proof, you can wait another ten years to get it — but that might be a bit late for some of you.

The work of Drs. Hellerstein, Gottheimer, Brunner and Rechnitzer, as well as our own studies, has shown as much as a three-fold reduction of fatal recurrences in patients who attend a rehabilitation program which contains an exercise component. Our own experiments have also led us to prefer walking and jogging as the mode of training, and LSD (long, slow distance) rather than "speed."

So that's it in a nut shell. We offer hard facts, hard work, and hard-line direction. In return, you get a second chance at life, and an opportunity to live it in a high state of physical fitness. But remember, your new lifestyle can only be maintained by constant effort. You can't build up a store of exercise or fitness that can be used over later months or years of sedentary living. Deterioration sets in within weeks of stopping training. So if you can't hack it, then don't bother starting. Exercise must become an integral part of your daily routine. The only way out is to obtain the letters R.I.P. after your name, and we don't intend to be handing out too many of those types of diplomas!

Stuart, Bill and Don, like many others, responded to the challenge. They entered the program, and began a new way of life.

The Origins of the Program

The remarkable escalation in the incidence of heart attacks, together with the realization that the survivors were still in peril from a fatal recurrence, led the author and his colleagues to the realization that something more than routine physician follow-up was required. If all the risk factors were to be covered, then a change in lifestyle was indicated. This cannot be achieved by a 30-minute visit with a physician every six months. Granted, such risk factors as high blood pressure, diabetes and high blood levels of cholesterol can be controlled by the regular visit to the physician, but the latter is only too ready to admit his failure in advising on such matters as diet, increasing physical activity, avoidance of excessive stress, and giving up smoking.

For most sedentary workers, increased physical activity can only be attained by an exercise program carried out in their non-working hours. To obtain advice from the physician on such a program is, as many patients will attest, notoriously difficult. The plain fact of the matter is that most physicians have not been trained to prescribe exercise. Increasing public and government interest in physical fitness programs is improving this situation slightly, but it is safe to say that the vast majority of physicians are still ignorant of this area.

Nevertheless, studies have shown that post-coronary exercise programs can be very effective in increasing cardiac efficiency by decreasing heart rate and myocardial oxygen consumption at a given workload. The training permits the muscles to extract more oxygen from the blood, thus reducing the amount of blood the heart has to pump for a given task. The trained heart muscle is more resistant to such unfavourable conditions as shortage of oxygen (a situation which arises when the narrowed coronary arteries are unable to supply an adequate amount of blood to a rapidly beating heart), or excess stress hormones (catecholamines) which are liberated into the blood stream in response to situations of high urgency. There is an increased feeling of well-being and a lessening of depression. There is often an improvement in chest pain, with many patients reporting relief from angina as they become fitter. These, and other benefits, are what one would expect to see in any individual who embarks on a training program. The encouraging thing is that having had a heart attack doesn't prevent you from obtaining these advantages.

A number of workers have reported that exercise programs reduced the incidence of fatal and non-fatal recurrent heart attacks in their patients. One of the longest studies has been carried out by Dr. Hermann Hellerstein in Cleveland, who found that deaths among his exercised post-coronaries amounted to only 1.9 per hundred patients per year. This compares favourably with the figure of 5.1 per hundred which he calculated for the non-exercising post-coronary population.

Dr. Daniel Brunner compared a group of 64 patients in his exercise program with another group of 65 post-coronary patients who had not followed any exercise regime. Over the period of a year, there were four recurrences and two deaths in the exercise group; the non-active group had nine recurrences and seven fatalities.

In a similar study by Dr. Peter Rechnitzer of Ontario, a group of exercise subjects were compared over a five-year period with a group of non-exercisers. The exercisers had a 1.3 per cent recurrence rate and a 3.9 per cent death rate, while the control group had a 27.9 per cent recurrence rate and an 11.8 per cent death rate. Dr. Gottheimer reported a 3.6 per cent death rate in a group of 1,100 male Israelis with coronary disease who followed an exercise plan; again, this is in marked contrast to a 12 per cent rate in a non-exercised group. Finally, Dr. Weinblatt reported no recurrences and no deaths over a five-year period in his exercise group, as opposed to a 4.6 per cent recurrence rate and 3.1 per cent death rate in a control group.

In terms of medical proof, we can only say at this stage that the work of these physicians is promising. Larger groups of patients, a longer follow-up, and more tightly controlled experimental factors are needed in order to satisfy all of the criteria necessary to come to a definitive conclusion. Once again, however, with coronary heart disease accounting for 40 to 50 per cent of the death rate in advanced countries, it does not seem unreasonable to examine this work and take from it whatever advantage may be offered to the current victim.

It was with this background in mind that my post-coronary program at the Centre was started. The aim was to offer positive advice and help, and by regular attendance to instill a set of health habits which could only do good. A pattern of exercise would be the main thrust, with additional factors being brought in as the program progressed.

As Medical Director of the Centre and prime mover of the project, I was convinced that its success would depend largely on the enthusiasm and quality of the initial treatment team. I was extremely fortunate in this regard. From my own staff came Johanna Kennedy, R.N., who assumed the role of co-ordinator. Professor Robin Campbell was loaned from the University of Toronto to work in the exercise testing laboratory.

Consultants were Professor Roy Shephard from the Department of Preventive Medicine and Biostatistics, University of Toronto, and Dr. Art Chisholm, Director of Cardiovascular Services at the University of Toronto's Sunnybrook Hospital. We were fortunate indeed in having Roy Shephard, an internationally recognized authority in exercise physiology, assume consulting responsibility for the exercise-testing protocol and the research aspects of the project. Art Chisholm, a cardiologist with a long-standing interest in exercise rehabilitation, provided not only expertise in his field but also those vital first few patients without which our plans would never have materialized. Johanna Kennedy brought to the position of co-ordinator outstanding organizational ability and also, as a result of her involvement as an administrator with the Canadian Track and Field Association, an intimate knowledge of the trials and tribulations and vicissitudes of the aspiring runner.

For we had decided to use running — or more correctly, jogging — as the exercise of choice. It was ideal for our purpose in that it required little in the way of equipment or expensive facilities, could be accurately prescribed in terms of intensity, duration and frequency, and was an excellent builder of endurance fitness. Today, seven years later, the treatment team has increased four-fold, and includes physicians, physiotherapists, occupational therapists, and physical educators; but happily the original founder members continue, more active than ever, and in expanded roles.

Post-coronary exercise programs are plagued by poor attendance and high drop-out rates. The patient's first flush of enthusiasm for exercise is often short-lived. He begins to find that regular attendance at the classes disrupts his social and business commitments. This problem is compounded in a large city, where he often has to travel long distances on traffic-clogged roads and highways. The answer is to reduce the number of weekly medically supervised sessions to the minimal compatible with training effectiveness and safety, and then have the individual work out on his own the rest of the week. After all, if he cannot be taught to exercise prudently when he is away from the watchful eye of the physician, how can he be expected to cope with the inevitable sudden physical stresses and strains of normal everyday living? Then again, if safe exercise rehabilitation programs are to become universally available, the logistics of the situation make it mandatory that medical staff be used for the maximum good of the maximum number; physicians, nurses and therapists are in short supply, and their services should be deployed carefully.

Thus it was decided that the group would exercise at the Centre under medical supervision only once a week. Since a greater frequency of training is needed for attainment of endurance fitness, four additional home workouts would also be required. This approach has worked very well, despite the opinion of many physical education authorities that at least two and probably three supervised exercise sessions a week would be necessary. The fact is that our patients have become fit and attend the weekly session with great regularity; indeed, the program has one of the lowest drop-out rates recorded. Interestingly, this system has now been adopted by the other six university centres which are taking part in the Ontario Multi-Centre Trial into the Effects of Exercise on Post-Coronary Rehabilitation, despite the fact that the original protocol called for three supervised exercise sessions a week.

Our program requires that all patients be referred by a physician. The referral documents, together with hospital reports and electrocardiograms, are carefully studied by the Centre's doctors to see if there are any absolute contra-indications to exercise. The patient is then brought in to the Centre for a complete examination. His height, weight, muscle power in arms and legs, and the thickness of the fat layers over various parts of his body are recorded. A medical examination, which includes a routine electrocardiogram, is carried out. Finally, the patient performs a sub-maximal exercise stress test as described in Chapter 3, either on the bicycle ergometer or the treadmill. The electrocardiogram is monitored continuously during this test, and expired gases are analyzed in order to estimate the patient's maximum oxygen consumption.

As a result of this test, the patient is placed in one of two categories: "uncomplicated" or "complicated." An uncomplicated test means that he has continued through to an estimated 75 per cent of his maximum heart rate without developing angina or any serious abnormalities in his electrocardiogram. The complicated case is one in which the subject did not finish the test because some evidence of cardiac ischemia supervened. A walking/jogging exercise prescription is now prescribed on the basis of the test result, the complicated cases being handled somewhat differently from the uncomplicated. The prescription states the specific distance to be covered and the time it should take. It calls for five workouts a week, one of which is carried out under supervision at the Centre.

In effect, then, each patient has an individual prescription based on his particular response to the stress test. Repeated stress tests show whether or not there is any improvement in fitness, and if there is, this leads to a new prescription; in this way, the patient progresses safely and at a rate based on his increasing level of fitness. Not infrequently, the complicated case, which initially may have a low starting level compared with the other patients, improves his performance on subsequent stress tests to the degree that he can transfer to the ranks of the uncomplicated.

Initiation into the program proper takes place after the first stress test. The patient attends a two-hour lecture, which deals mainly with the items covered in Part One of this book. This is followed on the next visit by a practical session dealing with the art of reading a stop watch, and taking a pulse count. Both of these procedures are of vital importance to the post-coronary patient who intends to exercise. If he is to interpret his prescription correctly, he must not only measure out the distance that he has to walk accurately, but he must also time his walk or jog equally precisely. An ordinary watch is not good enough for this purpose, and we always insist that before starting the program our patients purchase and become proficient in the use of a stop watch, which is also used to time the pulse count. Without a stop watch for guidance the patient tends to go too fast.

After these simple procedures have been mastered, each individual receives his prescription and carries this out on the Centre's track under the supervision of a therapist. If the trial workout results in the desired training heart rate, then the patient takes it away with him to carry out on his own until seen the following week. On the other hand, if the post-workout heart rate is too high or too low, the prescription is adjusted slightly to achieve the desired effect.

A typical supervised session starts off with a ten-minute discussion in which patients are encouraged to discuss problems they may have encountered with their home prescription. This affords an opportunity to educate the group into the do's and don'ts of exercise, the significance of various cardiac signs and symptoms, the importance and action of certain medications, and the trends of modern research into heart disease. There is a deliberate attempt to establish a free-wheeling type of atmosphere, and this enables full and frank discussion of various topics which would otherwise be suppressed in a more structured discussion: for example, sexual problems following the heart attack, the use of various "fad" diets, and the value of the current "cure" for heart disease constantly being reported in the lay press.

The discussion is followed by a 20-minute warm-up to music. The emphasis here is on simple flexibility exercises designed specifically for the middle-aged, and interspersed with walking and jogging. The group circle the exercise leader and at regular programmed intervals the music is interrupted by a 10-second characteristic low-pitched hum — a signal for the class to take a 10-second pulse count. These counts are then called out, thus giving the leader a "feel" for the individual's exercise response. Throughout the warm-up, and after each pulse count, an inquiry is made as to whether anybody is experiencing chest

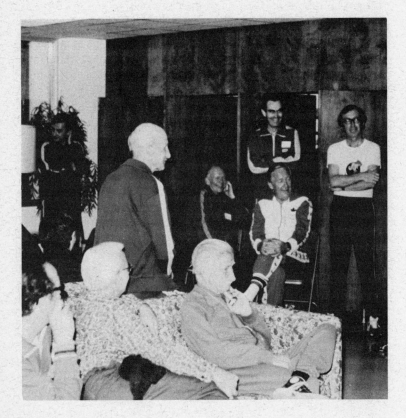

The post-coronary program in action: pre-exercise discussion; the warm-up; out on the T.R.C. track (each man is doing his own prescription).

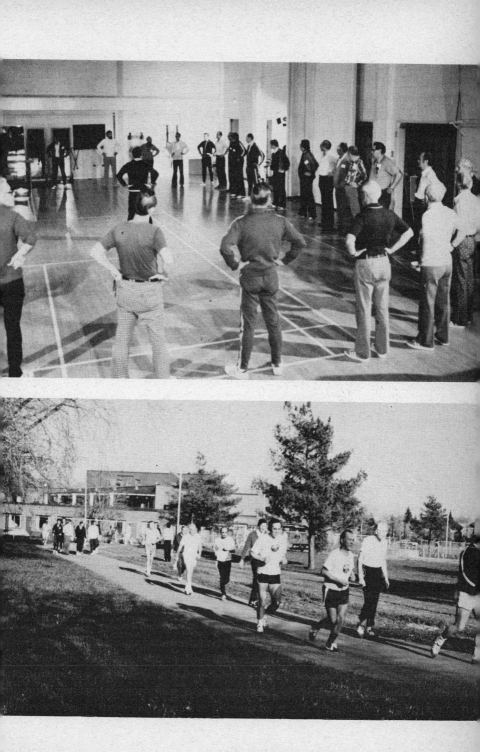

discomfort, skipped beats, vertigo or any other symptom. Again, this gives the supervising group an awareness of the individuals who are prone to ischemic symptoms. Marked problems during the warm-up will be an indication for a discussion with the patient, and possibly further medical assessment, including electrocardiograms. Opportunity is also taken during these warm-ups to teach the newcomers the style and technique of jogging.

It frequently surprises visitors to the program to find that I act as exercise leader in the warm-up. They seem both amused and intrigued at the spectacle of a middle-aged physician, clad in a baggy sweat suit, acting as a pseudo physical educator. My reasons are both medical and psychological. There is no better way to become familiar with your patient's responses to exercise than to take him through a warm-up. Untoward symptoms can be personally observed and noted. After two or three sessions of personal involvement you are in a better position to distinguish between the symptom-sufferers and the symptom-claimers — an important division when one is dispensing exercise therapy on the large scale. The "denier" of symptoms, the inept pulse-taker, the timid and frightened exerciser, the competitive type, are all stock characters in any post-coronary exercise class, and can be identified with more assurance by a trained physician — provided he is located where the action is, which in this case is on the floor of the gymnasium. Of course, he could stand and watch somebody else put his patients through their paces. But then how much more encouraging it is for the newcomer to take his first jogging steps "on medical orders," and from a physician who is not embarrassed to be attired as ridiculously as himself. Obviously not all doctors have the time or indeed the inclination to cavort around the gym with their patients; but I suspect more would be willing to do so if the benefits were drawn to their attention. Besides, what a spendid opportunity to get fit while on the job!

Patients are encouraged to discuss their problems openly rather than trying to corner the physician or nurse for a private tête-à-tête. We have found that most problems and symptoms are common to a large number of people, and therefore open discussion not only helps the individual who brought the problem up, but the many others who are having the same difficulty but are, at least in the early stages of their attendance, too shy to mention them. After the warm-up is over, the patients then proceed to carry out their individual prescriptions under the observing eye of the medical team.

All patients are required to keep an exercise log which they hand in every two weeks. This records their current prescription, the distance and time of each workout, and their pre- and post-workout heart rates. Once a month they record their resting heart rate; this is taken before they get out of bed in the morning, and the average of three morning counts is entered. The log also has space for noting any adverse symptoms experienced during a particular workout. The logs are read carefully by the treatment staff, and the distances, speeds and heart rates are carefully charted for each patient. In this way, progress can be easily gauged at a glance. Adverse symptoms are underlined in red and immediately passed through to the physician for his attention. If necessary, the physician will phone the patient to clarify some remark or even to suggest that the rate of exercise be reduced until he is seen at the next supervised session.

Our studies at the Centre have shown that the patient often feels a great improvement in mood and morale within weeks of starting the program. Nevertheless, a period of at least a year is required for more objective physiological benefits to appear. Ideally, two years is needed. However, while one is reluctant to discharge individuals from the program, the number of referrals has increased steadily over the years. This problem has been solved to a large degree by "promoting" patients when they have reached the satisfactory level to a group which attends the Centre only once every fourth week, and still later to another group which attends only every other month. These "post-graduates" are still expected to complete and return their exercise logs every two weeks, however, and these are reviewed as assiduously as those from the weekly attenders.

Due to the steady demand from out-of-town physicians, we have also instituted a home exercise program. The patient travels into the Centre for testing, is instructed in the execution of his prescription, and reports his progress by means of mailed-in exercise logs. Progressively heavier training workouts are prescribed as he gets fitter, and he returns for re-testing at six monthly or yearly intervals.

This book represents the final extension of the program. It is an attempt to reach the individuals with coronary heart disease who want to go on an exercise program but lack expert guidance. Obviously no book, no matter how well written, will substitute for personal supervision and contact, but it can help in the avoidance of the more dangerous pitfalls.

Over the years, the two commonest questions asked of me by doctors and patients alike are: what is a safe starting level of exercise, and how does one safely increase this to improve the training effect? Obviously, there is no single answer to either question. The starting level will vary with the individual, depending upon his initial state of fitness, the severity of his heart attack, his age, and the presence or absence of symptoms. Any increase in his training prescription will depend upon his response, expressed subjectively in his feeling of well-being and objectively in his heart rate response to the workout and to repeated stress tests. However, over the years, we have learned to streamline our exercise-prescribing technique and have developed a series of tables especially designed for cardiac patients. These, together with a set of progressing nomograms, should provide safe and effective guidelines for the intelligent layman. Used with the accompanying remarks on training techniques, they constitute a home version of the Centre program.

CHAPTER FIVE

So You Want To Exercise?

MOST coronary heart disease sufferers will benefit from a sensible exercise program. This includes individuals who have had a heart attack as well as those who experience anginal pain with exertion even though they have never actually had an attack. It also includes the middle-aged who exhibit any of the risk factors previously described (and that means most males over 40) or who have a high incidence of heart disease in their family. There are, however, some cases in which exercise is positively contra-indicated, either on cardiac or non-cardiac grounds. In others, there are relative contra-indications to exercise: situations in which exercise is possible, but must be modified and adjusted so as not to be harmful.

Cardiac Contra-Indications to Exercise

As I have said, these are few, and your physician should be your final guide. I shall, however, include a brief checklist here.

1. Recent myocardial infarction: Since the infarction scar takes six weeks to become firm, vigorous activity prior to that time may well result in an aneurysm, or bulging of the damaged area. This bulging occurs with each heart beat and, if large, constitutes in itself another contra-indication to exercise.

   Arthur P. is a case in point. He was discharged from hospital three weeks after his heart attack, and was advised to restrict his activities to casual walking for a further month before returning to his doctor for a check-up. Unfortunately, he became overly enthusiastic about the benefits of exercise and, through a combination of misinformation and misinterpretation, began to follow a self-devised running program. By the seventh week, he was forcing himself to jog between one and two miles over hilly terrain. Shortly after, he was readmitted to hospital with another attack. Fortunately, it was not fatal, but when he was later referred to me to ensure that any future exercising would be under supervision, he was found to have a large aneurysm of the heart wall. There is a strong likelihood that this was due to his premature vigorous running. One of my more depressing experiences was having to tell this man, who was still keen to exercise, that exercise therapy was now out for him, that anything more intense than a casual walk would be too dangerous.

2. There is no role for exercise in acute heart failure. In this condition, the heart is unable to pump the blood efficiently around the body. If the right side of the heart is affected, the blood tends to back-up in the general circulation, with resultant swelling from retention of fluid (edema) in the feet and legs. Left-sided heart failure causes the blood to back-up in the lungs, and this leads to excessive breathlessness in response to even the mildest physical activity. No matter which side of the heart is affected, exercise training aggravates the situation. Heart failure is a rare complication of coronary artery disease, but when it does occur, it is usually only in association with a severe myocardial infarction. Even then, healing of the infarct is often accompanied by complete recovery in pump efficiency, at which time exercise again becomes permissible.

3. As we have seen, a large aneurysm of the heart wall is a bar to exercise. Aneurysms may also occur in the walls of the large blood vessels (for example, the aorta), and their presence here also precludes vigorous training. There are, of course, cases in which small aneurysmal bulges are detected; here the question of whether or not to exercise becomes a matter of fine judgment. The benefits to look for may be psychological rather than physiological. In general, such individuals should not attempt to regulate their own

program, and skilled supervision by a physician is essential.

4. Patients with rapidly progressing anginal pain should not exercise. A marked change for the worse in the pattern and incidence of exertional pain may well be the warning of another heart attack. To exercise under these circumstances may well be to invite disaster.

5. The heart muscle can sometimes be involved in generalized infections, giving rise to a condition known as myocarditis, or inflammation of the myocardium (the medical ending "-itis" means "inflammation of"). This can occur in acute rheumatic fever or in diphtheria; viral infections such as poliomyelitis, influenza, and even infectious mononucleosis (glandular fever) can also affect the heart. Since exercise is always contra-indicated in acute infections, it is obviously even more dangerous when the infection involves the heart. While your physician will be the one to diagnose myocarditis and will certainly ensure that your physical activity is limited until the condition has cleared up, it should be stressed that mild subclinical myocarditis may be common in association with a number of viral-type infections. For this reason, I insist that all individuals on an exercise program stop training whenever they develop a heavy cold or an influenza-like illness. Exercise should never be performed in the presence of a fever, and to be on the safe side, the temperature should have returned to normal for a full seven days before working out again. Colds or flu which are accompanied by muscle pain and tenderness and a heart rate higher than normal are features suggestive of heart muscle involvement.

6. Grossly irregular heart action which is accentuated by exertion is a deterrent to training, especially if the electrocardiogram shows that the ectopic beats are emanating from more than one area in the heart. These "multi-focal" ectopics, which are aggravated by strenuous exertion, can on occasions lead to fatal ventricular fibrillation and exercise should not be undertaken until the condition has been controlled by suitable medication. Lesser degrees of rhythm irregularity can be compensated for by modifying the training regime; indeed, an increase in fitness will often reduce the incidence and severity of the condition. The occasional severe form will not respond satisfactorily, even to medication, and with

these cases, regular exercise can do nothing but aggravate the situation.

It should be stressed at this time that there are two types of irregularities that are benign. In the first, the condition is often present from youth. The irregularity, or skipped beat, is present at rest but disappears as the heart rate increases with exercise. The subject may or may not be aware of the occasional missed beat, and if he is, he usually describes it as a "palpatation" or a "hollow pause" felt in the chest. The second harmless type of irregularity occurs in the highly trained individual whose resting heart rate has fallen to very low levels because of the increased influence of the nerve which slows the heart, the vagal nerve — that is, training bradycardia due to increased vagal activity. This may be an indication of over-training (see later), and usually clears up in a week or two when the intensity of the workouts is reduced.

7. In certain types of valvular heart disease, especially those which lead to narrowing in the region of the aortic valve, exercise training is not advisable. Coronary heart disease does not affect the valves in this manner; rheumatic fever in childhood is the usual offender. Occasionally, the two conditions coexist, in which case one has to be guided by the severity of the valvular difficulty.

8. Recent cases of blood clots occurring either in the lungs (pulmonary embolism) or in the peripheral arteries, or veins (thrombophlebitis) should not be exercised. Physical activity may bring about further clots, or extension of the existing ones.

9. Repeated bouts of heart failure may, in the long run, give rise to a dilated enlarged heart. This will show up on the x-ray and, where the enlargement is gross, there will be no benefit from training. The stretched heart muscle has no reserve left and so is incapable of benefiting from even measured small doses of stress.

10. Many experts feel that exercise therapy is of little value in the condition of complete heart block. Here, the electrical conduction system between the upper and lower chambers of the heart is non-functioning, with the result that the two portions beat independently. Furthermore, an increase in heart rate does not occur when the subject exercises. In such

a condition, a pacemaker, or artificial rhythm conductor, is inserted. However, this merely brings the heart rate up to an average level and still does not permit it to accelerate in response to exercise. It is doubtful that patients with pacemakers will derive any cardiac training benefit; on the other hand, there is a suggestion by some workers in the field that training, while not being able to bring about the desirable bradycardia, will nevertheless result in an increased stroke volume. More research needs to be done in this area but, in the meantime, pacemaker patients should be limited to a walking program.

11. Most patients with high blood pressure do well on an exercise program. However, if the hypertension is very marked, and cannot be controlled by medication, then vigorous exercise is harmful in that it drives the pressure up even higher, and may even contribute towards brain hemorrhage.

12. Certain forms of congenital heart disease, especially those which are associated with bluish discoloration of the face and limb extremities (cyanosis) are bars to exercise.

Non-Cardiac Contra-Indications to Exercise

1. If you suffer from severe uncontrolled diabetes, you are best to avoid undue physical exertion. Milder forms of the disease are usually not a hindrance to training; in fact, the individual with marginal or latent diabetes may find that blood sugars approach normal levels with the attainment of fitness.

2. Exercise brings the body to a state of "arousal," and this may have untoward effects on the sufferer from epilepsy — on occasion increasing the frequency of attacks. The same applies to the related but much rarer condition of narcolepsy, in which the patient's seizures take the form of sudden uncontrollable bouts of sleepiness. One such individual was referred to my program but had to be refused when close questioning revealed a clear relationship between physical exercise and increased frequency of attacks.

3. Sustained exercise makes increased demands on the lungs, kidneys and liver. Therefore, certain chest conditions — for example, recent tuberculosis or recurrent spontaneous pneumothorax (entry of air into the chest cavity from rupture of a small "bleb" on the surface of the lung) — as

well as severe kidney or liver disease are obvious contra-indications to exercise.

4. The acute stage of various types of arthritis, such as rheumatoid arthritis or gout, are treated by appropriate medication and rest. Exercise will do more harm than good. However, during the quiescent phase, and provided the disease has not caused too much deformity by destroying bones and joints, suitably modified exercise programs will be beneficial. The more crippling type of osteoarthritis may be aggravated by running or jogging, and activities where the impact of body weight on joints is reduced, such as swimming, are more suitable. However, it is interesting to note that long distance runners have been shown to have a lower incidence of osteoarthritis in their hip joints than the population at large; this is due to the fact that movement keeps the protective cartilaginous lining of the joint surfaces healthy and well nourished. Our legs were meant for walking and running — not sitting and lying!

5. Chronic low back trouble is often exacerbated by jogging or calisthenics. Aggravating factors include obesity, running on an uneven surface, unsuitable running shoes, and sudden twisting movements of the spine. If a careful watch is kept for flare-ups, and activity is slowed with any suspicious symptoms, back strength should develop to the stage where a full program of jogging can be sustained without problem.

6. Anemia is a condition in which a lack of the protein hemoglobin in the blood causes an inadequate supply of oxygen to the organs and muscles of the body. In severe cases this results in fatigue, breathlessness, and sometimes anginal type pain on exertion. There are many causes for anemia, but among the most common are chronic loss of blood from a bleeding ulcer, bleeding hemorrhoids or excessive menstrual loss. Until the appropriate medical measures are taken to raise the blood level of hemoglobin to normal, exercise training is bound to be ineffective, since a vital link in the oxygen transport chain is defective. There is little point in the heart learning to pump blood more efficiently around the body if the blood itself contains an inadequate supply of oxygen.

7. There are a number of conditions, in addition to the above, in which exercise may be ill-advised. These include various

neurological, muscular and glandular disease which are relatively rare and, for practical purposes, need not be outlined here. In any event, the physician must be the final judge in these matters, and his advice and permission are essential for any patient with coronary heart disease who wishes to embark upon the training system outlined in this book.

Principles of Endurance Training

We have described the cardiovascular benefits of endurance training. Maximum oxygen consumption increases, the heart rate drops while its stroke volume improves, blood pressure falls, the oxygen-carrying capacity of the blood increases, and the muscles extract oxygen more efficiently from the blood stream. The endurance athlete's heart develops a greater blood supply and volume size. With all of these advantages (as well as such peripheral ones as reduction in the percentage of body fat, a drop in the level of circulating blood fats and stress hormones, and decrease in blood stickiness) is it any wonder that the long distance runner, swimmer, or cross-country skier rarely suffers from heart disease or sustains a heart attack? If you wish to develop the same degree of protection, then you must train in the same manner as these athletes — although not, of course, to quite the same degree. After all, you are not aiming to enter the Olympics, just to get some of the bonuses in terms of health and long life.

Training for endurance fitness requires the use of the large muscles of the legs or the trunk in a rhythmic fashion and on a regular basis. For our purposes, walking and jogging are the ideal activities. While I have no intrinsic objection to cycling, swimming, cross-country skiing or other similar endurance exercise, I feel that jogging gives as great, if not greater, returns of endurance fitness for a smaller investment of both time and money. The skill required to jog is minimal; the technique will be described later and can be learned in a matter of minutes. Special equipment is limited to a pair of good shoes and, if you want to go first-class, a sweat suit. You can jog almost anywhere — through parks, along roads or sidewalks, around neighbourhood school tracks. In cold weather, you can use the local Y gymnasium or you can try covered shopping malls, or even underground apartment garages. Opportunities are legion; the only basic requirement is motivation.

Although the principles of training are simple, we have to examine them more closely if we are to achieve success with our jogging program. It is generally accepted that in order to produce a minimal training effect in an unfit person, the intensity of training must be high enough to ensure that the heart rate reaches a certain level. How is this level established? Our own work and that of others have shown that endurance fitness results from training intensities equal to 50 or 60 per cent of your maximum oxygen consumption.

You may be interested in the manner in which this research is carried out. Large numbers of subjects are tested on the treadmill in order to establish maximum oxygen consumption, and also ascertain the running speed necessary to achieve it. It is a simple matter to calculate various percentages of this maximum speed, and note the heart rates for each speed. Training sessions resulting in heart rates less than those obtained at treadmill workouts that are below 50 per cent of maximum oxygen consumption are found to be relatively ineffectual in improving fitness. Ideally, an intensity of between 50 and 70 per cent of maximum oxygen consumption is needed to make a substantial gain; an intensity of jogging which is equivalent to only, say, 30 per cent of one's maximal oxygen consumption will likely be valueless in training the heart. Are there any upper limits to the desired intensity? Surprisingly enough, the answer is yes. To run at a speed which is 95 or 100 per cent of maximal oxygen consumption seems also to be relatively ineffective, largely because the activity cannot be sustained long enough to stimulate the development of endurance.

Thus, the optimum band of training speeds is narrow and, unless well advised, many individuals will jog at a pace which is either too slow or too fast for attainment of endurance fitness. The art of designing an efficient training program is to be able to match training speed to the immediate fitness and health status of the individual.

For the post-coronary patient, an even more important factor is the question of safety. While an activity level equal to 60 per cent of maximal oxygen consumption might be highly desirable from a training point of view, it could well, especially in the early stages of the program, exert excessive strain on a heart which is already suffering from an impaired coronary artery circulation. Not only that, it will probably prove too much for muscles, joints and bones weakened by years of inactivity. Most of us are grossly out of shape — even those who should know better! Recently a physician patient, when given his initial prescription requiring him to walk one mile in 20 minutes, admitted shame-facedly that he probably hadn't walked more than a quarter of a mile a day in over 25 years.

To sum up, then, the intensity of exercise must be sufficient to obtain a training effect, but care must be taken to see that it is within the tolerance of both the heart and the musculoskeletal system.

There are two other components to be considered in design-ing a training program: the length of the training session, and the number of times it should be carried out per week. With intensities in the order of 60 to 70 per cent, the duration of a workout should be at least 30 minutes, and our goal should be a 60-minute session. More intense levels of activity — say 80 or 85 per cent of maximum — may achieve the same training effect with shorter sessions, but the individual with coronary heart disease is better to hasten slowly.

There is another reason for preferring the one hour workout. The energy for short bouts of high intensity exercise comes almost entirely from the starches stored in the liver and muscles. Sprinters, football players, and ice hockey players, are "sugar athletes." Their bursts of physical effort are measured in seconds or minutes, and the fuel for their high-speed action comes from the quickly mobilized glycogen stores. The long distance runner, on the other hand, cannot rely entirely upon sugar stores, which begin to drop within 5 or 10 minutes of starting to run. By 30 minutes, glycogen provides no more than half the energy required, and from then on, the body begins to draw more and more on its fat stores (Figure 11). Have you ever seen an obese long distance runner? You probably never will. The duration of his training sessions are such that he burns all excess fat, with the result that his percentage of body fat is amongst the lowest of all athletes. It is duration rather than intensity, then, which burns off calories.

The implications for the patient with coronary heart disease are obvious. Not only will "long slow distance" keep his weight down, I have often thought it is not beyond the bounds of possi-bility that it could also reduce the size of the fatty plaques in his

Figure 11

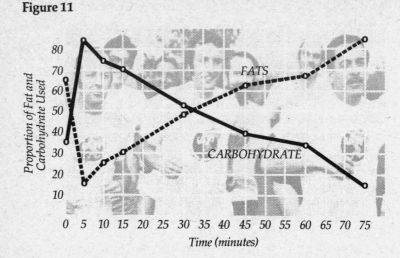

The Longer You Exercise, the More Fat Your Body Burns

arteries — provided, of course, that these plaques have not become calcified so that the fat is inaccessible. Recently my optimism has been rewarded by the findings of Dr. Ron Selvester and his colleagues in the Department of Cardiology at the famous Ranchos Los Amigos Rehabilitation Hospital, Los Angeles. They reported that six patients out of a group of forty in a one-year exercise program for coronary artery disease, showed a decrease in the size of the atherosclerotic plaques in their leg arteries. This is the first report of its kind ever made; let us hope it will be first of many.

As for the frequency of training, five times a week is ideal. Nowadays, the competitive athlete trains seven days a week, and not infrequently twice a day. Such draconian measures may well pay off in a situation where only yards and seconds separate the world's best and the third-rater. However, by the law of diminishing returns, one must expect a smaller improvement for every hour spent in training over and above a certain level. Individuals who train less than three times a week make minimal progress; those who average four or five times a week seem to do much better, and those with the time and motivation to train seven times a week show maybe an additional 1 or 2 per cent increase over that. Five times a week seems to be the answer, in terms of fitness payoff for time invested.

The Training Tables

I have developed these tables over the past seven years; they are the result of practical experience in the training of hundreds of patients with heart disease. Used sensibly, and in accordance with the instructions which follow, they will provide safe and effective exercise for the development of endurance fitness.

However, let me start with a word of warning. The aim is to provide a personal exercise plan. But you must remember that circumstances and individuals vary. Mindless adherence to these or, indeed, any other set of training tables, no matter how intrinsically sound they may be, could have unpleasant consequences in the presence of coronary heart disease. While improvement in general health and cardiac function is the usual response to a fitness program, from time to time the disease may become unstable. The warning signs and symptoms of such deterioration will be described elsewhere in this book; if they become apparent, the exercise prescription should be reduced immediately. Similarly, if you are having difficulty completing a prescribed workout, even though the guidelines indicate that you should be able to accomplish that particular level of activity, then do not hesitate to modify the requirements to suit your tolerance. If in doubt, consult your physician. Prudence takes precedence over enthusiasm when you are training a damaged heart!

With these precautions in mind, we will now take a closer look at the training tables reproduced in the Appendix on pages 291-93. They consist of three phases, each of which will be described in detail.

Phase 1 This relates your fitness level, in terms of maximum oxygen consumption, to a "starter prescription." Allowance is made for age; if you are over 45, your general physical condition is probably poor and the possibilty of atherosclerosis more likely.

If your initial maximum oxygen consumption (vo_2 max) is less than 16 ml/kg/min. (and we will see later how to measure this), then you should carry out a preliminary phase which lasts eight weeks. Actually, if you are overweight, or have been sedentary for many years, or suffer from musculoskeletal problems such as low back pain or mild osteoarthritis in your knees or hips, then it is not a bad idea for you to adhere to the eight week breaking-in period — even though your initial fitness may be higher than the specified level.

If your vo₂ max is higher than 16 ml., then the table will call for a three-mile walk, at a speed which varies with your level of fitness. The three miles should be approached in stages, walking one mile for two weeks, then two miles for two weeks, and finally the three miles, all at the prescribed speed. After that, of course, progression is made to the next level by walking the full three miles distance at a faster pace.

You should work out five times a week, and take two days' rest. It is immaterial whether these rest days are taken together, or split through the week; the choice is a matter of personal convenience, as well as the avoidance of cumulative fatigue.

It should be noted that the predicted maximum oxygen consumption levels used in Phase I were derived from the program's customary sub-maximal exercise stress test (see Appendix, p. 292). Ideally, your own initial level of fitness should therefore be estimated in the same manner. However, if this is not possible, a comparable test should be used; the step test described elsewhere in this book is a rough equivalent suitable in most cases.

Phase 2 This table progresses you through a series of steps which increase the intensity of the workout to a desired pace (10 minutes per mile if you are under 45, 12 minutes per mile if you are over 45), while at the same time decreasing the distance. When you achieve your desired pace, then the distance is lengthened to four miles, while maintaining the same speed. This is a crucial phase, and may take many months to complete. If you have heart disease, you should be particularly attentive to the possible development of such adverse symptoms as chest pain, extreme breathlessness, skipped beats, and light-headedness during the workout. These symptoms will be discussed again in the next chapter. If the condition of your heart is unstable, it is more likely to reveal itself at speeds faster than 14 minutes per mile (that is, a pace which requires uninterrupted jogging). At some point during this phase, fast walking develops into an awkward gallop, and becomes excessively strenuous; you will have to jog in order to complete the distance comfortably within the prescribed time. The precise level at which this occurs depends on your height and leg length, but in general takes place at the 15-minute mile pace.

When jogging becomes necessary, it is introduced into the workout in a specific manner. The instructions given to the

Centre patients are reproduced here, since they explain the method clearly.

So far your exercise prescriptions have been at a walking pace. This prescription may require some jogging in order to complete it comfortably within the required time. The transition from walking to jogging should be done in easy stages in order to avoid muscle, tendon and joint problems, and also to ensure a smooth acceleration of heart rate.

The procedure taught in this program is as follows: You should jog 10-15 second intervals spaced evenly throughout your prescription. You may find that a 15-second jog every half-mile will be sufficient. Or you may need to jog every quarter-mile in order to finish in time. *The pace should be only a little faster than your walk,* and the technique should be as you have been instructed in class. As you progress, go on adding quarter-minute jogging segments until you are jogging the last 15 seconds of each and every minute. In order to record your highest pulse, you should finish with a 15-second jog and immediately record your final exercise pulse.

As your prescription increases, gradually increase your jogs to 30 seconds. Eventually you will be jogging half the distance and walking half. From then on it is easy to progress to jogging the entire distance. By using this method you make the transition from walking to jogging in an orderly and safe manner.

Please note that during this transition phase we are interested in the highest heart rate achieved toward the end of the workout; therefore, please take and record your pulse *at the end of the final jogging interval.*

The jogging technique will be described in detail later, but at this stage it is sufficient to say that it should be relaxed, flat-footed and with short strides; the speed should be a little above that of a walk. Actually, I feel that the term "plodding" is more descriptive than jogging.

Phase 3   Here, you will progress to jogging six miles in 60 or 72 minutes, depending on your age. This goal requires about twelve months, and is well worth achieving. It puts you into the class of the long distance jogger, and brings all of the benefits we have previously discussed. Anyone who has managed to progress through the first two phases and is free from symptoms and signs should certainly attempt to finish Phase 3. Jogging for an hour a day five times a week may be time-consuming, but it pays off in terms of high-level cardiorespiratory fitness. From the ranks of the "one hour joggers" have come the post-coronary marathoners who so amply demonstrated the rehabilitative power of physical exercise.

How to Use the Tables

Determining your Starting Level   How fit are you? The only way to answer this accurately is to undergo a maximal or sub-maximal exercise stress test, as outlined in Part One of this book. This will give you a figure for your maximum oxygen consumption, expressed as the number of millilitres of oxygen your body burns each minute for every kilogram you weigh. Not only that, but the test will also show whether or not you develop electro-cardiographic abnormalities during training sessions. Such a test is, of course, highly desirable for individuals with coronary artery disease who wish to start exercising. It is mandatory for all patients entering my exercise rehabilitation program. If you are a would-be exerciser, and have a heart problem, then you should ask your physician to arrange an exercise test. If he doesn't do this procedure himself, then he should refer you to a physician who does.

What if there aren't any facilities for exercise testing in your area? There are a number of do-it-yourself tests, but these should only be carried out if you have had prior clearance from your physician to do so. They are a lot more strenuous than they look, and may even be dangerous for the middle-aged sedentary individual suffering from symptomless and so far undetected atherosclerosis of his coronary arteries. If you have had a heart attack, or suffer from angina pectoris or palpitations, and cannot be exercise-tested by a physician, I strongly advise that you start right at the beginning with Level 1 of the Preliminary Phase; in this way, you will assure your safety and, using the method described in the next section, will still be able to progress your training program in a rational and scientific manner. You may lose a few weeks at the start, but since getting fit and staying fit is a lifetime avocation, a few weeks here or there won't make much difference. Self-administered fitness tests can never have the accuracy of the laboratory evaluation. However, for the healthy individual, they provide a close enough approximation.

In general, there are two types of home tests; one based on the distance walked or run in a specified time, and the other on the pulse rate response to stair stepping. Of the former, the best-known examples are those devised by Dr. Bruno Balke, an authority in the field of exercise physiology, and Dr. Ken Cooper, author of the well-known book, *The New Aerobics*. They differ only in that Dr. Balke requires you to cover as much ground as you can in 15 minutes, whereas Dr. Cooper settles for 12 minutes. Maximum oxygen consumption is then calculated from the attained distance, using a formula. For further details of Dr. Cooper's test, you should consult his book. Dr. Balke's method uses the furthest distance you can run, jog, and/or walk in 15 minutes, expressed in metres (1 mile = 1609.354 metres); this is converted into metres per minute by dividing by 15, and your maximum oxygen consumption worked out from the formula: (speed - 133) x 0.172, added to 33.3 = vo_2 max. in ml/kg/min.

The problem with both these tests from our point of view is that they were designed primarily for healthy, young subjects. Furthermore, they are *maximum tests*, depending for accuracy upon a full-out effort. *Sub-maximum* testing is safer since it is tailored to the individual's age and/or weight, and sets the limit of exertion at approximately 75 per cent of maximum heart rate.

Sub-maximal Step Test

The following example of a sub-maximum step test is one devised by Professor Roy Shephard, and I am indebted to him for its use here. The procedure requires you to step up-and-down two 9-inch steps (total 18 inches — two staircase steps will do), to a count of 6. Start with the feet together on the ground, then left foot on the first step — count 1; right foot on the second step — count 2; left foot joins right foot — count 3; right foot on the first step — count 4; left foot on the ground — count 5; right foot joins left foot — count 6. The lead leg can be alternated every other minute to reduce fatigue.

The rate of stepping is important, since it will affect the energy cost of the test. We are aiming for an intensity of effort which is about 75 per cent of maximum; this will, of course, vary with age and body weight. However, the following tables give the appropriate tempo in numbers of steps per minute, as well

How to Estimate Your
Rate of Stepping, the Resulting
Energy Cost, and Target Heart
Rate from Your Weight and Age.

Rate of Stepping (steps per min.) / Energy Cost of Stepping (millilitres of oxygen)

Table A.1 MALE

AGE	Weight lbs. (kg.) 110 (49.9)	120 (54.4)	130 (59.0)	140 (63.5)	150 (68.0)	160 (72.6)	170 (77.1)	180 (81.6)	190 (86.2)	200 (90.7)	210 (95.3)	220 (99.8)
20 – 29	120 / 1570	120 / 1690	120 / 1813	126 / 2018	126 / 2143	126 / 2273	126 / 2398	126 / 2524	126 / 2653	126 / 2779	126 / 2908	126 / 3034
30 – 39	108 / 1437	114 / 1618	114 / 1734	114 / 1848	114 / 1962	114 / 2079	114 / 2192	114 / 2307	114 / 2423	120 / 2658	120 / 2781	120 / 2901
40 – 49	96 / 1304	96 / 1400	96 / 1498	102 / 1679	102 / 1781	102 / 1885	102 / 1987	102 / 2089	102 / 2193	102 / 2295	102 / 2400	102 / 2502
50 – 60	78 / 1105	78 / 1183	78 / 1262	78 / 1340	78 / 1418	78 / 1498	84 / 1679	84 / 1763	84 / 1849	84 / 1933	84 / 2018	84 / 2103

Table A.2 FEMALE

AGE	Weight lbs. (kg.) 80 (36.3)	90 (40.8)	100 (45.4)	110 (49.9)	120 (54.4)	130 (59.0)	140 (63.5)	150 (68.0)	160 (72.6)	170 (77.1)	180 (81.6)	190 (86.2)
20 – 29	96 / 974	102 / 1125	102 / 1229	102 / 1331	102 / 1433	108 / 1616	108 / 1724	108 / 1832	108 / 1942	108 / 2050	108 / 2158	108 / 2268
30 – 39	96 / 974	96 / 1070	102 / 1229	102 / 1331	102 / 1433	102 / 1537	102 / 1639	108 / 1832	108 / 1942	108 / 2050	108 / 2158	108 / 2268
40 – 49	84 / 877	84 / 961	84 / 1047	90 / 1198	90 / 1288	90 / 1380	90 / 1469	90 / 1560	90 / 1652	90 / 1742	96 / 1288	96 / 2038
50 – 60	60 / 684	60 / 744	60 / 805	60 / 865	60 / 925	60 / 986	60 / 1046	60 / 1106	60 / 1168	60 / 1228	60 / 1288	60 / 1349

Table B

Age (Years)	Heart Rate (Beats/min.)
20–30	160/min.
30–40	150/min.
40–50	140/min.
50–60	130/min.
60–70	120/min.

as the energy cost of this effort in millilitres of oxygen per kilogram of body weight per minute. They also show the age-related anticipated heart rate after three to five minutes of stepping — this latter figure is based on the normal sedentary population and is accurate to within plus or minus ten beats.

Having worked out the correct stepping rate for your age and weight, practice with a stop watch until you get the tempo, then step up and down for three to five minutes. Your aim is to attain your approximate target heart rate within that time. Immediately on stopping, take a 10-second pulse count.* With this figure, you can then calculate your maximum oxygen consumption by using the appropriate nomogram (Figures 14 to 17 pages 287-90).

A line joining your energy cost of stepping and your exercise heart rate will intersect the centre line at your estimated maximum oxygen consumption, expressed in millilitres of oxygen. Dividing this figure by your weight in kg. (1 lb. = 2.2 kg.) will give you your maximum oxygen consumption expressed in millilitres of oxygen per kilogram. min. Apply this figure to Phase 1 of the training tables, and you have your starting level of training. For example: Assume you are a 45-year-old male who weighs 160 lbs. From Table A you would need to carry out the step test at the rate of 102 steps per minute to burn 1885 ml. of oxygen per minute; which, for the average sedentary individual of that age and weight, would be equivalent to three-quarters of all-out effort. As a further check, the resultant pulse rate for that degree of effort is obtained from Table B, i.e., 140 beats per minute plus or minus 10 beats.

You now carry out the test at the required rate of stepping and, in the absence of excessive fatigue or adverse symptoms,

*See page 134 for instructions in taking accurate pulse count.

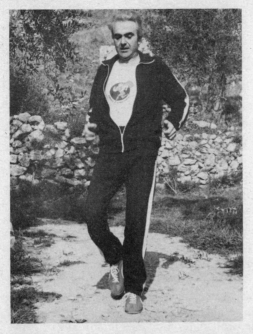

Running in Italy in spring (left). The active life: post-coronary marathoners in a friendly game of volleyball, Honolulu, 1974 (below).

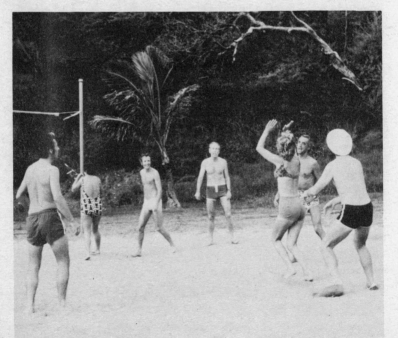

you continue for five minutes. At the end of this time you take your pulse, and let us say, for illustrative purposes, it comes to 150 beats per minute. Then, from Figure 16 you read off a predicted maximum oxygen intake of 2200 millilitres per minute (a line joining 1885 on the right column and 150 on the left column intersects the centre sloping line at 2200). You now divide your predicted maximum oxygen consumption of 2200 by your weight in kilograms (72.6 kg) and you obtain your vo_2 max. corrected for weight, i.e. 30.3ml/kg min. Applying this to the training tables would mean that you could start at Level 7 of Phase 1, or three miles in 45 minutes.

Sounds complicated? It isn't really, but if you find it a chore even to contemplate, then skip it and start at the Preliminary Phase, Level 1.

What if you develop chest pain or discomfort, extreme breathlessness, light-headedness, or other adverse symptoms before the five minutes are up? If this occurs, then stop immediately, and note your pulse rate. This will represent your maximum heart rate for training purposes. For safety's sake, you should obtain your doctor's permission before you start the exercise program. If he agrees that exercise can help you, then start at the preliminary conditioning stage of the tables, and be sure that your pulse rate during the workout remains at least 10 beats per minute below the symptom-producing level.

Two very important points! Your stepping rate must be as accurately timed as possible. The best way to do this is to use a simple metronome, the sort that piano teachers used to use. If you don't want to invest $10 or so to buy one then I'm sure you can borrow one from one of your musical friends. Just set the scale to the desired stepping rate, and merely keep in time with the beat. Secondly, pulse rate should be obtained *immediately* on stopping. Ideally, it should be taken during the last minute of the test, but this is very difficult to do. Instead, as you stop, take a ten second pulse count, and then multiply the result by six to give a full minute's count. Remember, the heart rate begins to drop pretty rapidly with the cessation of exercise, and if you delay as little as even 30 seconds in finding and counting your pulse, the result will not truly represent your heart rate in the final minutes of the test.

You may find that after two minutes or so of stepping you feel that you cannot continue for the plain and simple reason that your legs are too tired. This means that you are even less fit than the average sedentary person of your age and weight, i.e., the rate of stepping prescribed for you in Table A represents more than 75 per cent of *your* maximum oxygen consumption, and so you can't keep the pace up for more than a few minutes. If you take your pulse rate at the time that you have to stop, you will find that it is already well above target rate. Don't despair, try again the following day, but this time choose the tempo listed next lowest in the table, e.g. 96 instead of 102 steps per minute.

Finally, at the risk of being unduly repetitive, let me once again warn you against attempting this or any other self-administered test without the permission of your physician — especially if you have any of the symptoms of coronary artery disease. Paradoxically, those most curious to know their fitness level are the overweight, sedentary, obviously unfit members of the population — precisely those in whom atherosclerosis is likely to be present. Beware that curiosity doesn't kill the fat cat.

You are now in the position to choose a suitable starting level from Phase 1. If you do not know your fitness level, and suffer from heart disease, then start from Level 1 of the Preliminary Phase. If your fitness level has been measured, then it is a simple matter to use the calculated maximum oxygen consumption and apply it to the tables. For example, assume you are age 40, and were found to have a fitness level of 25 ml/kg/min. This would place you in Phase 1, Level 5 of the training tables, and would give a starting prescription of three miles in 48 minutes, five times weekly. You would start by walking one mile in 16 minutes for two weeks, and then increase this to two miles in 32 minutes for a further two weeks. At the end of this time, provided that you are not suffering any cardiac or musculoskeletal problems, you would proceed to your three miles in 48 minutes.

How to Progress Through the Tables

Having chosen a suitable starting level, we must now consider how you are to progress through the higher levels of Phase 1, through Phase 2 and then Phase 3, preferably without frequent repetition of time-consuming and relatively expensive laboratory exercise tests. We can achieve this by using our knowledge of the effect of training on heart function.

We have seen that endurance fitness is attained by exercising regularly at an intensity of about 50 to 70 per cent of maximum oxygen consumption. The problem is, oxygen consumption is not something which can be measured readily. Fortunately, however, there is a relationship between oxygen consumption and heart rate. Provided we know our resting heart rate and also our maximum heart rate, we can calculate a training heart rate which, as a practical field guide, corresponds to 70 per cent of maximum oxygen consumption.

Resting heart rate is easy to obtain. You merely take your pulse rate immediately on awakening in the morning, and before you get out of bed. As before, count the number of beats in 10 seconds and then multiply by six. This is much more accurate than obtaining a resting pulse after sitting still for five or ten minutes; too many extraneous factors such as a recent meal, emotional excitement, or recent physical activity can give a false result.

Maximum heart rate decreases with age, and varies substantially from one healthy person to another. The only way to assess maximum heart rate accurately is to carry out a maximum exercise test. However, since this requires all-out effort, it poses problems both in terms of motivation and safety. A more practical alternative is to use tables of average values for maximum heart rates at different age levels. Such tables are sufficiently precise for the safety of the post-coronary patient who is free from symptoms.

Thus, we have available the two essential pieces of information necessary to control progression in the training program: the actual resting heart rate, and the age-related maximum heart rate. Remember, however, that as you become fitter, you develop a training bradycardia; that is, both resting and working heart rates become slower. Eventually, the intensity and duration of the prescribed workout is ineffectual in obtaining the 70 per cent training heart rate. When this stage is reached, progression to a higher level is indicated.

The above basic principles have been used to devise a simple nomogram (A) which relates resting heart rate and age to a progressing heart rate. When the prescribed workout consistently fails to achieve the progressing heart rate for a period of two

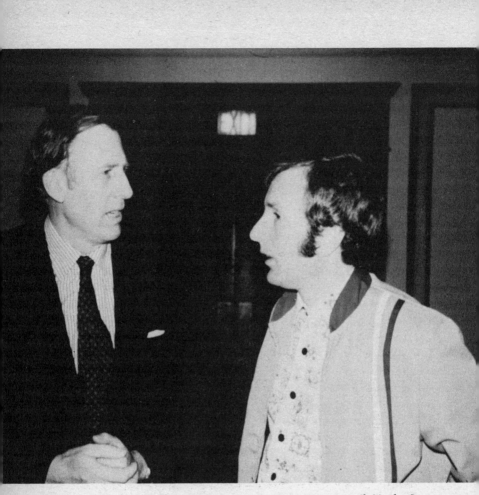

A unique meeting in Boston, 1975: Dr. Roger Bannister (left), the first man to run a mile in less than four minutes, and Herman Robers, the first man to be an official entrant in the Boston Marathon after having had a heart attack.

weeks, then the time has come to move up to the next level on the table. Say, for instance, that our 40-year-old who started at Level 5, Phase 1 (three miles in 48 minutes) had a resting heart rate of 68 beats per minute. To use nomogram A, he would take a piece of black thread and place it so as to join 72 on the resting heart rate column (values less than 72 can, for the purposes of the prediction, be ignored) and 40 on the age column. Where the thread crosses the centre line is his progressing heart rate: 130 beats per minute. Thus, when his pulse count in the

NOMOGRAM A
To Be Used for Calculating Your Progressing Heart Rate
For those who have completed a stress test without adverse symptoms or who are free from heart disease.

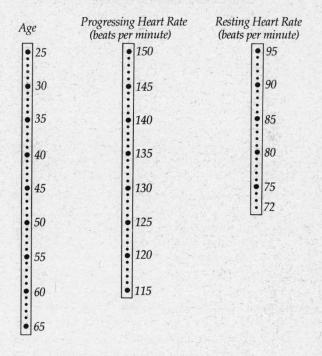

Age	Progressing Heart Rate (beats per minute)	Resting Heart Rate (beats per minute)
25	150	95
30	145	90
35	140	85
40	135	80
45	130	75
50	125	72
55	120	
60	115	
65		

A line joining your resting heart rate and your age will intersect the centre column at your progressing heart rate. Resting heart rates below 72 beats per minute should be charted at 72. To obtain your heart rate (pulse rate) and resting heart rate see pages 131 and 134-36.

10 seconds following his three-mile walk is at or below this level consistently for a period of two weeks (an average for ten successive workouts), he would be ready to progress to Level 6 (three miles in 45 minutes). The use of the nomogram, therefore, enables safe and effective progression without constant retesting. It gives you an element of objectivity in your training regime; instead of stepping up your program because you feel good, you can apply a physiological measure to validate your enthusiasm.

For the nomogram to be of maximal value, however, it must be used correctly. Not only must the post-workout heart rate be at or below the progressing heart rate *consistently* for ten or more exercise sessions but, moreover, progression to a higher level of effort should not be attempted in the presence of any of the signs of over-training such as excessive tiredness, palpitations (premature ventricular beats) or muscle aches and pains. (The latter will be discussed in more detail in the next chapter.) Your heart rate must be charted at the end of each exercise session in order to keep an accurate record.

Of course, the nomogram contains two other variables, age and resting heart rate. The majority of patients reach the end of Phase 2, or attain their maximum fitness potential, within a two-year period; therefore, once started on the program it should not be necessary to change their age level on the left-hand column. As for resting heart rate, this also drops with training but, as we have seen, the change is more variable than with exercise heart rate. For patients on a supervised program a new resting heart rate can be established at the time of each laboratory exercise stress test; failing this, you can obtain your resting heart rate every six months and adjust the right-hand column accordingly.

Obtaining Your Pulse Rate It is essential that the pulse rate be correctly obtained. So far, this has been taken for granted, but is such an integral part of a home exercise program that we will take the time now to discuss it in more detail. The pumping heart imparts to every large blood vessel an impulse which coincides with the heart beat. Physicians traditionally measure heart rate by timing the pulse of the radial artery in the front of the wrist just below the base of the thumb. The vessel is easily accessible in this position, lying just beneath the skin, and is easily felt because it can be steadied against the underlying wrist bones. Exercise physiologists tend to use the carotid pulse, the large artery in the front of the neck which can be felt on either side of the Adam's apple; this vessel pumps very vigorously during exercise, and for that reason is easier to obtain (except in short, thick-necked individuals when there may be some difficulty).

Whether you use the carotid or the radial pulse is probably unimportant, and will depend on whichever you find the easiest. If you use the carotid, then be careful not to press too hard with your palpating fingers, otherwise you will press on a structure know as the carotid sinus, and this will artificially slow the

Figure 12

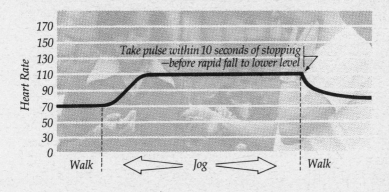

When to Take Exercise Heart Rate

heart rate momentarily. (As a matter of fact, simultaneous firm pressure on both sides of the neck over the carotid sinus may slow your heart rate to such a degree that consciousness is lost — a well-known tactic in karate!). Even though it may be more difficult to obtain the carotid pulse in some people, I usually try to train my patients to use this method of pulse counting; once mastered, it allows you to operate a stop watch in the other hand and so get an accurate count. If you are having difficulty in feeling the carotid pulse, it may be that you are instinctively throwing your head back, a movement which causes the carotid arteries to retract away from the front of the neck. If you want to feel the carotid pulse easily, then hold your head in the normal position, or even slightly tilted forward.

Having found the pulse, you must now count it accurately. Since you are only counting for 10 seconds, and multiplying by six, accuracy is essential. If you are as much as one beat out, then your one minute reading will be substantially in error. For uniformity's sake we have always told our patients to start counting zero, one, two, three, etc., the zero marking the commencement of the ten second count. Actually, I find it easier to repeat the word "five" a number of times as I watch the second hand of my watch approach the start point, thus: five, five, five — zero, one, two, three, etc. Somehow or other it gives me the correct rhythm for counting.

Why count for only 10 seconds? Ideally, we want to know what the heart rate is *during* the exercise session. As soon as you start to work out, your resting heart rate climbs, and within two or three minutes reaches a plateau which remains steady for as long as you exercise — provided, of course, that you maintain the same pace. It is the level of heart rate during the exercise session which we need to know. Since it is impractical to take the pulse rate while jogging, or even walking, we utilize the fact that it takes 10 or 15 seconds to drop from the plateau as soon as the exercise stops. Pulse rates, then, taken within 10 seconds of stopping jogging or brisk walking, are a fairly accurate measure of the heart rate during the workout. Thereafter, the rate drops off rapidly, and if you wait as little as 20 seconds to take your count, it will no longer be representative of the rate during exertion (Figure 12). Hence the need to be speedy and well-practised in this technique.

There is one exception to the rule of taking a pulse count precisely at the termination of the workout. During the transition period from walking to jogging, the pulse rate during the episodes of jogging is important, since it is highest then. Therefore, when you are in this phase, you should aim to finish with a 15-second jog and immediately record your final exercise pulse.

The Individual with Angina Pectoris or Related Symptoms

So far, we have been discussing the use of the nomogram to check the progress of the individual who, while he has heart disease, does not suffer from symptoms such as angina pectoris. In my program, I refer to him as the "uncomplicated exerciser." What of the individual who suffers from symptoms, especially when exercising? He falls into the category of the "complicated exerciser" and for him, there is a special nomogram. Into this category also fall those patients who have had a formal exercise test which has revealed the presence of such ECG abnormalities as severe ST segment depression or increasing extrasystoles. Here, our interest is not so much in fitness level as in determining the level of activity at which adverse symptoms or signs occur, and then formulating a training prescription which takes this factor into account.

This is no problem in a hospital-type program where regular stress testing can be carried out and an exact figure specified for the level of exertion at which cardiac problems develop. Such repeated testing is impractical, however, in a community-type home program. On the other hand, the use of average tables of maximum heart rates does not ensure enough accuracy for safety. A more individualized approach is required, and the obvious one is a simple record of the heart rate at which untoward symptoms or signs develop. Working on this principle, a second nomogram has been devised (B) which permits the choice of a suitable starting level of exercise for the patient with symptoms, and his subsequent safe progress through the various stages of the tables. Decision on the starting level of the tables requires rather more trial and error than in the uncomplicated case.

Assuming that symptoms develop during a stress test, either carried out in the doctor's office or at home, then note is made of the pulse rate at which these occurred. I refer to this as the maximum heart rate, symptom limited, or max. H.R.^{SL}. Using this figure, together with the resting heart rate (obtained as previously) then the training heart rate can be read from Nomogram B. A word of warning: If the difference between your resting heart rate and your max. H.R.^{SL} is 40 beats per minute or less, then you should exercise only under the strict supervision of a physician. As you can see from the nomogram, the spread between training and progressing heart rates would be small in your case, requiring careful, accurate monitoring — too delicate a job for the average reader of this book. However, if this proviso does not apply to you, a trial one-mile walk is then taken, at a pace which is considered brisk, but not so fast as to bring on chest pain, skipped beats, or undue breathlessness. The pulse rate is taken in the 10 seconds immediately following the walk, and is compared with the desired training heart rate. Depending on the result, the speed is adjusted to the nearest appropriate level in Phase 1, always erring on the side of safety: that is, keeping the intensity of exercise below the level at which symptoms of cardiac ischemia develop. It may take one or two sessions to select the desired pace, but with patience and care, it is surprising how accurate one can be.

The following example will illustrate the method. Assume you have a resting heart rate of 72 beats per minute. While being tested, you develop evidence of ischemia, say chest pain, at a

NOMOGRAM B
To Be Used for Calculating Your Training Heart Rate and Your Progressing Heart Rate.

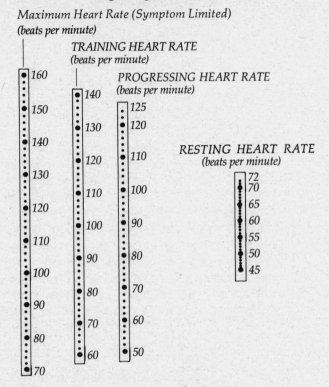

Maximum Heart Rate (Symptom Limited)
(beats per minute)

TRAINING HEART RATE
(beats per minute)

PROGRESSING HEART RATE
(beats per minute)

RESTING HEART RATE
(beats per minute)

For those who have <u>not</u> been able to complete a stress test because of the development of adverse symptoms or who have symptoms of coronary heart disease such as anginal pain, palpitations or breathlessness, etc. (see pages 129 to 130 and 137-39).

A line joining your resting heart rate and the heart rate at which your symptoms appear, your maximum heart rate (symptom limited), will intersect the centre columns at your training heart rate and progressing heart rate. Resting heart rates above 72 beats per minute should be charted at 72.

If the difference between your resting heart rate and your maximum heart rate (symptom limited) is less than 40 beats per minute, you should not attempt the training program in this book, except under medical supervision.

To obtain your heart rate (pulse rate) and resting heart rate see pages 131 and 134-36.

heart rate of 124 beats per minute. This means that you have a max. H.R.^{SL} of 124. From the nomogram, this will give you a training heart rate^{SL} of 110 beats per minute. You now go for a trial one-mile walk, choosing a level course, and keeping the pace slow enough to avoid chest pain or undue breathlessness. At the end of the measured mile, you discover that you have taken 20 minutes, and your immediate post-exercise heart rate is 108 beats per minute. This, then, is your starting level (Level 1, Phase 1 for an under 45-year-old) and over the next six weeks, you progress to two miles and then to three miles keeping the same pace of 20 minutes per mile. Using the same nomogram you can also tell what your progressing heart rate should be (in this example, 100 beats per minute). After each workout, you chart your pulse rate, and when this consistently fails to achieve 100 beats per minute for ten consecutive sessions, and provided you have none of the adverse symptoms mentioned above, then you progress to Level 2, Phase 1.

Not infrequently, a patient who initially shows evidence of myocardial ischemia during a test will, as he gets fitter, move into the category of an uncomplicated exerciser. This may take time, but nevertheless, for this reason, I feel that complicated cases should be exercise-tested every three months or so in order to have an objective measurement of improvement. When they can complete an uncomplicated test, then they can be progressed in accordance with Nomogram A. Complicated cases require much closer physician supervision than uncomplicated, and ideally should be enrolled in a formal post-coronary exercise rehabilitation class. In this way, they can be watched during supervised exercise sessions and monitored frequently during the workout.

In the early stages, the individual with symptoms during exercise will progress at a slower rate than his symptomless colleagues. This is to be expected, and should not be allowed to cause discouragement or depression. Above all, any temptation to progress faster than the tables indicate should be vigorously resisted. You cannot bully a damaged heart. This is one game where breaking the rules may mean more than the loss of a few yards or a touchdown; it may mean "game over" for the only player involved — yourself! So, have patience, and remember that if it took you twenty years to get out of shape, you can't really expect to regain your fitness in a few months.

CHAPTER SIX

Some Do's and Don'ts

Attainment of Fitness

There are a few basic facts about physical fitness which should be borne in mind. First, each of us has an optimal level of endurance fitness which is appropriate to our age, sex and genetic background. Once we reach that level, more intensive training will result in only marginal gains. By the law of diminishing returns, the improvement will be minimal in comparison to the time and effort invested. Mark you, if one is a world champion, the extra effort may be worth it, for even fractional advances may make all the difference between victory and defeat. However, for most of us, such slender gains are of little cardiovascular advantage.

Let me give you an example of what I mean. An international long distance runner, with a maximum oxygen uptake of 70 ml/kg/min. is averaging, say 70 miles a week in training. By increasing this to 90 miles a week, he might conceivably improve his oxygen uptake by a few millilitres (although it is more likely to help him by increasing the ease or degree of mechanical efficiency with which he runs, thus allowing him to go further and faster on the same amount of oxygen); this slight improvement may be sufficient to reduce his time by 20 to 30 seconds — which is probably all that separates the top ten men in the world in his event.

For us lesser mortals, the requirements are not so exacting. The training tables have been devised to progress you to a level which is suitable for your age and general tolerance. They are based on maximum oxygen consumption levels attained by patients on the post-coronary exercise program, and should, therefore, be well within the capabilities of the vast majority of readers.

Of course, there are always exceptions to the rule. For example, some will be unable to progress to the end of Phase 3 in the tables. They may stick at an earlier level because of adverse symptoms, failure to achieve the progressing heart rate, or fatigue after the workout. Does this mean that they are wasting their time training? Definitely not. They have attained what is the right duration and intensity of workout for them, at least for the time being, and can rest assured that if they continue to work out at this level, they will maintain their maximum potential.

A case in point is Charles W., an industrial chemist, who was one of the first patients on the program. He sustained a severe heart attack at the age of 58. For the first week or so after the attack, his condition was so serious that he was not expected to survive. Complications included multiple cardiac arrests, and almost complete failure of the heart to function as a pump. For days, he was kept alive only by the heroic efforts of the coronary care team. When he arrived at the Centre for exercise therapy, he was still troubled by an irregular heart beat, especially when he exerted himself. His exercise test revealed a very limited physical tolerance, poor fitness level, and many abnormalities on the dynamic electrocardiogram. Not surprisingly, Charles found it impossible to progress to the end stage of the training tables. As a matter of fact, he is still, after seven years, in the walking stage.

Has it helped? He thinks so, and I would most certainly agree. Forced into an early retirement by the attack, he worked out regularly, rarely missing a day. As his fitness increased, so his general tolerance improved, until eventually he was able to contemplate work again. However, with a new lease on life, he decided that rather than return to his old job, he would offer his services to Canadian Executive Service Overseas (CESO), an organization of Canadian executives who assist in the establishment of vital industries in the underdeveloped nations. Since then, he has travelled extensively in South America, the Caribbean, and the Far East. His exercise diaries have arrived from all parts of the world, and he has carried out his prescription walk in airports, around padangs, on board ship, in hotel corridors and, in fact, anywhere he can find a suitable space. So you don't have to run marathons to attain the fitness level right for you.

There is a misapprehension about the development of fitness which I think it is important to dispel. Most people believe that a training program, carried out regularly, results in a gradual day-by-day improvement in your physical state. In actual fact, I have found that this is not the case. If you are expecting progress in this manner, then you are in for a big disappointment. This explains why you plug away for weeks, or even months, without any apparent change, and then suddenly one day, you find the workout quite easy. At the same time, you will notice that your post-workout pulse rate has dropped a few beats or more. Or, you will discover that you have completed the distance a few minutes faster than ever before. At first you will doubt the watch itself, but when you repeat the performance the following day, you will realize that you have suddenly and almost miraculously attained a new level of fitness.

What has happened? One of the major effects of training is to open up new blood capillaries in the skeletal muscle tissue so as to be able to transport more oxygen to the working cells. These new capillaries, so small that they can be seen only under a microscope, do not form gradually. They "open up," almost like a budding flower seen under time-lapse photography, and in response to the stimulus of repeated and prolonged training sessions. The duration of their formative period obviously varies from individual to individual, and is dependent upon the type and nature of the training program. The thing to remember is that the plateau is an essential part of the process. Don't get discouraged because your condition appears to be static. In actual fact, the preliminary work of capillarization is continuing apace; the next day may see a great leap forward.

How to Jog

Recreational jogging for fun and fitness is reputed to have started in New Zealand. It was introduced by the world-famous track coach, Arthur Lydiard, who believed in marathon-type training for all his competitive runners, even his half-milers and milers. Since his protégés included such world champions as Peter Snell, is it small wonder that his training methods were imitated by coaches all over the world?

Apart from his interest in competitive track and field, however, Lydiard has always believed that physical fitness is the key to a happy and healthy life, and that slow long distance running is the best way to achieve such fitness. When Bill Bowerman, the highly successful university track coach from Oregon, visited New Zealand, he was amazed to find that jogging was the national pastime. Young and old, male and female, all were caught up in the business of running for miles through the countryside at a slow steady pace, often in groups, joking and talking with one another along the way. Lydiard persuaded Bowerman to join his group for a jogging session. For Bowerman, it was his moment of truth. Within a matter of miles, he was having difficulty keeping up with runners in their 60's and 70's; to make matters worse, he later discovered that one of the "oldsters" who accompanied him for most of the way had deliberately held back in order to provide the visiting American coach with company! When Bowerman returned to the United States, he immediately launched a movement to introduce recreational jogging. Today, his home town of Eugene refers to itself as "The Jogging Capital of the World," with thousands of the inhabitants jogging regularly.

The next major development was the introduction by Dr. Kenneth Cooper, at that time in the United States Air Force, of endurance-type running as the main component in the service's fitness program. He later went on to introduce the same program to the population at large, through the medium of his book, *Aerobics*.

Now we have the approach outlined in this book — the use of medically prescribed jogging and marathon-type training for the benefit of patients with heart disease.

Despite this impressive history, the technique of jogging still remains a mystery to many. It differs from running only in its speed of progression. In our particular context, jogging means running at a pace of 10 minutes per mile or slower. The action is simple; take short steps, about 2 to 4 feet in length, and always land flat-footed. The body should be erect, the shoulders and neck relaxed, and the head held naturally (if you fix your eyes

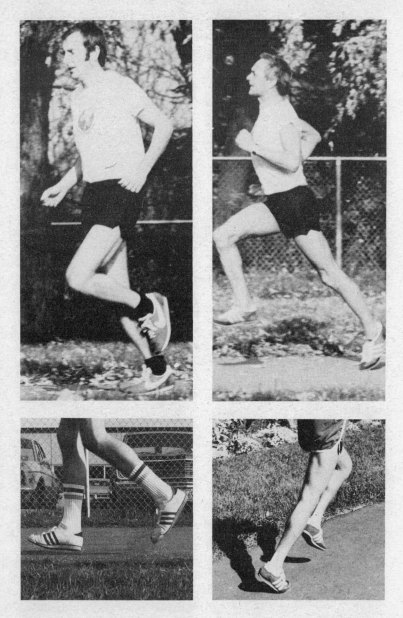

The right way (left) and the wrong way to jog. Note that the subject on the left is relaxed, the arms are carried at hip height and the body is upright. The close-up photo at the lower right shows good action for the youthful sprinter; but the close-up on the left shows the desirable style for the distance jogger, with a relaxed, flat-foot landing.

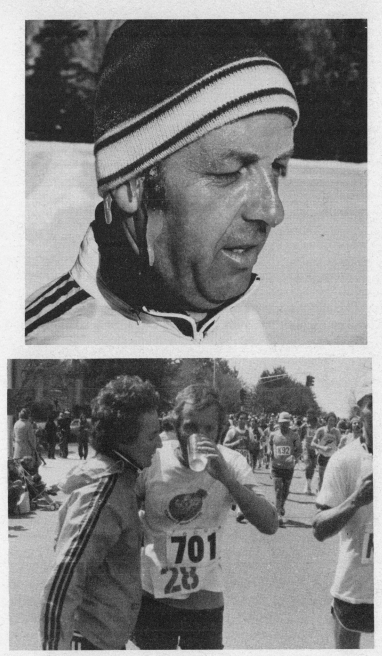

Winter training run.
Summer Marathon run.

on an imaginary spot about 30 yards ahead, this will give the correct head inclination). The elbows should be bent not quite to a right angle, so that the hands move backwards and forwards about the level of the hips; the more you bend your elbows, the faster your arms will swing back and forth, and this in turn will lead to an unconscious pick-up in the rapidity of your leg action and an undesirable increase in speed. The short stride and the flat-foot landing will ensure that your centre of gravity remains over the landing foot, thus preventing too much of a forward body lean, which is all very well for the sprinter or competitive middle distance runner, but plays no part in recreational jogging.

Middle-aged joggers should not try to emulate the running style of their teens. Running up on the toes, or practising an exaggerated heel roll, may have looked very impressive in the "summer of '42," but don't try it now — not unless you wish to develop a whole host of injuries which go by the impressive names of Achilles tendonitis, shin-splints, stress fractures, plantar fasciitis, tenosynovitis; need I list any more?

Equipment

You will need a *stop watch* for counting your pulse and also timing your workout. A deluxe model is very nice, and if you can persuade your family to give you one for Christmas or Chanukkah, so much the better. However, the majority of people in my class manage quite well with a watch which costs around $25, has a 30-minute dial, and is marked off in 1/5ths of a second. Pressing the centre winding-knob starts the timing mechanism, a second press stops it, and a third press returns it to the zero position. Incidentally, there is not much point in having an accurate stop watch if you haven't accurately measured the distance you are walking or jogging. If you are using the local school track, then don't assume that each lap is a quarter of a mile. As a matter of fact, a great many school tracks have been constructed in accordance with the space available, and may need five circuits to complete a mile. If you are working out on the road, you will get an accurate enough reading from a car odometer; I have rarely found these to be misleading — unless, of course, the hot rodder in the family has fitted your sedan with outsize tires!

Shoes are the most important item you will purchase, and you should not attempt to economize here. Just think of the number of times your feet will strike the ground when you are jogging five hours a week, week in, week out. Your feet require to be protected from the pounding they will receive, and it is precisely for this reason that special shoes have been designed for the long distance runner. While each manufacturer has individual variations, the following features tend to be common to all. They are relatively light, a pair often weighing less than two pounds. The sole is flexible but thick enough to absorb shock. It is frequently laminated, with layers of sponge rubber for shock absorption and high density rubber for stability. An arch support is usually built in, and the inner aspects of the tongue specially padded to protect the instep from the pressure of the laces. The upper is made of nylon or flexible leather, and the portion around the heel (the counter) is reinforced so as to grip the heel firmly and prevent it from wobbling from side to side as you run. Since the heel takes most of our body weight when we run, a special rubber heel wedge is often a feature and, to protect the Achilles tendon, or heel cord, the back of the shoe extends upwards in a soft padded tongue which adds additional support and prevents chafing.

Needless to say, no one shoe is ideal, and the individual will have to find the particular brand of running shoe which suits him best. At the time of writing, the major manufacturers in the field are Brooks, New Balance, Nike, Adidas and Puma. All of these manufacturers make a variety of shoes for runners. When you purchase, be sure to ask for a good "training" shoe. The so-called "racing flat" sacrifices some support for lightness, and while this is of value in an actual road race, this type of shoe is unsuitable for regular training.

A *sweat suit* is valuable, but not essential. A pair of slacks and a sweater will do just as well. It's purely a question of how natty you want to appear. Unless you live on the west coast, except for the summer months much of your training will be done in some form of garb which covers your legs and upper body. Therefore, a commercial sweat suit is probably the most convenient. My personal preference is for one which is made from a mixture of nylon and cotton, since this absorbs the sweat much better than a pure nylon suit. *Running shorts and T-shirt* are essential, but hardly represent a strain on the budget. While some runners like to run without *socks*, the majority prefer a light cotton pair in order to prevent blisters.

So you see, you don't require a mass of paraphernalia to embark on your training program, which means that if you are the sort of person who derives your greatest enjoyment from spending $300 or $400 on equipment for your latest whim, you should seek some more fashionable and likely less beneficial form of activity. You will never be able to blame jogging for that bank overdraft!

Over-training

Training is achieved by overloading the body to the point where it has to work just a little harder to accomplish a given task. Measured doses of stress are applied, regularly and over a prolonged period, so that eventually resistance to that stress develops. The art of scientific training is to apply just enough overload, or stress, to achieve the desired result but not so much that the organism is overstrained and breaks down. Over-training, or staleness as it is usually referred to by track coaches, is characterized by chronic fatigue, irritability, susceptibility to minor infections such as colds and boils, insomnia, loss of appetite, lack of concentration, and decline in inclination and ability to train. The competitive athlete who is suffering from staleness may force himself to continue training but his performance steadily declines despite all his efforts. The ultimate answer is to rest for one or two weeks, and give the body time to recuperate. This is dealt with more fully in Chapter 10 under the heading "Build-up *versus* Breakdown."

While such an exaggerated state of affairs is unlikely to occur in the post-coronary jogger, nevertheless it is even more important in his case that he recognize the signs and symptoms of over-training, since his condition demands that there be a finer margin of error in the training process. Be alert, therefore, for such signs as excessive muscle soreness, an increase in your resting pulse rate, undue tiredness persisting to the next training session, premature ventricular beats or palpitations, increasing angina, marked breathlessness, or light-headedness during exercise. These four last symptoms are evidence of myocardial ischemia, and their consistent presence during exercise suggests that the coronary blood flow is not keeping pace with the other training responses. Their presence contra-indicates progression to the next training level. Indeed, if they appear for the first time or become more frequent in response to an exercise prescription, you should reduce your prescription to the next lowest level.

Having said this, I should also add the rider that almost all post-coronary patients experience exercise-induced angina or irregularity of heart action at some time or other in their program. How much to permit becomes a matter of fine judgment based on experience, and if you are not enrolled in a regular cardiac exercise class, then you should consult your physician on this matter.

Before blaming the prescription entirely for an increase in symptoms, you should consider whether or not you are under unusual business stress or are working prolonged hours. The typical post-coronary exerciser is usually enthusiastic and con-scientious, and he often tries to maintain the prescribed level of exercise even during busy spells at his job. The result is that when he is at work he worries that he won't have time to carry out his exercise prescription, while during his workout he is worrying that the time spent in training could have been spent at work. I have learned to beware of various occupations at certain times of the year: for instance, accountants towards the end of the financial year, and departmental store workers during the Christmas season. At these times of stress, an exercise pre-scription which under normal circumstances is carried out easily and without symptoms may give rise to angina at the end of a long and worrisome day. The obvious solution is to cut back the exercise prescription until the work pattern returns to normal.

What if the high stress pattern of employment looks like becoming permanent? The answer again may be to reduce the level of training. But, in the long run, it may be better to take a serious look at the job itself and your attitude towards it. Are you giving to your job more than your employer expects? Are you trying to carry out a job for which you lack the necessary aptitude? An honest answer to these questions may be very self-revealing.

Perhaps you should also re-examine your sleep habits. Chronic lack of sleep seems to be a feature of modern urban living. The long journey home from the office to the suburbs usually means a late evening meal, often followed by watching television until the early hours of the morning (have you noticed how late all the best shows start?). The occasional late night is inevitable, but don't make a habit of it and expect to reap the benefits of training. And don't assume the running program is making you feel overly tired when you haven't bothered to adjust your sleep pattern so as to allow for your additional energy expenditure.

From time to time, one of our joggers who has developed a relatively high level of fitness may experience premature ventricular beats on exertion. These are probably due to the high vagal tone which accompanies a training bradycardia, and usually clear up completely after seven to ten days' rest from training. In such cases, irregular beats do not have serious significance, and I find they occur even in fit long distance runners who are free from heart disease. However, this does not apply to the post-coronary exerciser who develops ectopic beats in response to activity in the early stages of training, and before he has had the opportunity to become truly fit. In these circumstances, they should be taken more seriously.

In the initial stages of the exercise program, it is almost inevitable that you will develop painful ankles and knees, Achilles tendonitis or inflammation of your heel cord, sore feet, and other relatively minor muscle tendon and ligamentous injuries that follow walking and jogging after years of inactivity. While not serious, they are a nuisance and can have an adverse effect on your motivation. A careful warm-up as described below can help but, once again, if the problem persists throughout a complete workout, or is felt between workouts, then a complete rest is indicated. Usually a week is sufficient, but if the trouble recurs on returning to exercise at the end of that time, then you should see your physician who will probably prescribe a course of physiotherapy. Close adherence to the tables, as well as the technique of jogging previously described, will reduce such injuries to a minimum. Remember also that dehydration from jogging in very hot weather can contribute to minor muscle tears, so drink plenty of fluids as advised. Our program's incidence of injuries over the years has been negligible, despite the fact that we are dealing entirely with the middle-aged sedentary individual who hasn't exercised for years.

A pleasant feeling of physical relaxation and tiredness should follow a suitable workout. In many cases, there is an immediate post-exercise sense of exhilaration (for this reason, some people prefer to workout in the morning or early evening rather than just prior to going to bed). Excessive fatigue may be defined as tiredness which is still present after a good night's sleep. It is usually accompanied by muscle soreness and pain and is a sure indicator of over-training. It may not be apparent after one or two exercise sessions, but the build-up from three or four sessions on consecutive days will make it obvious.

Usually after a workout, the pulse returns to its resting level within two hours; this may take a little longer on a hot and humid day. However, a fast heart rate (tachycardia) that persists for four hours or longer suggests that the workout has been too intense.

If you ever find that you are dreading your next workout, then this is a sure sign of over-training. A fit individual usually looks forward to the workout either as a relief from work-a-day tensions or out of sheer animal spirits. In the early stages of the program, you may not be quite this enthusiastic, but you shouldn't actively dislike the thought of training. If you do, then the exercise prescription is too ambitious and should be reduced.

Excessive irritability is not a symptom to treat lightly. In our experience, it may even herald another heart attack. Your wife may be the first to notice it, and it may be so marked that she takes the trouble to mention it to your family doctor. She may comment that you are "becoming impossible to live with again," thereby implying that you are beginning to act similarly to the way you did before your initial heart attack. In a situation like this, it is essential that you look at your overall work and domestic situation in order to find and, if possible, minimize the cause of stress. In any event, your level of exercise should be cut drastically until the problem is corrected. If you are compulsive, you may resent this; but I am insistent with my patients that the exercise be reduced until at least I and the cardiologist have had a chance to assess the overall situation.

For those who are hooked on exercise, and are jogging five or six miles in an hour, the recognition of over-training may be difficult. The explanation for this may lie in Dr. Hans Selye's famous theory of stress. The application of mild and healthful stress produces both a feeling of elation and euphoria which may last for some hours, and also a change in the body's mechanism which makes it more resistant to that particular form of stress. However, if the stress, or training stimulus, is continued to excessive levels, then specific resistance develops at the cost of generalized resistance; in other words, the highly trained runner becomes extremely resistant to the fatigue of running, but less and less resistant to concurrent infections or mental stress. This may well be the explanation for the high susceptibility of world-class athletes to food poisoning, dysentery, and even such disease as poliomyelitis. In any event, while the loss of generalized resistance may be obvious to the trained observer such as the physician or the coach, it is often hidden from the athlete by the short-lived sense of well-being which follows each training session. Thus, he may be losing weight, becoming more irritable, and developing many of the other symptoms described above; but each time he works out he feels great for two or three hours and so falls into the trap of repeating the training sessions in the hope that his overall condition will improve.

If you Suffer from Angina

If you suffer chest pain on exertion, then you should slow your pace until it goes away. If this does not work, then stop, and wait for it to disappear. As soon as this happens, start to walk again at a pace slow enough to prevent it recurring. Some individuals can "walk through" their angina, but I caution against this in the early stages of the program until you have become thoroughly familiar with your exercise response.

Use of Nitroglycerin On occasions, you may have to take a tablet of glyceryl trinitrate or some similar medication during the workout in order to remove the pain. An alternative is to take the medication ten minutes or so before your training session. I am frequently asked if this in some way reduces the effectiveness of the training. The answer is no. The fact that it enables you to complete your exercise session is, in itself, proof of its value. As you become more fit, you will find that the angina occurs less and less frequently, until eventually you are able to carry out a full workout without the necessity of medication. While on the subject of glyceryl trinitrate tablets, I should correct a common misapprehension. Your heart does not become accustomed to them, neither does their frequent use in any way aggravate your condition; in point of fact, they should be taken as often as required. It is surprising how many patients are reluctant to seek relief from nitroglycerin because of some imagined ill effect.

Warm-ups   Angina often occurs during the early part of the workout, and can frequently be obviated by practising a warm-up. This means spending five to ten minutes walking at a pace slower than the prescribed intensity, or performing a series of light flexibility calisthenics until your body breaks out into a light sweat. As soon as the sweat appears, you are then warmed up and may commence your prescription. This is very important for angina sufferers, and frequently works just as well as a nitroglycerin tablet. If your prescription is still at a low level, then you can enhance your warm-up at even slower speeds by wearing a sweater under your track suit in order to accelerate the stage of perspiration.

Exercise after Meals   Exercise should never be carried out within two hours of eating a heavy meal. This is particularly important for angina sufferers, since the digestion of food requires an extra supply of blood to the intestines, thus depleting the coronary circulation. In a situation where the coronary arteries are already narrowed, the loss of even a small reservoir of blood in this area can give rise to myocardial ischemia.

If you are an early morning runner and don't like running on an empty stomach then by all means have a roll, cup of coffee, or glass of orange juice before sallying forth; but don't try to trundle through the streets topped up with bacon and eggs, or corned beef hash.

A Flat Course   Hill running may be great training for competitive athletes, but it should be avoided by those with heart disease. It will certainly aggravate a tendency to angina, since the energy expended in running up a slope is a great deal more than that required to cover the same distance at the same pace on the flat. Consequently, all of the distances listed in the tables are assumed to be on a flat course. A slight gradient is permissible provided it is relatively short and is compensated for by an equal length of downhill course. Ideally, however, all of your workouts should be on the flat. If hills are unavoidable, then reduce your speed accordingly.

Effects of Weather   Some patients are particularly bothered by angina in the cold weather. We are not sure why this is so, but there are two current medical theories. One is that the cold air irritates the large air passages in the lungs, and causes a reflex spasm or narrowing of the coronary arteries; if the calibre of these vessels is already reduced as a result of atherosclerosis, then the additional narrowing may result in critical shortage of blood supply to the myocardium, and thus ischemic chest pain. The provision of a simple cold weather face mask (see p.215 which "pre-heats" the inspired air works successfully in the majority of patients.

The second theory is that exposure to intense cold causes a marked rise in blood pressure, and this adds to the cardiac workload; the oxygen requirements of the myocardium increase and, in individuals in whom the coronary circulation is already compromised, this leads to ischemia and angina pectoris. If this is indeed the mechanism, then it provides an explanation for those patients who find that their tolerance to cold increases as they get fitter, for since training reduces blood pressure and myocardial oxygen consumption both at rest and at exercise, it would tend to counter these tendencies in cold weather. From a practical point of view, however, and for those who are in the early stages of training, I advise the use of the jogging mask, and the taking of glyceryl trinitrate before the workout.

Interval Training   Assuming that your angina is so severe that you find it impossible to walk or jog continuously for the time prescribed, don't despair; there is another method you can use for training which I have found to be very effective. This is known as interval training; in its modified form, it consists of brisk walking for 15 to 30 seconds at a pace just below that which brings on the chest discomfort. Walk casually for a further minute, and then repeat the brisk walk for another 15 to 30 seconds. In this way, cover a mile, always staying below the level of effort which brings on the pain. You will eventually find that you can extend the distance to two or three miles in this way, with only infrequent episodes of discomfort.

Warming-Down

"Warming-down" is equally as important as warming-up for the heart patient. It is dangerous to stop exercising suddenly, because blood tends to pool in the legs, with the result that there is insufficient return to the heart. This causes a precipitate drop in the pumping force, and the coronary circulation is adversely affected. So, spend 5 or 10 minutes winding down after your exercise session, moving around and gradually letting your body return to its resting level. Many so-called "exercise deaths" occur after the exercise session is over and when the individual has returned to the locker room. It could well be that lack of a warm-down was a contributing factor in these cases.

While on this topic, a caution should be sounded against having hot showers immediately after a workout. This can be potentially dangerous, since the heat of the shower dilates the blood vessels in the skin, reducing the flow through the coronary circulation. This, following on an exercise session, may prove too much for the individual with coronary artery disease, and may lead to complications. So I advise all patients to wait 10 or 15 minutes after exercising before taking a lukewarm shower.

Smoking

We have seen earlier that cigarette smoking seems to be associated with a high incidence of sudden death, and my personal experience confirms this. Although the number of fatal recurrences in our exercise group over the past seven years has been very low, the majority of these have been heavy smokers.

Smoking and exercise do not mix. The plain facts of the matter are that the smoke you inhale from your cigarette, cigar or pipe contains small amounts of carbon monoxide. Not only is this a poison, it is a very selective poison. It displaces oxygen from the hemoglobin molecule in your red cells, and so immediately reduces the effectiveness of your oxygen transport system. Furthermore, traces of the drug nicotine in tobacco smoke, by releasing the stress hormone nor-epinephrine into the blood stream, cause the blood pressure and heart rate to increase and the small blood vessels in the skin to constrict, thus making the heart muscle work harder than it needs to.

So if you smoke, you are defeating the whole purpose of endurance training. No matter how efficient your heart may become in pumping blood around the body, no matter how effectively your muscles learn to extract oxygen from the blood, it is all pointless if the blood is unable to carry its full quota of oxygen. Some authorities go so far as to say that for the smoker to undertake an endurance training program is a complete waste of time. While I would not subscribe completely to that statement, I do feel that the smoker has to devote a good deal more time in training to achieve the same effect. Three of his workouts are probably equivalent to one of the non-smoker's in terms of fitness payoff.

Before leaving this subject, I should draw your attention to the obvious fact that carbon monoxide is carbon monoxide, whether you inhale it from your own cigarette or somebody else's. Non-smokers who breathe the smoky atmosphere of night clubs, or share an enclosed space such as a car with a smoker, probably have high blood levels of carbon monoxide. The moral? If you stop smoking, try to persuade your relatives and friends to do likewise.

Medication

Certain medications which are used in the treatment of coronary artery disease cause a drop in the heart rate, both at rest and during exercise. Currently, the most commonly used are those belonging to the group known as Beta-blockers. They act by blocking the nervous stimulus to acceleration, and so reduce the work of the heart. For this reason, they may be very valuable in the treatment of anginal pain. The most commonly prescribed of these substances goes under the trade name of Inderal (Propanolol).

While small doses of Inderal may not affect heart rate, larger doses invariably do so, and this has to be allowed for in the training program. Individuals who are taking Inderal may have resting heart rates in the 50's, with a concomitant reduction at all levels of exertion right up to maximum. Attempts to achieve heart rates, either during exercise testing or workouts, based on age-related tables may be fraught with disaster. For this reason, I place all patients taking Inderal or a similar substance in the complicated category, and use Nomogram B for establishing both training heart rate and progressing heart rate. Even this is not entirely satisfactory, since our method of evaluating a training effect (the development of a training bradycardia), is being influenced by a pharmacological agent rather than by physiological change. Another problem that I have found in attempting to train patients who are taking Inderal is the difficulty of predicting the onset of fatigue; the individual suddenly becomes tired during a workout and then has to stop within a matter of 30 seconds or a minute. As one patient put it, "I find I poop out very quickly and without much warning."

Inderal is cleared fairly rapidly from the body, but this is a drug which should not be stopped suddenly. Recent reports indicate that a gradual reduction in dosage is advisable if untoward effects are to be avoided. Incidentally, this is a point to bear in mind if you are one of those foolhardy individuals (of whom I have come across more than a few) who, without consulting their physician, stop their medication when they are "feeling good."

Another commonly used medication which affects the heart rate is Digitalis. This has been used by physicians for many years, being derived originally from the leaf of the common purple foxglove; its main purpose is to strengthen the heart's action. It differs from the Beta-blockers, however, in that while it may reduce the resting heart rate, in the dosages usually taken it does not appear to have much effect on the working or maximum pulse level. For this reason, it is less of a problem in a fitness program, although allowance must be made for the fact that it can produce a resting bradycardia, and this should not be confused with the effects of training. Digitalis accumulates in the body, and it may take as long as two weeks after its use is discontinued for its effect on the heart rate to disappear — an important factor if the physician stops the drug temporarily for the purpose of checking progress by means of an exercise test. Digitalis can also cause a false depression of the st segment of the electrocardiogram during an exercise test.

Isometric Exercises

Not so long ago, this type of physical activity became very popular as a method of building muscle size and strength. Its proponents reported major gains in these parameters by merely devoting a few minutes a day to isometric muscle contractions. The validity of these claims is not our immediate concern. On the other hand, the role of this type of exertion in the training program of the heart patient is very pertinent. The plain fact of the matter is that isometric exercises are entirely contra-indicated for this group. They are not conducive to endurance fitness, and, even more important, they may have a harmful effect on the damaged heart.

Let me be more specific. An isometric muscle contraction is one in which the muscle contracts without shortening, or shortens only to a minimal degree. For example, the normal action of the biceps muscle in your upper arm when it contracts is to bend your elbow. If maximal contraction is carried out while at the same time flexion of the elbow joint is prevented, then the biceps muscle will not bunch up in the usual manner of "making a muscle"; you have achieved an isometric contraction of your biceps. Examples of isometric effort in everyday life are straining to raise a jammed window, or trying to lift a suitcase which is too heavy for you, or attempting to push an automobile which is stuck in the snow. This type of muscle action, as opposed to the "isotonic" movement in which the joint is allowed to move and the muscle to shorten, causes a precipitant rise in the diastolic blood pressure and a marked increase in the pressures within the chambers of the heart. If the heart wall is scarred from a previous heart attack, and if the coronary blood circulation is impaired as a result of atherosclerosis, then the results of such pressure increases can be dangerous. Lifting of heavy weights is, for this reason, prohibited as a training endeavour or a recreational sport. Straining to lift heavier and heavier loads may well build the body beautiful, but the isometric element involved makes it an avocation suitable only for those with the healthiest of cardiovascular systems.

A sad case reported by Dr. Bruce of Seattle may underline my point even more emphatically. A patient of his on a post-coronary exercise program seemed to be doing quite well, but then sustained a second and fatal heart attack while water skiing. The likely cause of death, in the opinion of Dr. Bruce and his colleague Dr. Pyffer, was the deleterious change in cardiac pressures brought about by the intense isometric action of gripping the tow bar.

Another example of the adverse cardiovascular effects of an isometric effort is found in Lord Moran's book on Sir Winston Churchill:

> Washington, December 27. "I am glad you have come," the P.M. began. He was in bed and looked worried. "It was hot last night, and I got up to open the window. It was very

stiff. I had to use considerable force and I noticed all at once I was short of breath. I had a dull pain over my heart. It went down my left arm. It did not last very long, but it has never happened before. What is it? Is my heart all right? I thought of sending for you, but it passed off."

Sir Winston was obviously an astute observer of clinical symptoms. He was describing typical angina pectoris as a result of excessive load on his heart and coronary vasculature. He was lucky not to have had a heart attack; in which event, the course of world history might have been radically altered by an isometric muscle contraction.

Certain types of power calisthenics contain an isometric-like component and are to be avoided. Among the most popular of these are "push ups" and "chinning the bar," proficiency in both of which seems to be a measure of fitness, if not masculinity, in the North American male. An additional problem with these, and indeed all isometric exercises, is that the uninitiated tend to hold their breath while carrying them out. While this may seem to enhance performance in terms of power of lift or number of repetitions, it introduces another element of danger for the person with heart problems. A not uncommon sight in any gymnasium is an exerciser slowly going blue in the face as he attempts to strain himself to the limit. This is due to the fact that in holding his breath, he has closed off his windpipe, and in the course of his exercise is forcing the air in his lungs against the closed valve. This state of affairs is referred to in physiological circles as the "Valsalva manoeuvre." Its effect, like that of the isometric muscle contraction, is to throw a heavy burden on a heart already severely taxed by the particular exercise which is being carried out. Hence power calisthenics, or any physical activity which encourages the Valsalva manoeuvre, is off limits for the individual at risk.

Does this mean that you must go about your daily activities in constant fear of holding your breath or inadvertently carrying out an isometric muscle contraction? Of course not. As a matter of fact, the more endurance fitness you develop, the stronger your heart will get and the more it will be able to resist such stresses and strains. My point is that you should be aware of the dangers of these types of exertions, should not practise them on a regular basis, and certainly should not include them as part of your training program.

The Use of Saunas and Steam Baths

Many people derive a sense of physical and mental well-being from the regular use of a steam bath. In recent years, the North American continent has seen a great rise in the popularity of the sauna, with the result that a significant number of high-rise apartments and even private dwellings now contain this facility. Consequently, I am frequently asked by the post-coronary patient if exposure to such extremes of heat is permissible on safety grounds. My interpretation of the limited number of studies which have been carried out on the effect of exposure to the heat of the sauna or steam bath on those with cardiovascular disease suggests a cautious approach.

Both normal and post-coronary patients have been found to develop electrocardiographic evidence of myocardial ischemia while in the sauna; these changes took the form of ST segment depression and frequent ectopic beats. They did not occur to anything like the same extent when these same subjects were exercised to an increased heart rate level equivalent to that attained in the bath. The reason for this seems to be that excessive heat, like emotional stress, releases into the blood stream a type of hormone which may have adverse affects on the myocardium. Potentially dangerous falls in blood pressure have been reported (especially when the subject is in the sitting position) with resultant decrease in coronary blood flow.

As a result of these potential hazards, one investigator has suggested that the middle-aged subject, and especially the sufferer from coronary artery disease, seek the cooler type of bath (temperature range 60°F. to 70°F.), or limit his stay in higher temperatures to five minutes; adopt the customary Finnish posture of lying down rather than our more usual one of sitting up, thus improving coronary blood flow; does not use the steam bath to "sweat out" symptoms which might well be the early portents of coronary artery disease (for example, "muscular" chest pain, excessive fatigue, "bursitis" in the shoulder); and, above all, does not, out of a false sense of pride, attempt to "tough it out with the fellows" if he feels himself getting dizzy, breathless, or developing an unpleasant thumping of his heart.

Sticking with the Prescription

Do not be overly ambitious. The coronary-prone individual is apt to over-estimate his capabilities and push himself to the limit.

Not infrequently, he works on the principle that if something is good for you, more of it is even better. Apply this dictum to a medication, and you may pay with your life.

Exercise training in the presence of heart disease is no less critical a prescription. I am constantly having to warn individuals about trying to go too fast. The lengths to which people will go to avoid this advice is a never-ending source of amazement to me. Intelligence and education have nothing whatsoever to do with it; the most unlikely subject, often one who should know better, will attempt to break through the tables and achieve a personal best every time he works out. Witness the remark of a well-known cardiologist who has himself had by-pass surgery for coronary artery disease, attends the program regularly, and is in every other way a model patient. His exercise diaries showed an increasing escalation of his three-mile pace, and when asked for the reason replied: "I thought the whole point of training was to push yourself at each session." While this may be justified in training Olympic athletes (although Oregon's Bill Bowerman alternates heavy and light training sessions with his highly successful track men), it hardly makes sense for the middle-aged heart patient. Adherence to the tables and the method of progression will, in almost every case, assure safety, as well as a desirable training effect.

A Beneficial Addiction

Anyone who exercises regularly will tell you that they experience a feeling of exhilaration after each session — or, to put it in the modern venacular, a "high." By the same token a layoff, even for a few days, will often result in a "downer," with symptoms of depression, anxiety or irritability. The more regular and intensive the training program the more marked the reaction to layoffs.

This urge to continue training is often so powerful that from time to time it will override common sense and lead the individual to persist in running throughout a period of heavy business or social commitments, or despite musculoskeletal injuries or attacks of flu which would obviously respond better to rest than physical activity. Small wonder that the sedentary onlooker refers so scathingly to the "fitness nut."

For many years I have recognized this compulsion to train in young athletes, and now I find it to be just as evident in the middle-aged jogger. It has all the hallmarks of a true addiction.

But, you say, isn't that a bad thing? Not really. Provided you are aware of the compulsion and can leaven enthusiasm with common sense, then addiction to physical activity can be desirable.

How can this be explained? Well, a pair of medical researchers, Doctor Malcolm Carruthers and Doctor Peter Taggart, both of London, England, have put forward a fascinating explanation based on their own experimental work. They explain that stress situations such as rock climbing, parachute jumping, public speaking, acting, racing driving, et cetera are accompanied by emotional stress, the main components of which are anxiety, aggression and even aversion. These reactions cause the adrenal glands (two small bean-sized organs which lie above the kidneys), to release into the blood stream two similar stress hormones called epinephrine and nor-epinephrine. Both substances, in high concentration, lead to a rise in blood pressure, an increase in blood sugar, and an elevation of blood cholesterol.

None of these changes are particularly desirable in the unfit sedentary individual, especially if he has heart disease. However, epinephrine and nor-epinephrine have a side effect which makes them attractive to the human body; they stimulate the pleasure centres in that primitive part of the brain known as the hypothalamus, possibly by liberating a substance recently discovered and known as endorphin. This substance is apparently released from brain cells when the body is subjected to physical or psychic stress. In small amounts, its effect is to give rise to a mood of satisfaction and pleasure. However, when given in greater quantities, it "freezes" both mind and muscle producing a state of stupor and muscle rigidity very similar to that found in the mental disease schizophrenia. Could it be that a "natural" amount of stress ("natural" in the primitive sense of the word) such as occurs when the body is exercised, results in the correct amount of endorphin being released and thus producing amongst other things, a pleasurable mood, or "high"? Which explains why the racing driver, the rock climber, or the actor all derive enjoyment from constantly recreating tense and anxious situations for themselves. Vigorous physical activity, such as jogging, releases the same substances and therefore results in the same desire to recreate the pleasurable stimulation. However — and this is the crucial point — vigorous sustained exercise does not bring about the same consistent rise in blood sugar or blood cholesterol which is associated with the more sedentary thrills. This is because it causes the body to burn sugar and fat as fuels. Here, then is one beneficial addiction in which you can indulge yourself with safety!

Concurrent Infections

You are now aware that a number of viral-type infections can involve the heart muscle. The effect may be transitory, lasting only a matter of days or weeks. It may pass unnoticed by the patient, and leave no permanent damage. However, strenuous physical activity should be avoided during this time. Although severe viral myocarditis is relatively rare, mild forms of the condition may exist much more frequently than we suspect. Since a visit to the cardiologist is hardly justified every time you develop a fever, we work on the rule that it is better to be safe than sorry, and advise against carrying out the exercise prescription if you are suffering from any flu-like illness. To be further on the safe side, you should not work out until a full seven days have elapsed after your temperature has returned to normal.

Some time ago, a patient on our post-coronary exercise program collapsed while running on a community indoor track. Facilities for resuscitation were not available, and he was dead on arrival at hospital. An autopsy was not carried out, but it is probably safe to assume that he had sustained a further heart attack. His case was unique in that he was the first patient to suffer a myocardial infarction, fatal or non-fatal, during exercise, since the program started in 1968.

Naturally enough, I enquired carefully into the circumstances of his death, hoping to learn something which would be of benefit to the rest of the group. The salient features which emerged were as follows. In his 40's, he had always been hard-working and ambitious, with a high sense of responsibility. For six months or so prior to his death, he had been working on a special project in his job. This required him to put in many hours of overtime. Despite this, he had made no concession to his training program, putting in five workouts a week in spite of the fact that he must have been feeling overly tired. He then developed flu. He didn't seem to be able to shake this, and it dragged on for two or three weeks. Again, he refused to cut back on his running, despite advice to the contrary by his colleagues on the exercise program who, like him, had been frequently admonished on this point.

Finally, it emerged that he had been exceeding his exercise prescription, and running at a pace a good deal faster than he was required to.

None of these facts appeared on his exercise log. There is no proof that any or all of these factors contributed in any way to this individual's death. It may well be that his second and fatal attack would have occurred in any event, and irrespective of whether he was running, sitting at his desk, or watching television. And yet, one cannot help but wonder whether, had he adhered to the precautions outlined in this chapter, the outcome might have been different. The point to bear in mind is that all of the above advice is based on practical experience in the training of many post-coronary patients. The rules have been formulated in response to their reactions, both adverse and favourable, to the exercise regime.

How Much Do You Weigh?

While obesity is less suspect than was previously thought as a risk factor in heart disease, it should still be considered an additional hazard for the post-coronary patient. Excess fatty tissue means excess work for the heart. Not only that, but overweight is consistently associated with a higher mortality from diabetes, hypertension, strokes, chest infections, digestive problems, kidney disease, and accidents. With a heart problem already, who needs the rest?

Body weight doesn't necessarily give a true measure of the amount of fatty tissue a person possesses. A heavy-boned or well-muscled individual may well be heavier than his slight-built counterpart, and yet not be obese. For practical purposes, however, and in our present-day affluent society, excess weight invariably means excess fat. There are a number of methods of estimating your percentage of body fat. One of the most accurate is under-water weighing, a laboratory procedure which has little practical application for the man on the street. However, you can obtain a reasonable estimate of your fat layer by pinching up the skin and fat over your abdomen an inch or so below your navel and parallel to the skin creases. Ideally, the distance between your finger and thumb should no more than half an inch. The fat fold over the back of the upper arm, half way between the tip of your shoulder and the tip of your elbow is more convenient to measure; this should be no more than 1 inch (1^1/$_2$ inches in females). In the laboratory, these assessments are carried out using special skin calipers and taking the average of eight skin folds, but such refinements are unnecessary for most purposes. Another way of estimating your obesity factor is to use the Ponderal Index. Divide your height in inches by the cube root of your weight (in lbs.). Here are some cube roots, to save you frantically searching for your calculator:

100 – 4.64	125 – 5.00	150 – 5.31	175 – 5.59
105 – 4.72	130 – 5.07	155 – 5.37	180 – 5.65
110 – 4.79	135 – 5.13	160 – 5.43	185 – 5.70
115 – 4.86	140 – 5.19	165 – 5.49	190 – 5.75
120 – 4.93	145 – 5.25	170 – 5.54	195 – 5.80

For example, if you are 5'8" tall and weigh 160 lbs., then you obtain your Ponderal Index by dividing the cube root of 160, (i.e., 5.43) into 68, or your height in inches, to give 12.5. The lower the index, the higher your amount of body fat. If it comes to less than 12.2, then your percentage body fat is over 30 per cent and you should start reducing.

It is customary in our society to assume that as one gets older, one "puts on a little weight." Mothers and wives, through generations of teaching, are made to feel that their sons and husbands should have a well-fed and plump appearance. The middle-aged Englishman of the eighteenth century was considered both handsome and dignified only if he were portly — all very well when leanness was a mark of poverty and malnutrition, but hardly applicable to our twentieth-century well-fed Western world. There is no earthly reason why anyone should weigh more at 45 than he did at 21. Competitive long distance runners, hardly an unhealthy breed, frequently have a body fat of less than 10 per cent. Ideal weights are hard to define. One rough calculation is to double your height in inches and add 10 per cent of the sum. A much more scientific approach has been taken by the American Society of Actuaries who studied the mortality rates of half a million insured individuals over the period from 1935 to 1954. The inference to be drawn from their data was that if you are of medium build, then the closer your weight is to the table on page 210, the more likely you are to achieve a normal lifespan.

If you do need to reduce, you should use a combination of dietary restriction and exercise. I do not intend to deal with the subject of diet, since this book is primarily concerned with exercise training. However, I have included some comments under a later section on Long Distance Running on p. 182 which I think are pertinent.

Alcohol Intake and Exercise

There is much uncertainty in the minds of the public about the effects of alcohol on the heart. Many can remember when the physician prescribed a daily ration of brandy or whisky for the post-coronary patient on the premise that it was a cardiac stimulant and dilated the coronary vessels. There is little to condone that practice today. On the contrary, recent evidence indicates that alcohol depresses heart function by decreasing the contractile force, or pump efficiency, of the myocardium, especially when it is the seat of ischemic changes or scarring from coronary artery disease. The amount of alcohol needed to cause this adverse effect in heart patients is quite small: in one study, just two ounces of Canadian whisky. There is also agreement among the experts that the heart muscle cells may suffer permanent damage from prolonged alcohol consumption, leading to the condition of alcoholic cardiomyopathy. Another practical consideration is the one of body weight; alcoholic beverages are high in caloric value, so you can scarcely expect to lose weight on a diet of cottage cheese, lettuce and double martinis!

For all of the above reasons, you should consider carefully whether or not to consume alcohol. If you have serious cardiac problems, you'd be better off on the wagon. Chances are, however, that if you are capable of exercising, you're capable of drinking, but in moderation — no more than a shot of liquor daily ($1^1/_2$ - 2 ounces) or two bottles of beer, or a glass of wine.

Just as you shouldn't drink and drive, so you should never drink before jogging, especially if you suffer from heart disease. Not only is your heart less likely to be able to cope with the additional stress, but your judgment of pace and distance is probably impaired, as is your ability to count your pulse and interpret such warning signs as angina or light-headedness. If you must drink, then do so in moderation, and *after* your workout.

Physical Conditions

Don't underestimate the effect of running into a head-wind. It has been shown that an athlete weighing 134 lb. and running at a 6-minute mile pace on a still day expends approximately 6 per cent more oxygen in the face of a light, 10 m.p.h. wind; to put it another way, he will have to put out the effort of a sub-5-minute mile pace! A 40 m.p.h. wind jacks the oxygen cost up by over 40 per cent. When you are talking oxygen increments of that order, you may be getting into a situation which is beyond your maximum oxygen consumption. Of course, I realize that you wouldn't deliberately set out to jog into steady gale force winds, but you can sometimes misjudge the wind force when the conditions are gusty. The trick is to back off if you notice yourself getting unusually breathless and tired on a windy day. Allowing for the wind resistance, the slower time will be giving you the same training effect anyway.

The best surface to run on is a smooth one. The hardness or softness doesn't really matter; your shoes should take care of that factor. An uneven surface increases the effort of running considerably, driving up your oxygen consumption and heart rate accordingly, and sometimes giving rise to anginal pain which would otherwise not occur. Some athletes feel that it is easier to run on a grass surface, and will seek one out if they are trying to nurse a leg injury. In my experience, this only makes matters worse, since beneath the deceptive green covering, the underlying ground is often rutted and uneven, making each stride a hazard and increasing the stress on tendons and ligaments. If possible, then, do your training on the road or on a track with a good surface.

Participation in Other Sporting Activities

When can I play tennis? What about golf? Is badminton okay? How about swimming? These and other similar questions are asked of me constantly by post-coronary patients who are on the exercise program. I try to answer each one individually, taking into account the patient's state of training, age, severity of heart attack, and presence or absence of symptoms. If you are working out in accordance with the training tables in this book, then you can use your achievement of the various levels as a rough guide to your ability to participate safely in a number of recreational physical activities (see table on page 296).

While some of these recreational physical activities may be more enjoyable than jogging, they are harder to quantify in terms of energy expenditure and cardiac work. If you are good at a game, then you will perform it with greater skill, or to put it physiologically, with a higher degree of mechanical efficiency. Thus your oxygen consumption will be lower throughout the game than if you were a less proficient player. A poor swimmer will expend more effort threshing across the pool than his skilled counterpart will in an apparently lazy workout covering two or three miles. The squash player with twenty years' experience will finish a game hardly perspiring, while his sweating novice opponent may have just had the match of his life.

Actually, this is a problem with skill games, as a recent physician-patient of mine discovered to his cost. He had played squash for over twenty-five years and was so good that his daily workouts at the Y over the past five or six years had given him little if any training effect. The result was that when he was fitness tested, he scored no better than the average sedentary male of the same age.

Other variables in recreational sports include difficulty in pacing oneself, the effect of emotion and excitement, as well as extraneous factors peculiar to the game itself — as for example, the isometric component involved in gripping the golf club or the ski-tow bar, or the late nights (and possibly the hip-flask conviviality) associated with club curling.

CHAPTER SEVEN

Fads, Facts and Fallacies

OVER the years I have developed the habit of holding 15- or 20-minute informal chats before each exercise session, answering patients' questions and discussing the implications of recent studies and experiments on heart disease, fitness and related subjects.

The following are some of the topics most commonly brought up in these sessions. I hope they will clarify a few of your own problems, or even correct some of the half-truths, fallacies and prejudices with which the exercising heart patient is surrounded.

Sexual Activity after Myocardial Infarction

In a recent survey of 160 of our post-coronary patients, it was found that precisely half reported a reduction of sexual activity since their heart attacks. The main reason given was a fall-off in desire. A smaller number said that they were frightened of suffering another heart attack during intercourse, and a few actually reported adverse symptoms such as palpitations or angina pectoris during the sexual act.

The individual who becomes apathetic towards sex after his attack frequently shows high levels of depression and anxiety. He has lost some confidence in his masculinity and doubts his ability to function again in his role as head of the family. His reluctance to seek full satisfaction in sexual relations is perfectly understandable under these circumstances. As his confidence returns (and this often occurs with increasing physical fitness), the situation usually rights itself.

But what of the individual who is frightened of sexual intercourse because of its possible ill effects on his heart? Is there any justification for his fears? Should he adopt special precautions during the sex act, and if so, what should they be? How long after his heart attack should he wait before resuming a normal marital relationship?

The answers to these questions may have been provided by your cardiologist, but I find that many of the patients referred for rehabilitation have not been so lucky. Beyond being told that they should "wait about a month" before resuming sex, they have been given little guidance in this area. The reason is not hard to find. There has been minimal research carried out into the effects of coitus on the damaged heart, and medical literature contains little on the subject. It is for this reason that we are now carrying out studies on this aspect in order to add to our knowledge in this important but neglected field.

The sex act results in cardiovascular responses very similar to those induced by exercise. There is a rise in heart rate and blood pressure, as well as an increase in rate of breathing. So far, the most detailed study of these responses has been carried out by Dr. Hellerstein of Cleveland, Ohio, a leading figure in post-coronary exercise rehabilitation. In summary, he found that the cardiac cost of intercourse was modest, with increases in heart rate about the same as that observed in climbing a few flights of stairs, or walking briskly around the block. As a matter of fact, much higher heart rates may occur during angry discussions at work! ECG monitoring of fourteen subjects during the sexual act showed that a small number developed changes compatible with cardiac ischemia (ST segment depression and ectopic beats), but these particular individuals experienced similar adverse signs during their usual occupational activities; in other words, coitus did not have a disproportionately higher stress effect.

Hellerstein's conclusions were that the vast majority of post-coronary patients can safely indulge in sexual activity without fear of excessive cardiovascular strain. Most of the subjects in his study were average middle-aged, middle-class individuals who had been married for a number of years. There are grounds for believing that intercourse with a younger or less familiar partner may lead to more profound physiological changes, with much higher increments of heart rate and blood pressure and so greater cardiac stress. Extra-marital intercourse may well provide these ingredients, and since it may also be accompanied by a bout of excessive food and alcohol intake, might well be dangerous. It is probably in these circumstances that the occasional coital death occurs — a death dramatic enough to become more colourful in the retelling, and so needlessly frighten the more conservative, "non-swinging" members of society!

Are there then any precautions to be taken after a heart attack? Sufficient time should be allowed for the infarction scar to form before indulging in intercourse. This means at least six weeks after the attack, and probably eight weeks to be on the safe side. If you suffer from angina during coitus, then try taking glyceryl trinitrate before commencing the act. Symptoms such as angina or ectopic beats may be relieved by changing your position. In the male-dominant position, much of your body weight has to be supported on your arms; this amounts to isometric exercise, and as previously noted, will lead to a disproportionate increase in blood pressure and cardiac workload. The affect is enhanced if the duration of the act is prolonged. Therefore, if you are bothered by symptoms, you might find it advantageous to try the side-by-side position or the female-dominant.

A proportion of my patients said that while they themselves were not apprehensive about having sex, their wives were unduly anxious. I have corroborated this on many occasions, both by questionnaire and frank discussion of the matter with wives. A fearful partner can put the husband at a disadvantage, and even increase his own doubts and uncertainties. In a situation like this, a knowledgeable family physician can be of great help.

To sum up, then, you are ready for sexual intercourse as soon as you can go for a brisk walk, or climb two flights of stairs without difficulty; this usually means about eight weeks after your heart attack. The chances of intra-marital coitus damaging your heart are remote and the sense of well-being associated with a normal marital relationship far outweigh the mythical dangers. If you suffer symptoms, then try taking glyceryl trinitrate or changing your position. Finally if you find the frequency with which you desire sex is diminished, then for goodness sake, don't panic. Everyone's reaction to an illness is different, and there is no need to develop a complex merely because you don't feel like performing as frequently as you did before your attack.

Depression Following Myocardial Infarction

Our own studies, as well as the work of others, have shown that a significant number of heart attack survivors are extremely depressed as a result of their attacks. Actually, one-third of the group we analyzed demonstrated this finding. Psychological testing and interview showed that, in addition to being depressed, they also have extreme tendencies toward hysteria and hypochondriasis — the so-called "neurotic triad." This state of affairs was only evident after careful evaluation; it was not obvious to the onlooker. As a matter of fact, neither the patient's wife nor his physician had even suspected it. When confronted with the evidence of the psychological assessment, the unhappy individual invariably admitted his melancholy. The tragic thing is the frequency with which he felt that he was unique. A typical remark was, "I envy the other guys. They seem to have accepted the fact that they've had a heart attack, and they never seem to worry about it. So what can I do? I'm scared stiff I'll have another one, but I can't admit it to anyone. So I play along, kibbitzing with the rest, and pretending that life is a big joke."

Despite this facade, the depressed heart patient is very much lacking in confidence. He demonstrates less initiative at work, and is reluctant to make important decisions. He procrastinates, hoping that time will solve his problems. At home, he leaves more and more responsibility to his wife. Often this is in complete contrast to his pre-attack personality. This change was so marked in one patient that his wife, before leaving for a holiday, wrote him a note in which she abjured him to pull himself together, and revert to the strong-minded man she had married who had consistently called the shots for both of them. The trouble is that this is easier said than done. It takes time, a lot of patience and understanding, and sometimes the skill and advice of a professional.

Whether the depression is entirely due to the heart attack, or whether it is part of the patient's personality which has merely been brought to light by the illness is a moot point. There are some who believe that the depression is endogenous, and may indeed be a factor in actually causing the attack. If this is so, then psychotherapy may be advantageous not only in relieving the depression, but possibly in helping to prevent another heart attack. On the other hand, if the condition is entirely exogenous, then it should disappear with time and as general health improves.

In either case, there is little doubt that great benefit can be derived from an exercise rehabilitation program. Fitness improves the quality of life, and brings with it enhanced self-confidence and improvement in morale. Our depressed patients have gained considerably from the exercise program. However, we have learned to take a slightly different approach with our depressed as opposed to our non-depressed patients. The latter have little sense of insecurity; psychological testing reveals that they are abundant in self-confidence. Ambitious, driving, and over-competitive, they deny adverse symptoms and are obsessive in adherence to their exercise workouts. They are constantly matching their performances with those of others and setting themselves harder and harder goals. They are inclined to exceed their exercise prescription and have to be observed carefully in order to see that they do not do too much, or ignore the indications for a reduction in training intensity.

A depressed person is just the opposite. He tends to be overly protective, frightened of exerting himself too much, doubtful of the program's value, pessimistic about his own chances of improvement, and inclined to do less than the prescription calls for. He allows any number of trivial happenings to deflect him from his exercise session, frequently complains of leg muscle stiffness, or vague discomfort in the chest, and constantly seems to be searching for an excuse to drop out. He needs encouragement, reassurance, and a high degree of persuasion to see that he keeps on exercising at a suitable level. He is helped by observing the success of other post-coronary joggers who are obviously doing so well, and if he can just stay with it long enough to start feeling the benefits of fitness, he is well on the road to recovery.

Do you recognize yourself as belonging to either of these two groups? Whichever group you identify with, there is plenty to read, digest, and benefit from in these pages.

Dietary Supplements

This is indeed a tangled web, spun by researchers, evangelists and ignoramuses alike. Nevertheless, the subject warrants consideration and so, without fear or favour or more ado, here are some thoughts for your consideration.

Vitamin E Few subjects arouse more passion in medical circles than that dealing with the possible therapeutic value of this substance. The proponents of Vitamin E therapy angrily denounce their antagonists as being short-sighted, and accuse them of deliberately ignoring the evidence of innumerable case histories in which large doses of Vitamin E have been of value in heart disease, leg ulcers, skin infections and a whole host of other conditions. The opposition, however (and that probably includes the bulk of the medical profession), counters with the argument that there is a paucity of controlled clinical trials demonstrating that Vitamin E therapy is of any value, that deficiency states occur only rarely, and that Vitamin E is obtained in sufficient quantities from a normal diet without requiring to be supplemented by further intake. The battle has raged since Evans and Bishop of California discovered the substance, also known as tocopheral, in 1922. Present in large amounts in wheat germ and green leaves, its absence from the diet of laboratory rats was shown to cause sterility and a peculiar condition in which the muscles become swollen and weak.

In this brief section, it would be impossible to discuss all the pros and cons of Vitamin E therapy, and in any event, we are interested only in its real or apparent effects on heart disease.

The current rationale for the use of Vitamin E in the treatment of atherosclerosis is based on the theory that the present epidemic of coronary artery disease is largely due to a deficiency in this vitamin, resulting from our modern diet. The milling and purification of flour and other foodstuffs has led to the elimination of Vitamin E, it is argued, so that we now need to supplement this factor artificially. Among its reputedly beneficial effects are a reduction in the tendency for blood to clot, a dilation of peripheral blood vessels, and a reduction in the oxygen requirements of the tissue cells. Unfortunately, none of these properties has been consistently demonstrated by laboratory trials. In point of fact, the theory that coronary artery disease is due to inadequate amounts of Vitamin E, or indeed any other substance, in modern foodstuffs is still very much that — a theory.

When faced with the question whether or not it is advisable to take for therapeutic purposes a substance which has not as yet received the universal blessing of the medical profession, I am forced to fall back on two questions: Is it safe? And, is it expensive? Certainly, no toxic effects from the use of large doses of Vitamin E have ever been recorded in human beings. There have been occasional reports of side effects in rats, including increased deposition of cholesterol in the large blood vessels. I am told by a good physician friend of mine who prescribes Vitamin E for many conditions, that it should be used with caution in patients with high blood pressure, at least in the initial stages of treatment; and that it is contra-indicated in patients with certain types of valvular disease of the heart.

A recent article in the *Journal of the American Medical Association* has linked high intake of Vitamin E with a drop in the body's Vitamin K content. Vitamin K helps blood to clot, and so it is just conceivable that tocopheral, in destroying Vitamin K, may reduce the likelihood of thrombosis occurring within the coronary arteries. A more immediate implication of this finding, however, is that patients who have been placed on anticoagulant medication ("blood thinner"), after their heart attacks, might well be cautious about taking non-prescribed mega doses of Vitamin E for fear that the cumulative effect will result in excessive bleeding.

With the above proviso, I think we can conclude that Vitamin E is safe; but it is not cheap. However, if you have to cut down your smoking in order to be able to afford a year's supply of Vitamin E capsules, then it is money well spent.

Before leaving this contentious subject, I should make the point that I do not advise any of the patients on my exercise program to take Vitamin E. From questioning them, I know that a small minority do. On the other hand, just for the record, none of the individuals who have taken part in the marathon runs described elsewhere in this book have used Vitamin E as part of their training program.

Vitamin C This substance is essential for the manufacture of collagen, the base substance which acts as a cement for much of the tissue and organs of our bodies. It occurs naturally in citrus fruit such as lemons and limes. James Lind, a physician in the British navy in the eighteenth century, empirically deduced that its absence led to the condition of scurvy. In the days of sail, long sea voyages meant that the crew would go many months without fresh fruit or vegetables. The result was that they frequently became ill with a disease which was characterized by fatigue, bruising of the skin, and a tendency to bleed easily from the gums and mucous membranes. These are the classical symptoms of scurvy, a disease which was the scourge of the British navy for hundreds of years before it was found that the addition of fresh fruit, such as limes, to the diet had a preventative effect. It was this insistance on limes in the British sailor's food store which led to his countrymen being referred to as "Limeys." It was not until 1932 that the specific protective agent in the lime was isolated in the form of Vitamin C; two years later it was first synthesized.

Recently, there has been renewed interest in Vitamin C for a number of reasons. The world-famous scientist and Nobel Prize winner, Dr. Linus Pauling, has advocated the therapeutic use of large doses of Vitamin C to help the body's defence mechanisms against infection. Once again, this subject is obscured by controversy. Time and time again, you will come across the arguments for and against the use of so-called mega-vitamin therapy. Orthodox medical teaching has established minimal daily requirements for all of the vitamins known to man. It has also identified a number of clear-cut and relatively easily identifiable conditions which result if these minimal daily requirements are not met. For those of my readers under the age of 40 who would like to have some first-hand knowledge of the obvious ways in which these conditions can occur, I suggest you talk to some Second World War veterans who were Japanese prisoners-of-war; they will be all too well acquainted with the results of Vitamin B shortage. Scurvy, beri-beri (lack of Vitamin B), rickets (Vitamin D), night blindness (Vitamin A), are all examples of gross deficiency in vitamins. The mega-vitamin advocates, however, maintain that disease entities exist which are less dramatic and obvious in appearance, and are caused by a chronic partial shortage of dietary vitamins. This, they feel, is due to modern methods of food refinement and the addition of artificial food preservatives which tend to destroy the natural vitamin in the food. They aim to correct these conditions by supplementing the diet with large doses of the vitamin in question.

Their arguments are still tenuous, and valid scientific data to prove their point are still lacking. Nevertheless, to be fair, while large numbers of misguided, ill-trained enthusiasts and outright cranks are advocating all sorts of vitamin therapy for a host of conditions, both real and imagined, an increasing number of reputable physicians and scientists are devoting their attention to a careful study of even the most apparently outrageous claims.

The opinion of an individual such as Dr. Linus Pauling cannot be ignored. Others, such as Professors Terry Anderson and Harding le Riche, both of the Department of Preventive Medicine and Biostatistics, University of Toronto, are proceeding with carefully controlled and fascinating studies into the value of mega-vitamin therapy as well as the possible harmful effects of modern diet.

To return to Vitamin C. It is not too surprising to find that some researchers have claimed coronary artery disease to be a Vitamin C deficiency state. Their argument is that adequate quantities of this substance in the body will protect against atherosclerosis, possibly by reducing blood cholesterol levels. Again, there is no proof that this is so. However, there are certain facts about Vitamin C which are worthy of note. High levels of physical stress will result in a depletion of the body's stores of Vitamin C. Thus, an exhausting long distance run such as a marathon race, or two or three nights without sleep, will deplete our Vitamin C reserves. Now it is an interesting fact that our bodies cannot manufacture Vitamin C; we must obtain it from the environment, either in natural or synthetic form. Consequently, it is reasonable to argue that individuals who are under high physical stress will require increased doses of the vitamin. Another point to bear in mind is that smoking and alcohol both destroy Vitamin C.

With these facts in mind, it does seem reasonable to take Vitamin C as a supplement when you are under physical stress. In our context, this would include heavy training. The man who is jogging three or more miles five days a week would be included in that category. I recommend to my patients who are running five to six miles an hour, five times a week, that they take 500 mg. daily. If they are running longer distances, then I recommend higher dosages. I consider such a level of training to be stressful, and I have found that the incidence of muscle and tendon injuries in my joggers has been minimal. It is difficult to prove that this is the result of their Vitamin C intake without undertaking a large and expensive clinical trial, but I think that the proven role of Vitamin C in the formation of healthy connective tissue makes my assumption a reasonable one.

What about the cost and the safety factors? Of all the vitamins, surely Vitamin C must be the cheapest, so that does not constitute a problem. On the matter of safety, there are one or two provisos. The body can only store so much ascorbic acid in the tissues, and any excess is excreted in the urine. This tends to make the urine acid, and some authorities have stated that this could lead to the formation of certain types of kidney stones. While this is a remote hazard, it can be reduced by maintaining an adequate fluid intake. Further, stone formation seems to me to be likely only when the intake of the vitamin is truly massive.

The influence of high dosage is probably also a factor in a more cogent objection, namely that the body becomes accustomed to high Vitamin C levels, and if the high dosage is suddenly withdrawn, then a mild type of scurvy may occur. Again, this seems unlikely with dosages in the order of a half a gram to a gram; even so, I recommend that the long distance jogger reduce his intake gradually over a week or two if for some reason training is reduced.

Finally, a recent preliminary report indicated that ingestion of half a gram or more of ascorbic acid may destroy some Vitamin B_{12} in the serum and in the body stores. Since B_{12} plays an important role in the formation of blood cells, it should be taken into consideration when considering Vitamin C therapy. The study was carried out on a group of paraplegic patients who were taking one gram of ascorbic acid daily by prescription in order to keep their urine acid and thus free from infection (a chronic problem with this type of patient). Their reduction in B_{12} blood levels was not sufficient to have serious consequences, but possibly the results warrant taking additional B_{12} along with the Vitamin C.

"Bulk" Diets Dr. Dennis P. Burkitt has suggested that a number of diseases which are characteristic of modern Western civilization may be due to a lack of bulk in our diets. In addition to appendicitis, cancer of the large bowel, ulcerative colitis, and various venous disorders, he also includes diseases associated with cholesterol metabolism. Of the latter, coronary heart disease and gall stones are undoubtedly the commonest.

The basis of his argument is that the past hundred years has seen a steady fall in the fibre content of our foodstuff, especially flour. The daily fibre intake from bread is now reduced to about a tenth of the level it was in the early part of the nineteenth century; packaged cereals, also poor in fibre, have replaced the high-fibre breakfast of porridge or oats. The effect of this lack of roughage in food is to reduce the weight and bulk of the fecal stools, and to increase the time of its passage through the intestine.

Primitive peoples who still eat high residue diets pass large bulky stools, which pass through the intestinal tract in 35 hours or so, as opposed to 70 hours in those on a Western diet. In these individuals, diseases of the intestine are rare, as are such conditions as varicose veins, deep vein thrombosis, and hemorrhoids.

Of even greater importance, the presence of a high fibre content in the feces seems in some way to be connected with low serum cholesterol levels and the relative absence of ischemic heart disease. The mechanism for this is uncertain. Burkitt himself is careful to point out that a high residue diet may be only one factor in the causation of these various conditions, but his opinion is worthy of respect. How do you increase the fibre content of your diet? Merely by adding two heaped dessert spoonfuls of unprocessed bran to your diet daily. You can take it in the morning mixed with your usual breakfast cereal, or can mix it with juice and have it with lunch. It's cheap, and it can do you no harm.

Is Sugar Deadly? Doctor J. Yudkin, Professor of Nutrition and Dietetics at the University of London, attributes the rise in atherosclerosis to an increase in the consumption of refined sugar. He points out that refined sugar, whether from cane or beet, is a relatively recent addition to our diet, only appearing in great quantities on our tables within the last hundred years. Already, however, the per capita consumption of this substance in the United States and Britain is an amazing one hundred pounds annually, if you count the sugar content of cookies, cakes, white bread, soft drinks, jams and other spreads, breakfast cereal, and so on.

According to Doctor Yudkin, experiments show that a high sugar intake is harmful for a number of reasons. First, it represents an inordinate intake of so-called "empty calories." Since it is an unnatural foodstuff the calories it provides are unaccompanied by vitamins or any of the other nutrients found in natural sugar sources such as fruit. Furthermore, in sugar-sensitive individuals it leads to a derangement of the body's ability to adjust its own blood sugar level, and this in turn can predispose to a variety of ills, of which atherosclerosis is but one. Finally, it is partially addictive in that the more you take the more you want.

The atherosclerotic effect of sugar is brought about by increasing blood cholesterol levels and enhancing blood stickiness. For more details you can read Doctor Yudkin's book, *Sweet and*

Dangerous, which explains his theory in lay terms.

Doctor Ancel Keys of Minneapolis, who blames a high content of animal fat in our diet as the chief cause for heart disease, has taken issue with Doctor Yudkin's hypothesis, pointing out that the relationship between high sugar intake and heart disease breaks down in the cases of the South American countries and also Sweden, areas with high sugar consumption and relatively low incidence of heart disease. Furthermore, Doctor Keys' own experiments have failed to show an elevation of blood cholesterol levels as a result of diets containing as much as 40 per cent sugar. Needless to say, Professor Yudkin has rebuttals for both arguments, and there is no doubt that his theory is an intriguing one. On balance, however, I would have to say that at this time it has relatively few adherents.

The Hard and Soft Water Controversy   A number of epidemiological studies have noted that there is a higher incidence of deaths from heart disease in those areas where the water is soft. Hard water flows over rocks rich in the mineral dolomite, and so contains larger amounts of magnesium and calcium. A low level of either or both of these substances in the tissues may, it is argued, affect the rhythm of the heart and, if this organ is already the seat of a disease such as coronary atherosclerosis, predispose to cardiac arrest.

Dr. Andrew Shaper, a research worker for the United Kingdom Medical Research Council, in an article published in 1974 in the *Journal of the American Medical Association*, describes how the death rate from cardiovascular disease in Monroe County, Florida, was found to have dropped considerably after the water supply had been changed from a soft to a hard water source. Residents of the hard water areas, both in America and the United Kingdom, have been variously reported to have lower blood pressures, lower heart rates, and lower blood cholesterol levels than their soft-water fellow citizens.

Whether it is the calcium or magnesium in the water, or both, which exerts a specific protective influence against death from circulatory disease is, in our present state of knowledge, impossible to say. Researchers from England and Finland have found that areas in which the soil is rich in both these minerals have a low heart disease rate.

Professor Terry Anderson of the University of Toronto, has

verified that the populations of soft water areas have a lower magnesium content in their muscle tissue (including their heart muscle) than residents of hard water areas. Since the hearts of persons who have succumbed to a heart attack are also found to have abnormally low concentrations of magnesium, he feels that his findings are compatible with the belief that waterborne magnesium exerts a protective effect. He also proffers the fascinating hypothesis that the basic problem is due to the critically low levels of magnesium in the highly refined Western diet, with the hard water inhabitants receiving just enough to avoid a heart muscle deficiency state.

Despite what might appear to be impressive evidence, most workers in the field are quick to point out that the whole matter is still very much open to question. Certainly there is insufficient data to warrant altering the water supply of the nation, or of advocating that physicians prescribe oral calcium or magnesium for their heart patients.

Long Distance Running

The theme of this book is the value of endurance training in post-coronary rehabilitation. More specifically, the beneficial effects of LSD or long slow distance. Why is it necessary to work out for an hour at a time? After all, hasn't a recent popular book on fitness extolled at length the benefits which accrue from a mere 30 minutes of exercise weekly (a gospel with a built-in appeal for a population conditioned to looking for the instant solution to everything)? Why should you have as your goal the ability to run five or six miles? The answer is simple; instant fitness, if such a thing exists, is about as durable as instant art, or instant music, or instant scholarship. Unpopular and unpalatable as it is, the fact remains that no one becomes proficient at anything by practising a mere 10 minutes a day. If you intend to achieve a worthwhile state of cardiorespiratory fitness, then you have to impose some degree of overload, either in terms of intensity or duration, on your cardiovascular system. Since your heart has some degree of damage, the intensity component has to be limited. Duration, on the other hand, has a much wider margin of safety.

Slow jogging for up to an hour has a number of benefits to offer. It is an excellent way to relieve tension and anxiety. Problems have a way of solving themselves during the workout, largely because they are seen in perspective. Jogging permits only a superficial, holistic type of thought; minutae and trivia recede into the background, leaving only the important high points for consideration. You no longer miss the wood for the trees. There is also the ego-building factor. The first time you complete five or six miles, no matter at what speed, you know you have set yourself apart from the majority of your fellow men. You are no longer "the guy who had the heart attack."

The psychological benefits of long distance recreational jogging should not be underestimated. In fact, we now have reports from psychiatrists who recognize its value in the treatment of mental illness. Dr. Kostrubala, a psychiatrist practising in Los Angeles, has formed a long distance jogging group for his patients, and carries out group therapy during training sessions. He reports considerable improvement in his patients as they become fitter. This has been the experience of many depressed, tense and anxious individuals after starting a distance jogging program — so much so that if they miss a few training sessions, they often notice the build-up of tension again.

The physiological gains are also immense. After half an hour of steady exercise, you begin to fall back on your stores of body fat as fuel. Fatty acids are burned, and the body relies less and less on its sugar stores. In addition to the metabolic advantages in terms of blood lipid levels, the actual caloric expenditure is considerable. A 160 lb. man running for an hour at a steady 10-minute mile pace will burn 600 calories. This, repeated five times weekly, means that he will burn 12,000 calories a month — which equals 3 lbs. of fat. The surprising fact is that caloric expenditure is more dependent upon the distance you cover and your body weight than upon the speed of your run. For example, a fit young athlete may run five miles in 30 minutes, while you may take 50 minute for the same task. You are burning less calories per minute (10 calories as opposed to 18 calories, to be precise), but since you are running for a longer period of time, you both finish up even. The heavier you are, the more energy you need to keep your bulk on the move, and so the more calories you spend.

You never see an obese long distance runner. I believe that he burns his body fat more efficiently than the sedentary person and this is borne out by experimental work. Not only that, but I find he automatically tends to eat less starchy and thus less fattening foods. He shuns sweet desserts. He avoids rich cuts of steak, usually heavily marbled with fat. Animal fat is easy to store, but hard to burn; vegetable fat is much more readily used, and maybe this is why the long distance runner tends to prefer it. Many long distance runners tend to adopt the same dietary habits. Is it by accident or design? One cannot help but wonder if the body naturally chooses the foodstuffs most suitable for its needs. And maybe it is not coincidental that the runner's diet happens also to be the one most suitable for the prevention of atherosclerosis.

Before leaving the subject of body weight, mention should be made of the work of Mayer, who ascribes the relationship between appetite and weight to the activity of an appetite centre in that primitive portion of the brain known as the hypothalamus. He believes that in sedentary individuals, this control centre becomes inactive with the result that the nice balance between appetite and body weight is lost. Fat stores increase, but appetite remains high. Obesity encourages less activity, less activity leads to even less energy expenditure, and so even greater fat storing. In this way, the vicious circle continues. Finally the fat person may indeed come to eat less than his slim colleague, but he still continues to get fat.

Cinephotography has shown that obese subjects in a girls' camp were consistently more sluggish in all physical activities. For example, during field games they moved around as little as possible, and during swimming practice they rested much more frequently than their slim, active friends. A physical activity program reactivates the control centre in the brain, restores the balance between food intake and energy expenditure, and ensures the success of a sensible, moderate reducing diet.

Many of us require a goal to aim for, and recreational joggers are no exception. For those of us who spend a major portion of our spare time plodding through the streets and parks, the ultimate distance is 26¼ miles — the marathon race. Merely to have completed such an exhausting trial, at no matter how slow a speed, is a triumph in itself. The aim is not to race against anyone. We leave that for the fleet-footed athletes who disappear from sight at the sound of the starting gun, never to be seen again by those of us who make up the rearguard. Our needs are few; merely to be privileged to leave with the pack at the starting signal, and lucky enough to be able to cross the deserted finish-line on our feet — three, four, five or even six hours later. With such simple wants, how can we be denied?

Let us be certain of one thing, however; like most things in life, the travelling is often more rewarding than the arriving. By that I mean that it is the training needed to ensure successful completion of the marathon that confers the benefit. There is no magic in the race itself from a health point of view. Thus, I cannot agree with my good friend, Dr. Tom Bassler, the Los Angeles pathologist, who believes that anyone who completes a marathon race in under $4^1/_2$ hours is immune from a heart attack for the next five years. (He excludes smokers.)

The so-called "Bassler imperative" seems to be not only an exaggerated claim, but also a totally unnecessary one. We have discussed the undoubted physiological benefits to the heart which accrue from endurance training. We have looked at the evidence in favour of exercise as a preventive measure in coronary heart disease. We have considered the sense of exhilaration and well-being which accompanies the trained state. To make any greater claims is to destroy the force of our arguments to date. This I will concede; the lifestyle associated with marathon-type training is hardly likely to contain too many heart attack risk factors. On the other hand, completion of a marathon run is no guarantee of immortality.

One of our patients who, some three years earlier, had finished a marathon run in five hours, died in his sleep. Autopsy failed to show any evidence of recent coronary thrombosis or myocardial infarction; it must be assumed that he had suffered a cardiac arrest. He was a smoker, and in the five or six months immediately prior to his death, had increased his cigarette consumption considerably. Running does not permit you to flaunt all of the other risk factors — especially when you have already had one or two previous heart attacks and know that the dice are already loaded against you.

For those who are interested in marathon running, I have discussed the matter in some detail and included suitable training tables in Chapter 10.

More and more doctors are appreciating the value of jogging, although I must say that their numbers are still miniscule when viewed in terms of the profession as a whole. Nevertheless, there is now an active group of physicians and allied health professionals who have formed the American Medical Joggers Association. Under their neurologist president, Dr. Ron Lawrence, they have championed the cause of jogging for health. They encourage their members to take part in long distance road races, including marathons, and schedule their medical meetings around such events as the Boston Marathon, the Mission Bay Marathon, and the Honolulu Marathon. The papers given by the members are invariably stimulating, and ample time is allowed for frank and free-wheeling discussion. The tone of these meetings is friendly and frank, without the scientific constraints which are customary in many medical conventions and which, at times, have a rather stultifying effect on verbal interplay. It is strange to attend a medical meeting where practically all of the members go for a jog after the day's proceedings, and wind up the whole affair by entering a marathon race. The post-marathon dinner is a euphoric affair, with each member discussing step by step his experiences during the race held earlier in the day. Equally unusual, there is a noticeable absence of smoke and liquor to accompany the proceedings! The members of the association now exceed 2,000, with a significant proportion of them Canadians. They include the Honolulu cardiologist, Jack Scaff, who is a keen jogger himself, and who introduced the Cardiovascular Division into the First Honolulu Marathon in 1973, having been stimulated by the example of the Toronto men in Boston nine months earlier. Dr. Tom Bassler, referred to earlier, is also a member, as is the author.

Another medical group which has long recognized the value of exercise in cardiovascular disease is the American College of Sports Medicine. This group is considerably larger than the AMJA, and consists of physicians, physiologists and physical educators who are interested in the scientific and medical aspects of sports. The association journal, *Medicine and Science in Sport*, frequently contains articles on exercise therapy, and the annual meeting invariably has a section dealing exclusively with exercise and coronary heart disease. The members of this association are growing rapidly, and this signifies the burgeoning interest in the subject. The emphasis here is more scientific than that of AMJA, with heavy stress on experimental work, both laboratory and clinical.

For the reader who has never been involved in an exercise program before, and who on reading this book intends to start exercising, I hope the above will provide the necessary motivation. If nothing else, it should at least indicate to him that he is anything but on his own. There are thousands of us out there in the street, so come on out and join us! A wave of the hand, and a short "Hi" as we pass in the night, and you've been initiated.

Exercise and Heart Surgery   Surgical treatment for coronary artery disease is now a feasible proposition for select cases. Earlier procedures included attempts to revascularize the ischemic heart tissue by implanting into the heart wall a substitute vessel for the ineffectual coronary artery (the Vineberg operation). The terminal portion of an artery supplying blood to the chest wall is used. Results were not too satisfactory, and so the search continued for other techniques. Today, the most commonly used is the saphenous vein coronary by-pass. In essence, this procedure consists of removing a piece of the large vein from the patient's thigh and grafting it between the aorta and the diseased coronary artery. This allows blood to flow from above the narrowed portion of the coronary artery, through the graft, and into the distal healthy portion. One, two, or all three coronary vessels may be by-passed in this way. There is one proviso; the distal portion of the vessel beyond the block must be healthy enough to allow a reasonably effective blood flow. Ideally, then, the vessel to be operated on should be almost normal except for a single discrete area of narrowing. Also, the general condition of the heart muscle should be good; a new blood supply will be of little avail to a myocardium which is already extensively scarred from previous infarcts or long-standing ischemia.

What is the situation with regard to by-pass surgery and exercise therapy? Are these two approaches to be looked upon as alternatives, or are they compatible? I believe that exercise therapy has a wider application than surgery, and it makes more sense for the vast majority of patients. For those individuals in whom surgery is inevitable, then exercise training, both pre- and post-operative, can be a very valuable adjunct. Patients who have already been on an exercise program, have failed to progress and then been operated upon, seem not only to be better operative risks, but also have a better mental outlook towards recovery. I have this on the very good authority of Dr. William Bigelow, Professor of Cardiovascular Surgery in the University of Toronto, and one of the pioneers in his field.

It stands to reason that individuals who have been trained, even to a limited degree, are going to have a more efficient oxygen transport system than if they had remained entirely sedentary. Their muscles are stronger, and their lungs function more effectively, with the result that they can be mobilized more rapidly after the operation, and so are less susceptible to many post-operative complications. They are also keen to get back to exercising again, and have a higher morale. One of the long-term complications of by-pass surgery is blockage of the graft so that blood fails to flow through it. This occurs in as high as 10-15 per cent of cases. It is too early to say, but one might even hope that the stimulus of exercise following surgery might help to reduce the incidence of this unpleasant event.

Barring complications, by-pass patients can start exercising three months after surgery, and if I had my way, I would insist that all such patients be offered an exercise training program. The logic of such advice seems to me to be inescapable. The unfit, overweight, cigarette-smoking, high-risk middle-aged patient who has had a by-pass and doesn't change his lifestyle remains the same unfit, overweight, cigarette-smoking, high-risk middle-aged patient — with a by-pass! The tip of the iceberg has been removed, but nothing has been done for the underlying residue of danger. The disease is still present, and will continue to progress unless something is done to stop it. It is not unusual for follow-up angiograms, taken twelve and eighteen months after by-pass surgery, to show marked atherosclerotic narrowing in hitherto unaffected branches of the coronary tree. All the more reason, then, that the by-pass patient, now free from angina, should take advantage of a training program and obtain true functional benefit from the surgery.

Cardiovascular surgeons have made strides of a magnitude undreamed of as recently as ten years ago. But I wish they were more aware of the value of post-operative rehabilitation. While there are many in the Toronto area who do refer their patients for such a service, I am sure their numbers are small in the overall picture. A paper delivered at the annual meeting of the Canadian Cardiovascular Association reported on the results of a follow-up carried out on patients who had received heart-valve replacement surgery. While the procedure had resulted in an improvement in their cardiac function, only 10 per cent had increased their physical activity as a result; 66 per cent were less active than before, and 34 per cent were unchanged. Only 52 per cent were employed, whereas prior to the surgery 78 per cent had been working.

The author of the paper concluded: "In general, patients were found to have incomplete information about prescribed diets and medications and received little guidance concerning their level of activity during and following convalescence." She went on to recommend that "an ongoing hospital teaching program be established to prepare the patient to return home. An active vocational rehabilitation program in the community should also be established to encourage the patient to return to a level of activity that is consistent with his post-operative functional status."

Amen to that!

CHAPTER EIGHT

The Woman in the Picture

In the Foreground

Heart disease has little respect for sexual equality. It singles out men, maiming and killing the male without regard for the current laws prohibiting sexual discrimination! We are not sure why this should be so, unless it is yet another example of what my old physics teacher used to refer to as "the general cussedness of nature." After all, the liberated woman of today is often as sedentary, obese and tense as her male counterpart; she eats as much animal fat, sugar and "denatured" bread; she drinks as much alcohol, soft water and coffee; she smokes as many (if not more) cigarettes; her heart and coronary arteries differ in no significant way from that of the male. Despite all this, she suffers about one-tenth the incidence of heart disease as her male counterpart. When and if she does have a heart attack, it is more likely to be associated with a history of heart disease in the family, or the presence of high blood pressure, or a diabetic condition. For this reason, some research workers have argued that coronary artery disease in the woman is a separate entity; in other words, a different disease from the one presently afflicting men in such great numbers. Of course, it may be that, as yet, it is too early for the full effects of sexual equality to be felt. Possibly by the 1980's, the hard-driving, heavy-smoking, sedentary female executive will be sharing equal time in the coronary care unit with her male colleague.

Currently, it is presumed that the presence in the body of female hormones in some way protects against the full onslaught of atherosclerotic heart disease. This theory seems to be borne out by the fact that post-menopausal women have about the same number of heart attacks as men of the same age (recognizing, of course, that the incidence in males is declining during the fifth, sixth and seventh decades). Further support for the as yet tentative hormone theory may lie in a recent report published in the *British Medical Journal* which indicated that heart attacks were considerably more frequent in a group of women who were taking the birth control pill, which acts as an artificial regulator of female hormone levels. Only time will tell whether or not this was a coincidental finding. In the meantime, we are left with the fact that the pre-menopausal woman who is free from a family history of coronary artery disease, is not diabetic or hypertensive, stands in much less jeopardy from a heart attack than a male of the same age.

If, on the other hand, she possesses any of the unfavourable characteristics mentioned above, then, in addition to seeking medical advice, she should adopt a lifestyle which is free from the risk factors discussed in this book. She should avoid smoking, practise discretion in eating fatty foods, and keep physically active. If she is interested in jogging, there is no medical reason whatsoever why she should not carry out the program outlined here. Unfortunately, it is still considered unusual for a middle-aged female to don a sweat suit and jog through the streets of our towns. If she is a trifle obese into the bargain, then her embarrassment is compounded. Fortunately, things are changing. The girl athlete is no longer considered a rare phenomenon. Swimming, track and field, volleyball, tennis, are but a few examples of sports in which the ladies' events are as exciting as the men's, and in which the top level of competition is surpassed by only the most exceptional male performers. Today, women race all distances up to 1,500 metres on the track, often at a faster pace than the male Olympic champion of twenty or thirty years ago. More women are entering marathon races, and even the Boston Marathon now permits females to enter officially; indeed, Dr. Van Acken, the famous German coach and physiologist, maintains that a woman's metabolism is better adapted to feats of endurance than a man's, and he forecasts that women may one day out-perform men in distance running. Men may continue to dominate those activities requiring pure muscle power and speed, but the day might come when a suitably trained woman captures the world long distance running, swimming or cross-country title — and, if the appearance of many of our present-day lady athletes is anything to go by, without sacrificing anything in the way of grace, beauty or charm.

For the moment, however, ladies of the coronary-risk generation are often stuck with the Amazon image. If they partake in any physical endeavour which makes them huff, puff or sweat, their femininity is suspect (unless that endeavour be sexual intercourse, which is of course always exempt from male criticism!)

There are other difficulties which beset the novice female jogger. Unlike her husband, she can rarely expect to have her breakfast waiting on the table when she returns from her early morning run. It is more likely that she will be expected to get up all that much earlier so as to prepare both their meals. The same applies to supper. What about the daytime? Well, housework and children's meals seem to occupy most of that.

How then is it possible for the busy housewife to jog regularly? One way is to accompany her husband on his workouts. If a running track is used, both parties can be "together" even though jogging at different speeds. A circular road circuit will achieve the same effect if each lap is no longer than half a mile, and if one jogger goes clockwise and the other counter-clockwise. That way, you pass each other twice every lap — possibly a safety factor in some neighbourhoods when jogging in the evening. As a matter of fact, few joggers enjoy training with someone step by step and side by side. Each finds a comfortable pace, and rarely will two individuals feel the need to slow down or pick up the speed at precisely the same time. Furthermore, jogging alone is half the fun; it provides you with the opportunity to collect your thoughts and sort out your problems, free for once from the distractions of modern life such as radio, telephone and television. For this reason, "company" for the jogger usually means sharing the decision to start the workout, getting ready, and setting out together. Remember, it's twice as hard for two people to miss a training session as one!

If your husband doesn't jog, that shouldn't deter you. You should make up your mind that you are going to find the time, whatever the cost. Within weeks, you will begin to feel, act and look younger, shapelier and more relaxed. You will be able to do more work and feel less tired during the day, and you will sleep more soundly during the night. And if your husband doesn't then decide to start jogging himself, I'll be very surprised.

The woman jogger should use the training tables exactly as described, with the same age division and precautions. You may not wish to progress beyond the three-mile distance, although there is no earthly reason why you shouldn't if you are prepared to devote the time. I recall when my cardiac marathoners were out on a training run a few years back, we first met a middle-aged lady jogger proceeding leisurely along the same park track. Our next encounter was when we watched her finish a determined and gallant last in her first full marathon race. At 55, Judy Kazdan, a hobby jogger of eight years duration, has finished five marathons, the latest being the World Masters Championships held in Toronto in August 1975. She runs on her own and occasionally with her husband, trains herself, and finds the time to be a "housewife" besides.

In the Background

Every so often, I devote a full evening to giving a lecture to the wives and girl friends of the men on the cardiac rehabilitation program. The talk, illustrated by slides, lasts for one and a half to two hours and covers much of the information contained in this book. After coffee, the questions start. With anything from 80 to 100 women assembled, the queries are many and varied, and the session usually lasts for a further two or three hours. I try to answer each questioner as honestly and as carefully as I can, pointing out that in matters of judgment, as opposed to fact, my response has to be based on my personal opinion, which in turn is based on my experience with the program as well as my interpretation of the experience of others.

The purpose of the meeting is to help these women help their husbands. It attempts to do that by giving them some knowledge of the disease which has come to exert such a large influence on their husband's and their own lives, and by providing them with direct answers to questions which they have never had the opportunity to ask previously. Since the husbands are not present at the meeting, the wives can be as frank as they wish in expressing their fears, doubts and concerns. For instance, I find that for many wives the interpretation of symptoms is often a problem. Should every ache and pain be taken seriously? Or should an apparently trivial complaint be handled with firm reassurance, thus helping to build up self-confidence? How much normal work around the house should be permitted? Should lifting be allowed?

Some of these questions are too individual to be answered in general terms. Others have been dealt with elsewhere in this book. However, the following paragraphs are based on the questions most often asked by the concerned partner, and hopefully will be of help.

Overcoming Despondency   It is now accepted that rehabilitation should start as soon as the patient gets out of the coronary care unit and returns to the general ward. The hour-to-hour battle to save his life is over, and the time for healing has begun. For the moment, the patient is glad just to be alive, but as the days pass, that feeling of relief is replaced by one of despondency. The mind is plagued by doubts and uncertainties, all revolving around the ability to be able to do all of the things which were part and parcel of everyday life before the attack. As one patient said to me, "I wanted to get out of the hospital, and yet I was scared to go home. Activities which I had always taken for granted now became a first; the first time you walk up the stairs, you wonder if it's safe, and you breathe a sigh of relief when you get to the top of the flight and nothing happens. The first day you mow the grass, or clean out the basement, or go back to work, it's the same feeling — will you make it? It's as if you're trying to pick up the pieces of your life again, and never being sure if they'll fit together properly this time."

Of course, a good post-coronary rehabilitation program helps to overcome much of this fear. No program, however, can help as much as a well-informed wife. What, you say, can I do? First of all, take a positive approach right from the first hospital visit. Don't avoid discussing the future. The vast majority of heart attack patients return to their previous jobs. If your husband's is the exceptional case, it still does no harm to discuss alternatives. To make small talk and steer away from a topic as important as future work plans is a great mistake; to the depressed patient, it can only mean one thing — there is no future to discuss. Even if he doesn't feel inclined to pursue the subject in great detail, he will thank you later for displaying such confidence.

When the day comes for your husband to return home, don't make the mistake of one of my patient's wives who automatically picked up his suitcase and carried it to the car. That one action, well-intentioned as it was, put the seal on all his fears. Four years later, he still sees it as his most humiliating moment. Better to have let him offer to carry it himself (after all, how much personal belongings can you accumulate during a three-week stay in the coronary ward?); or if lifting has been entirely prohibited by the physician, make some remark to the effect that you are obeying doctor's orders, which means lifting is out, for the time being. The main thing is to avoid being over-solicitous. Exercise sensible precautions, but don't fuss. No doubt there is an increased element of risk in certain physical activities, but then driving an automobile isn't exactly 100 per cent safe these days, and no one can live his life completely immune from risk. Besides, until recently, the tendency has been to exaggerate the dangers of physical effort for the heart attack patient. We now know that many of the things that he will want to do are perfectly safe.

In the first few months after the attack, there is often a reluctance to make decisions. This is perfectly natural, and is just another manifestation of the depressed mood. Eventually, the situation rights itself. Just be patient, and whatever you do, don't get into the habit of making all the decisions in the home. If you do, you may well find yourself stuck with the role of decision-maker permanently. Every so often, give your partner the opportunity to regain the initiative.

How to React to Symptoms Symptom-claiming is not unusual in the early days following the attack. It is an expression of insecurity, and represents a need for reassurance. It may last a matter of months only, but it can be a real trial for the wife who never becomes quite inured to a succession of frightening complaints of chest pain, numbness in hands, dizziness, and so on. Often the symptom complex is similar to the one which heralded the initial attack, and it is difficult not to push the panic button and call the physician on every occasion. However, each wife knows her own husband, and very often will have an instinctive feeling for the true state of affairs; as likely as not, it will be safe for her to follow that instinct and give him the reassurance he is seeking. If, on the other hand, she is not all that sure of herself, she will usually learn from the first few false alarms.

Is it not better to be sure than sorry? Within reason, yes. However, a man cannot spend half his life running in and out of the doctor's office or the hospital emergency department. If he is to live a normal life, he must learn to exercise judgment and maturity in assessing the significance of various symptoms. To get into the habit of requiring an electrocardiogram every time he gets an ache or a pain is to follow the path to cardiac neurosis — in my experience, one of the most difficult of all conditions to cure. The ironic thing, of course, is that the electrocardiogram is by no means infallible. If this preoccupation with symptoms persists beyond a six-month period or so, and shows no signs of responding to simple reassurance on your part, then it should be mentioned to the family physician or the cardiologist. Psychiatric treatment may be indicated to relieve the condition before the pattern becomes set.

Once again, it should be borne in mind that reluctance to make decisions or to take responsibility, as well as exaggeration of symptoms, are merely expressions of depression, a not uncommon reaction to a heart attack in a certain personality type. Depression recedes with time, although since the trait is probably inborn, it never disappears entirely and may reoccur in response to some other misfortune. Frank depression, accompanied by a mournful, long expression, is rare. The depressed individual is more likely to cover up his real feelings, and feign a cheery, jocular mood. In many cases, his act is good enough to deceive even those closest to him, including his wife. However, the underlying mood cannot help but express itself in the more subtle ways already described.

There are certain symptoms which should be taken seriously, since they may herald a recurrence. Complaint of severe pain in the chest, left arm or jaw and which is accompanied by pallor, sweating and alteration in pulse rate is classical; it will be underestimated by only the most ineffectual or callous observer. Such a picture demands urgent medical attention, and precious time should not be wasted "waiting to see if it will go away."

An analysis of the patients referred to the Toronto Rehabilitation Centre showed that a high proportion of them had six hours or more warning of their attack. The manner in which the attack started varied (see Figure 13), but pain in the chest or arm was the commonest. Since the survival rate is highest in those who receive medical care quickly, the recognition of warning signs is of paramount importance. The problem is compounded by the tendency for some men to deny that the symptoms they are experiencing are those of a heart attack. Blame is usually laid at the door of the gastro-intestinal tract. Beware the severe attack of "indigestion" which lasts more than half an hour, does not respond to simple antacid medication, and is made worse by lying flat.

There are other indications of impending trouble which, although less dramatic than chest pain, should nevertheless be heeded. In some ways, they may be more important, since they may antedate the attack itself and so allow more time for preventive action. Foremost among these intangible and often vague signs is excessive fatigue. Tiredness which is not relieved by a good night's rest should be considered suspect in the recent post-coronary patient, and search should be made for the cause. A heavy workload or an overcrowded social itinerary is usually the culprit, and steps should be taken immediately to adopt a more sensible and relaxed routine. Dr. Nixon, cardiologist at the Charing Cross Hospital in London, places great emphasis on irascible mood as an ill-omen, and I agree entirely with him. Frequently, the wife is the first to recognize the onset of a cantankerous, irritable manner which was so typical of the first attack. Both fatigue and irritability may be the result of a return to the old, driving, overcrowded lifestyle, with its business and financial worries, impossible work schedule, and absence of physical activity and recreation. In short, a repetition of the very set of circumstances which probably triggered the initial acute attack.

Preventing Another Attack Recognition of dangerous symptoms is one thing; preventing them from appearing is a far more worthwhile goal. What positive steps should you take to help your partner keep from having a further attack? It can be expressed in a phrase: "Assist him in his efforts to change his lifestyle." His previous way of life contained the seeds of his attack. He has been given a chance, maybe his last, to alter the situation. This means a suitable diet which is low in cholesterol and animal fats, a physical fitness program, a veto on cigarette smoking, and moderation in both work and play.

Figure 13

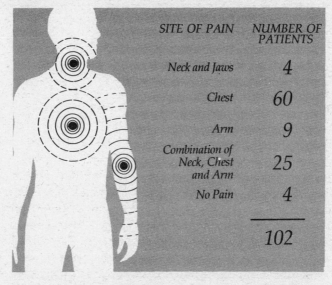

SITE OF PAIN	NUMBER OF PATIENTS
Neck and Jaws	4
Chest	60
Arm	9
Combination of Neck, Chest and Arm	25
No Pain	4
	102

The Sites of Pain in Heart Attack as Reported by 102 Patients Referred to the Centre's Post-coronary Exercise Program

Sounds easy? Well, maybe. It's no use applauding these aims and then getting irritable because this new lifestyle precludes some of your favourite social engagements and habits. After all, if he has to jog in the morning, he may not exactly relish a late party the night before — even if it is with that delightful Jones couple you feel you "owe" it to. He may want to go to bed around 10:00 p.m. or so, without that 11:00 p.m. nightcap which he used to look forward to so much. He may object to your smoking, especially if he is suffering the tortures of the damned trying to give it up himself! He will be learning to say no to things which he really doesn't want to do (or knows he shouldn't do), instead of always saying yes to every request, trivial or otherwise.

As the wife of one patient put it, "Bill isn't the same anymore. He used to be so kind and thoughtful, and took me wherever I wanted to go. Now, he says he isn't going anywhere just because he has to. Last week, he refused to go to my cousin's wedding. Sometimes when we have company and it gets late, he just excuses himself and goes to bed at 11:00 p.m."

Bill has had two heart attacks, is now a dedicated jogger and is fitter than he has ever been in his life. My guess is that if he keeps on playing it so smart, he'll live out his normal lifespan.

You will need to accommodate to this new partner. The more accommodation needed, the more you can console yourself with the thought that the rehabilitation is proceeding successfully. You may have to arrange mealtimes so as to fit in with exercise sessions. Don't nag because you have to keep food hot while you wait for him to come back from his jog. If you can't jog with him, then take the trouble to acquaint yourself with the distance he has to go and the time it should take, and then plan accordingly.

If you feel that this is a chore, just think of Mrs. R. whose husband had a heart attack when he was 29 years old.

"Certainly Herman's running is time-consuming," she related at a recent meeting of the Ontario Heart Foundation. "In fact, our daughter was two years old before all three of us ever had Sunday dinner together; Herman was always out training with the cardiac marathoners. But that's a small price to pay to have him alive and healthy. Besides, we were only married two years before his attack, and the picture looked so bleak, that we decided that it would be irresponsible of us to start a family. However, he improved so much on the running program that we changed our minds."

Herman R. has run six marathons in the past two years, his fastest being in 3 hours, 11 minutes. In 1975, he was the first heart patient ever to officially enter the Boston Marathon, where he placed 1,500 out of a field of 2,500 and returned a time of 3 hours, 20 minutes. Three months after that, in August 1975, his second daughter was born.

Part of the new lifestyle will include sensible weight control, and here you may have to change your previous notions of what the well-fed man should look like. Just glance at the table of ideal weights in the Appendix (p.295). Your natural reaction is one of horror, right? Most women react the same way. The fact is that you have been brainwashed, likely by your own mother, to accept that your man should be pleasantly rounded and should always look "well-fed." Admittedly, he might have got away with two helpings of dessert if he had been physically active, but until he achieves that state, your extra calories will only thicken his midriff, puff out his jowls, and clog his arteries. Get used to a slim, even scraggy, mate — unless, of course, you can't bear him to look younger than you.

If you are to play an intelligent role in the rehabilitation program, you should take the time to read this book carefully. Master the training tables, understand the method of progression, and become familiar with the signs of over-training. Learn how to use a stop watch, and check your husband's jogging times. Have him complete a daily workout diary, and check to see if he is going too fast or too slow. Discuss his progress with him and congratulate him on each upward step he makes in the tables. Encourage him when he plateaus, and keep his spirits up when he seems to stick for too long a time at one level.

In short, aim to be his mentor and his coach, remembering that no one can really consistently train themselves; from time to time, everyone needs the objectivity of an informed onlooker, one who will not only urge them on to greater heights, but one who will also apply the brakes when the signs call for it. As the "coach" of a cardiac athlete, you have additional responsibilities. Never forget that this particular jogger has a scar in his heart, and that excessive enthusiasm or competitiveness is uncalled for and even dangerous. The name of the game is health through fitness, not fitness for competition.

As your man's condition improves, there will be a simultaneous improvement in his symptoms, including angina and tolerance for heavier physical work. Eventually, he will be carrying out physical tasks which are far beyond the level of his pre-attack capabilities. This may in itself cause problems. He may wish to discontinue the prescribed medication. Most of the time, this is all to the good, but try not to let him do this before he checks with his physician. I am constantly having to remind my patients of this.

Another side effect of increasing fitness is the desire to take up new and sometimes more strenuous leisure activities, such as camping, sailboating, backpacking, cross-country skiing. Often allied with this is an increased interest in the simpler pleasures; walking in the rain, a good novel, a fall outing on foot to catch the colours.

Can you adapt to this? I still recall with crystal clarity the bemused tone with which one of my earliest "successes" described his wife's reaction to his newly awakened yearnings. "You know what she said, Doc?" he intoned sadly. "I wish you hadn't changed. We were so happy when you were the way you used to be."

The "way he used to be" was over 300 lbs. in weight and every weekend spent in front of the television set downing a succession of 12-packs. The fact was that his wife couldn't cope with the new 165 lb. man of 45 who now wanted more from life than a succession of lost weekends. The result? They parted.

Then there was the 36-year-old executive who carried out his jogging prescription after work three nights a week at the local Y, and came home to a wife who went out of her way to make him feel guilty because she couldn't accept that anything other than work should delay him from coming home to her. How did they solve the situation? They also parted.

Such cases are in the minority, but they and others like them actually happened. I would be less than honest if I failed to emphasize that the successfully rehabilitated man may not be the man you married. In a minority of cases, the new version may not be to your liking. If this is so, then the outlook can be grim. Fortunately, the opposite is usually the case. The wife is happy beyond words to see her husband regain the healthy outlook on life which he once had before the lure of so-called "success" got to him.

Before closing, let me touch on a delicate subject. If you have read the early chapters, you will have noted that the life expectancy of the individual who has had a heart attack is less than normal. Maybe the adoption of a new lifestyle will correct that; if we didn't think so, it would hardly be worth the effort. Nevertheless, the unpalatable fact of your partner's possible early death may be hard to live with. Yet this is a fact of life, which may help to put my whole argument into perspective. Don't dwell on the negative side. Accept the odds, then make up your mind to reduce them to a minimum. You cannot live your life by statistics, otherwise you would take no risks at all. Get on with the business of living, and may you both live happily ever after.

Part Three

Write the vision, and make it plain upon tables, that he may run that readeth it.

Habakkuk 2:2

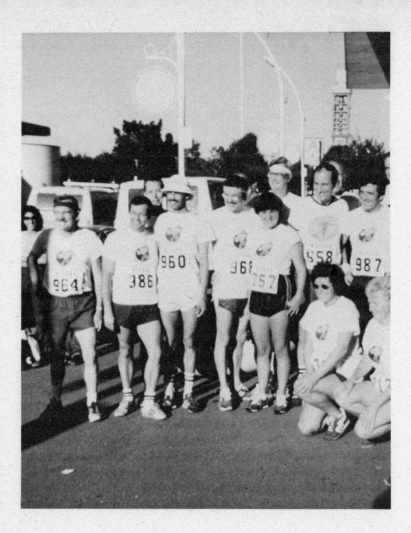

CHAPTER NINE

Loping and Coping

IN recent years there has been an increasing interest in the healthy, active lifestyle and the adoption of many of the principles advocated in this book. People are becoming more concerned with the positive attainment of health, rather than merely the cure for disease. This may well be why in the United States, coronary artery disease, although the major killer and likely to remain so for some years to come, has recently started to decline in incidence at the rate of about 1.5 per cent a year.

Part of the movement of accepting the responsibility for one's own health maintenance is the tremendous growth in the number of middle-aged individuals who have taken up jogging. More power to them! Some are happy to stay at two or three miles, three times weekly; others aspire "just once," to finish a marathon. Some are perfectly healthy; others may have coronary artery disease and not know it. Some are cautious; others are imprudent and reckless. All of them can, I feel, benefit from the advice and information contained in this chapter and the one that follows.

No one's life is problem-free, and the jogger is no exception. Time is precious, and the conscious decision to spend some of it on regular jogging sessions may meet resistance from unsympathetic family or friends. Excessive zeal may lead to injuries, minor in the overall scheme of things, but sufficient to put a temporary halt to your workouts, lead to a chorus of "I told you so," and make you miserable and mad with the world. The air around you may be so thick with gasoline fumes and industrial pollution that you wonder if you wouldn't be better off to buy a stationary bicycle. You are bombarded with contradictory advice about jogging shoes, dietary supplements and a whole host of "essentials" for the jogger. You pick up the paper one morning to find jogging is *the* road to health and fitness, only to read the next day that the middle-aged jogger is dicing with death.

The veteran jogger will have learned to roll with the punches, temper enthusiasm with common sense and use a mixture of guile, deafness of convenience and sheer indifference in order to keep family, job, friends and himself together — and still jog! He can probably teach you the tricks of the trade — if he has the time. Otherwise, you are going to have to learn the hard way. Hopefully some of the topics covered in this chapter will set you thinking in the right direction.

Injuries

Let's face it, jogging is a safe sport. Compared with football, ice hockey, English rugger and the like, it's pretty tame. The ancient Irish game of hurling (reputedly the fastest field game in the world and without doubt the most dangerous-looking) makes jogging look about as perilous as threading a needle; no badly smashed bones, dislocated shoulders, eight-inch lacerations, fractured skulls, broken noses, tendons and ligaments shredded like crab meat. And yet, even the gentle game of golf can give rise to the painful condition of "golfer's elbow." Swimmers can develop "swimmer's ear," a rather painful exzema of the ear canal. Prolonged knitting can result in a tenosynovitis, or inflammation of the wrist and finger tendons. I cannot think of a single physical recreation, no matter how mild, that does not carry with it the possibility of injury. Nevertheless, you should be aware of some of the more common injuries which can occur so that you can recognize them in their early stages and take swift corrective action.

Cause of Injury   Jogging injuries are self-inflicted wounds. They are due to carelessness, vanity, unwarranted enthusiasm, over-estimation of one's capabilities, or just sheer stupidity. This may sound harsh, but time and time again when confronted with the forlorn victim pouring out his tale of woe and demanding instant relief so that he can quickly return to his hobby, I can usually elicit a history of excessive speed, duration or frequency of workouts — all without adequate build-up. Frenetic training on hills, not making due allowance for headwinds or rough ground, allowing one's shoes to wear so badly that they no longer provide adequate support or protection, are all examples of the sort of thing I mean. Some joggers are more susceptible to injury than others because of congenital structural weaknesses in their feet or knees, but these cases are relatively rare, and even they can avoid problems if they use care and moderation.

There is little excuse for the health jogger to hurt himself. Unlike the competitive runner, there is no element of pressure or urgency in the workouts, no running against the stop watch, no need to teach the body to ignore the intense discomfort of muscle-screaming fatigue; this is the lot only of those whose talent and temperament have destined them for one goal and one goal only, to be first across the finish line. Such heroics are not for us. The name of our game is cardiovascular fitness and health, and this can be achieved quite adequately without the risk of bodily insult. That is the first and most important principle you can learn.

Essentials of Treatment   Jogging injuries rarely occur dramatically. A sprinter or a jumper who tears a muscle in full flight will often collapse like a shot rabbit, clutching the injured leg wildly. Muscle tears in joggers are comparatively rare. Injuries are usually the result of chronic over-use. The feet of a relatively short-striding jogger will hit the pavement about 1,500 times for every mile covered. As the mileage goes up, so does the possibility of injury. Pain is invariably the warning sign. When it occurs during the run, it is a signal for you to slow down and evaluate the situation. Where is the pain located? Is it sharp or aching? Have you experienced it before? Does it feel similar to a previous injury? If slowing your pace removes all trace of discomfort, then gradually pick up your speed again and note what happens. If all is well, then chances are you have merely experienced one of the countless and transitory inconsequential musculo-skeletal aches and pains which are the lot of every sportsman. A return of the pain at a quicker pace, however, is a clear signal to back off and finish the workout at the pain-free level. If the same thing happens on the next workout, then accept the fact that you have an injury, relax, and skip the next two or three training sessions.

Seems obvious? Well, maybe it does, but it is surprising how many joggers adopt the opposite approach. Their motto is "When in doubt, run it out." With such a philosophy, a relatively minor injury, which would respond quite well to a few days' rest, is aggravated to the stage where it becomes chronic and requires not only prolonged rest, but often professional treatment. The vast majority of joggers' problems can be detected by the alert jogger at a stage early enough to respond to rest. If rest doesn't work, then a cause for the difficulty must be found and appropriate remedial steps taken.

Let me give you a simple example. Today, as I write this chapter, I have just returned from a 10-mile jog with a group of my post-coronary marathoners. We had six inches of fresh snow last night. Despite this, the sky was blue, the sun was warm and our usual route through the park adjoining the Centre was a delight. On the other hand, this was the first snow of the winter, and our legs have not, as yet, toughened to the countless unaccustomed compensatory movements needed to keep one's balance. Our captain, Harry B. has had trouble in the past with his knees. After five miles, he noticed a slight discomfort in the left knee. Immediately, he slowed and then, after half a mile, walked back to the safety of the ploughed pavement where he finished his workout on an even surface. Had he continued to soldier on with the rest of us, there is a strong likelihood that he would have let himself in for a lengthy layoff and a time-consuming period of physical therapy treatments. As it is, I have no doubt that he will be jogging again tomorrow, free from complaint. After eleven years of jogging, he knows that prevention is a good deal easier than cure.

Assuming that a period of rest has not been successful, then usually the next stage in treatment is one of a number of *physiotherapy* treatments, some of which can be employed by the jogger, others which need professional application and then usually only after the condition has been diagnosed medically. Cryotherapy, or the therapeutic application of cold, is often used in the initial stages of an acute injury to relieve pain and reduce swelling. It can also be used over a chronically inflamed tendon, such as in heel cord (Achilles) tendonitis. Cold is applied in the form of a commercial cold pack or, more usually, by massage with an ice cube. The ice is held in a towel and then applied directly to the skin over the painful area. Care should be taken to see that skin sensation is normal to start with, that you are not one of those individuals who is hyper-sensitive to cold (the skin becomes red, "wealed," and swollen within minutes), and that the area has not been frostbitten at any time in the past. The ice is used in a circular or back-and forth movement over the skin, which first feels cool, then burns, and then after about three minutes, begins to ache. Finally, the area becomes numb. Ice massage should not be used for longer than five minutes and can be repeated morning and evening, and after workouts.

Therapeutic heat often relieves discomfort and increases circulation to the affected part, thus accelerating the healing process. Superficial dry heat can be administered by use of a heating pad (caution: severe burns have occurred as a result of people falling asleep while the heating pad is still on), or an infra-red heat lamp (for maximum effect, the feeling should be one of comfortable wamth, *not* excessive heat; the lamp should be about 1½ to 2 feet away from the area being treated and the treatment time should be about 20 to 30 minutes). Examples of moist heat applicators are the so-called wet pack or hydrocolator. These are canvas packs which contain a heat-retaining substance; they are placed in boiling water, heated to a temperature of 160° F., wrapped carefully in a towel so that they do not burn the skin, and placed carefully over the painful area. If you have never used one before, it is advisable to have your physician or physiotherapist demonstrate their use first.

Contrast baths are excellent for foot and lower leg injuries. To carry this out properly, you will need two buckets, or plastic waste baskets. Half-fill one with water at a temperature between 55° and 65° F., the other with water at a temperature between 95° and 100° F. Place the injured leg for 3 to 5 minutes in the hot water and then for 1 to 2 minutes in the cold; alternate for about 30 mintues and remember always to start with the hot and end with the hot. Small whirlpool baths are also useful for lower leg injuries, although one should recognize that dangling the leg in a whirlpool for 30 minutes or more can sometimes aggravate the condition by giving rise to gravity-induced swelling. Individuals who suffer from diabetes or restricted circulation to the lower limbs should not carry out any of these self-prescribed procedures without first seeking the advice of their physician.

A deeper form of heating can be achieved by the use of machines which generate high frequency electrical currents. The three commonest deep heating currents used today are short wave diathermy, microwave diathermy, and ultra-sound; all have to be used with great caution since there are situations and conditions in which they can cause unpleasant and sometimes quite serious side effects. Specialized training is required for their use, and they should be applied only by a suitably qualified professional. They can, however, be particularly valuable, either used singly or in combination, for treatment of deep-seated tendon or joint injuries.

Massage can be used to relieve pain, increase blood supply, reduce swelling, and both stretch and soften tendons and scar tissue. There are numerous techniques, the commonest being light or deep stroking, kneading, or deep friction. I find that the last is particularly valuable in the treatment of a chronic Achilles tendonitis. Briefly, the foot on the affected side is held in the relaxed position with the toes pointing down so that the tendon is loose and mobile. Then, using the straight middle finger reinforced by the index finger on top of it, pressure is applied over the painful area of the tendon just above the heel bone and a side-to-side sawing motion is carried out for about 10 to 15 minutes. By then, the tendon will feel quite numb but free from discomfort. The treatment is repeated every second day for about a week or so. For the treatment to be effective, the painful area must be very accurately defined so that the treatment is given precisely. The movement of the massaging fingers must be across, or at right angles to the direction of the tendon itself, and great care must be taken to see that the massaging finger and the skin over the tendon move as one so that it is the fibres of the tendon itself which are being massaged and not the overlying skin. Failure to observe the final point will lead to reddening and damage to the skin itself. A physiotherapist familiar with the technique can readily teach you so that you can carry it out on your own.

Medication   The most common non-prescription medication likely to be used by the injured jogger is acetylsalicylic acid, more frequently referred to as ASA or aspirin. Aspirin is primarily an anti-inflammatory drug. Its pain-relieving property is not all that powerful, and yet the public tends to see it purely and simply as a pain reliever. In point of fact, aspirin is often the drug of choice to reduce a high temperature or take the redness and swelling out of inflamed joints. It is therefore a useful drug for the over-use syndrome frequently met with in joggers. The chronically inflamed knee or Achilles tendon will often respond well to a combination of rest, physiotherapy and aspirin.

The drug comes in two strengths, 300 mg. and 600 mg. and, under normal circumstances, the average individual can easily tolerate up to 1,200 mg. daily. Like all medications, however, there are side effects. The most prominent is irritation of the lining of the stomach. If you have an ulcer, beware of taking aspirin. You can get enteric-coated aspirin tablets which pass through the stomach and dissolve in the intestine, but even these are likely to aggravate a peptic ulcer. Remember that aspirin makes you sweat and may make you susceptible to dehydration if you are continuing to exercise in the very warm weather. It also destroys Vitamin C, so you might be wise to increase your intake of that vitamin when you are on aspirin therapy. Finally, it has a tendency to make your blood less sticky. If you are on blood thinners (so-called anticoagulants) you should consult your doctor before using aspirin. Barring these precautions, you will find that, from time to time, aspirin will give considerable relief for sore joints or tendons.

Other anti-inflammatory agents include phenylbutazone (Butazolidin), oxphenbutazone (Tandearil), indomethacin (Indocid), ibuprofen (Motrin), naproxen-sodium (Naprosyn) and cortisone. All these medications are obtainable by prescription only, since they can have adverse side effects. Another prescription drug which is neither anti-inflammatory nor a pain-killer is sometimes prescribed in sports injuries. This is methocarbanol (Robaxin). Its action is to relieve the muscle spasm which is often secondary to a joint or deep tendon lesion. The spasm is really a protective mechanism, an attempt on the part of the body to reduce the mobility of a moving part. Muscle spasm is not always beneficial, however, sometimes giving rise to its own particular form of pain, or by persisting too long, preventing the joint from regaining its full range of movement after the underlying problem is cured.

Therapeutic exercise   This plays a large role in the treatment and prevention of sports injuries. It is prescribed most frequently to improve mobility and/or strength. Range of motion exercise can be either *passive*, in which the therapist moves the relaxed muscle or joint without the help of the patient, or *active*, in which the patient performs the work entirely unaided. The active type is the most frequently used in sports medicine. The commonest form of active range of motion exercises is *stretching*, the purpose of which is to restore or achieve normal range of movement or alignment in a joint.

Strengthening exercises can also be divided into two types. There are the *isometric* exercises, in which the muscle is contracted but the joint which it helps to move is held motionless. A further refinement of this is to force the contracting muscle to work against an added weight. An example of this is the so-called "static quadriceps hold," where the patient keeps the knee joint in the fully extended position by contracting the thigh muscles, while at the same time, the therapist applies appropriate weights to the foot. This manoeuvre is particularly valuable if you are dealing with a situation where you want to build up the strength of the anterior thigh muscle (quadriceps) while at the same time not aggravating a painful knee condition by bending and straightening the knee joint too much. *Isotonic* exercises build strength by having the muscle contract, but at the same time allowing the joint to move. This is usually carried out against the resistance of a weight and, since the weight is increased as the patient's tolerance permits, the procedure is known as *progressive resistance exercise.*

Over-use injuries, when not due to excessive zeal, are often the result of either inappropriate or badly worn *shoes*, or *gait defects*. For this reason, I usually ask the injured patient to jog or walk once around the track while I observe him. Badly worn shoes are a frequent cause of trouble. Heel wear tends to cancel the advantages of the heel raise. A worn sole exposes the front of the foot and the bases of the toes to excessive pounding. All materials deteriorate with time, and it should be no surprise that the nylon and rubber composite in the shoe lose some of their resilience and flexibility with the passing months, especially after being exposed to conditions ranging all the way from sun-baked pavement to snow-covered parkland. A 30-mile-a-week jogger, even if lightfooted, is probably ready for new shoes every twelve months. When you do buy a new pair, don't forget to break them in properly. I usually take four to six weeks to do this, using them for only one workout the first week and then wearing them for an additional workout every five to seven days or so. No matter how well the new shoes fit, no matter how comfortable they feel, they are never quite the same as the old ones and will require minor adjustment of gait to accommodate to the differences in weight, balance and resilience.

While the subject of jogging shoes has been written about ad nauseum, it does no harm to mention some of the features we should be considering when choosing a new pair. Weight is important. If they are too heavy, they can give rise to a form of shin splints. Too light, and they start to come apart and wear excessively in a few months. The only way to be sure is to try them on, and remember that the heavier you are, the more sturdy the shoe you will require. The heel should be sufficiently raised, probably about three-quarters of an inch, and the outer layers of cushioning should be sufficient to break the shock of landing, but not too spongy, otherwise you will develop soreness in the lower calf. Once again, the amount of heel cushioning you require is dependent upon your body weight. The exaggerated heel flare which was so common a few years back proved to be valuable when running on soft ground or fresh snow, but was much more than the foot required when jogging on hard pavement. The result was excessive mobility in the knee joint, with resultant increase in knee injuries. So, avoid the excessive flare, and choose one which is more modest. The heel counter, or back of the shoe, should be made of a firm material and should fit the heel snugly enough to prevent side-to-side movement. A sloppy-fitting heel counter or one that is made of a soft flexible material puts excessive strain on the heel cord and is a common cause of Achilles tendonitis. A good shoe has a sole and shank which is flexible in the heel/toe direction but has a fair degree of torsional rigidity, thus allowing the foot to bend, but not to twist. The degree of inside padding in the shoe is a matter of personal preference, but the built-in arch support which is now standard in all jogging shoes should at least fit the natural contours of your own arch. Finally, make sure that the toe box is sufficiently spacious to accommodate your toes without cramping; the tip of the big toe or longest toe should be about one thumb's breadth from the end of the shoe; if you have high flexed toes, they should not rub against the top of the shoe. A marathon jogger's feet will swell during the 26-mile jog and if the shoes do not allow for this (not infrequently the swelling amounts to half a size), then expect to finish with blackened toe nails.

By watching the jogger in action, or even while he is walking, you can detect a number of defects which are characteristically associated with the more common over-use injuries. In the normal stride, the leg and foot pass through the *swing* phase (when the foot is in the air), and the *stance* phase (when the foot is in contact with the ground). The stance phase can be divided into three stages — heel-strike, mid-stance and toe-off. Our major interest is in the stance phase. The heel should strike the ground slightly to the outside of a vertical line drawn through the centre of the heel bone. Proof that the heel-strike is correct can be found by inspecting the jogger's shoes. The maximal point of heel wear should be about a half an inch to the outside of the mid-line. As the body's centre of gravity moves forward and over the heel, weight-bearing continues along the outer aspect of the foot to the base of the little toe. This is the stage of mid-stance. Finally, as the heel leaves the ground, more weight is taken in sequence by the heads of the fourth, third, second and first metatarsals — that is, the bases of the fourth, third, second and big toes. At the time of take-off, then, most of the body weight is over the base of the first and second toes, the area commonly known as the ball of the foot. If the gait is normal, inspection of the shoe will show the maximal area of wear in the sole to be the outside edge and the area just over the point where the first and second toes bend up during toe-off.

The precise mechanics of gait are, of course, a great deal more complex than I have described. For the detection of simple gait disorders such as are associated with the more common jogging injuries, however, a knowledge of the basics will suffice.

To begin with, however, it is important to understand what is meant by the terms *pronation* and *supination*. Since there is a tendency at the moment to ascribe practically all jogging injuries to defects in gait or malalignment of the feet, these two terms have been working overtime. In essence, they both describe the position of the feet in two extremes of rotation around an imaginary axis which extends from the centre of the back of the heel through the full length of the foot and out through the tip of the second toe. Inward rotation of the foot around that line is termed pronation; outward rotation, supination. You can observe these positions on your own feet by carrying out the following manoeuvre. Stand with your feet about 18 inches apart, the toes pointing forward; without sliding your feet, rotate your upper body as far as it will go to the left. Your right foot is now in extreme pronation, with the inside border, or longitudinal arch, touching the floor and the heel bone canted outward. The left foot has assumed the position of extreme supination, with the outside border of the foot jammed against the floor, the longitudinal arch high and withdrawn from the floor, and the heel bone canted inward.

Pronation and supination should not be thought of as twin evils. As a matter of fact, the foot is in slight pronation during the heel-strike portion of the stance stage, and then becomes supinated through the stages of mid-stance and toe-off. So pronation and supination must occur if the gait is to be normal. When the foot is in the pronated position, it is mobile, with all the joints flexible and loose. In the supinated position, joint motion is more limited and the foot is rigid. It is this ability to flow easily from a supple to a rigid position that imparts to the normal foot its amazing versatility. Not only is it capable of supporting the entire body weight concentrated through its small surface area, but it can also act as a fulcrum over which that weight shifts safely and smoothly.

Excessive pronation is the cause of a number of injuries to the foot, the bones of the lower leg and the knee. The feet are frequently in the "ten-to-two" position, toeing outward in the standing position and also in walking and jogging. The heel strikes the ground on its outside edge rather than just half an inch or so lateral to the centre line, and the feet have a flat appearance. When viewed from behind in the standing position, the heel cords, instead of bisecting the heel, appear to be displaced inward. This is because the heel bone itself is tilted outward. A glance at the shoe shows much more wear to the outside of the heel than normal.

Excessive pronation may be due to abnormalities of the muscles or joints of the foot itself, so-called fixed pronation. Or it may be the result of malalignments elsewhere in the leg, in which case it is known as compensatory pronation. You can demonstrate the most common form of compensatory pronation by carrying out the following experiment. Stand with your feet about 6 inches apart, the toes pointing forward. Then, with the ankle completely relaxed so that the foot droops down and the knee held straight, raise one foot off the ground by a "shrugging" action of the hip. Now rotate the hip outward; the leg and foot will follow suit. A short step with this leg will result in the foot striking the floor in an exaggeratedly pronated action. This exercise shows that if you hold your hip externally rotated you will have a marked pronated gait and will suffer from all of the difficulties associated with it. What is the cause of the externally rotated hip? In the vast majority of cases, tightness or shortening of the hamstrings and external rotator muscles which straighten and externally rotate the hip joint. The cure for this type of compensatory pronation is to carry out stretching exercises for the shortened muscles. There was a time in my distant youth when army physical fitness instructors and the like taught that the correct way to stand and walk was with the toes pointing slightly outward. The hip joint, of course, had to follow suit and also rotates outward. After a number of years, the hip joint muscles which normally carry out this rotatory action become shortened, and so we now have a permanent case of compensatory pronated gait.

There are two causes of excessive pronation which one comes across from time to time. If you ask the jogger to stand up straight with knees touching and find that he can then not place his heels together, he is displaying evidence of knock-knee deformity. The effect of this on the feet will be to bring the inner borders closer to the floor, thus exaggerating pronation. A jogger who can stand straight with heels together but then has a wide space between his knees is suffering from bow legs. The bow-legged individual again has to pronate both feet excessively to get the inner borders of his feet to the floor.

Excessive supination of the feet is much rarer than excessive pronation, and is usually found in the individual with a high arch. The supinated foot is a locked and rigid structure which transmits the shock of heel-strike abruptly to the bones of the lower leg and knee. Small wonder that the deformity is associated with fatigue fractures of the foot and leg. Protection from this should be sought in shoes which have good interior padding and more than the average degree of resilience and softness in the sole and heel. Jogging over rough uneven surfaces should be avoided.

Whether the pronation or supination deformity is fixed or compensatory, its ill effects can often be counteracted by the use of modifications to the shoe. These can either be *external* or *internal*. The commonest type of external modification is the heel wedge, which is placed on the inside or outside edge of the heel, depending upon the deformity being treated. Basically, the wedge is intended to restore the heel bone from its tilted position to a more vertical one. Obviously if the heel moves inside the shoe, then the wedge is of little use. Other examples of external modifications are sole wedges, transverse bars at various points on the sole, and "raises" of different heights. However, the internal shoe modification, or *orthotic,* is frequently used. We seem to have reached a stage where the jogger without an orthotic feels underprivileged. There are five basic types of internal shoe modification commonly prescribed and made by the orthotist. They are the longitudinal arch support, the metatarsal arch support, the internal heel wedge, the heel bar, and the internal heel lift or pad. The longitudinal arch support is most useful in the treatment of excessive pronation. Such inserts can be either soft (made out of moleskin, orthopedic felt or piano felt), semi-rigid (made out of cork, leather, fibreglass and flexible plastics), or rigid (made out of rigid plastic and acrylic). These orthotic devices can be transferred from shoe to shoe, but the rigid, and sometimes the semi-rigid, types are made from a casted model of the foot and can be very expensive, costing anywhere from $100 to $250. The rigid ones take some getting used to, and many joggers have difficulty tolerating them unless they are extremely accurately fitted and made. Obviously, not all cases of pronated foot require a rigid orthotic device. In many cases, the semi-rigid type will do, and if you want to save money, you can always try the type of arch support obtainable in any drug store first; it usually costs less than $10. The grossly deformed foot which is the source of recurring injuries, however, will inevitably require custom-made orthoses.

Finally, let me again stress that jogging technique is all-important in avoiding injury or reawakening an old one. The pace should be comfortable, the body erect and the stride short. If you visualize your foot landing flat rather than with an exaggerated heel-first or toe-first strike, then not only will the foot behave normally, but your speed will be more controlled. A loose arm carriage with the elbows bent to about 30° or 40° short of a right angle (so that the hands are held at about hip level), relaxed shoulders and neck muscles, and the head erect — all contribute to a controlled jogging posture which is free of strain and tension and less prone to bodily hurt. At the time of writing, close to 3,000 post-coronary patients have passed through the Toronto Rehabilitation Centre's exercise program. They have logged over a million hours of walking and jogging. The incidence of injury is extremely small, and I can number in single figures the patients who have been forced out of the program through an injury which was resistant to treatment. Yet the average age of the men is 48, the women 53. The program has its fair share of individuals with pronated feet, histories of back trouble, old football knee injuries, all the wear-and-tear problems to which joints are prone with the passing years. The low incidence of injury is due entirely to a combination of careful jogging technique, insistence upon suitable jogging shoes, and a training procedure which stresses slow build-up over a period of many months.

Common Jogging Injuries and Related Medical Problems

Runner's Knee   This is not a medical term, but has been coined in recent years to describe pain in the knee which afflicts some long distance runners. In a typical case, pain is experienced usually over the inside but sometimes over the outside of the knee joint. The pain comes on anywhere from three to ten miles into a jog, and can be severe. There is rarely any redness or swelling present, but pressure over the painful area will usually elicit discomfort. On occasion, the complaint will be of pain under the kneecap. In severe cases, the pain is brought on not only by running, but also by anything which causes the front thigh muscles to contract strongly — for example, doing a full squat or climbing stairs.

The knee joint is a complex structure and obviously the causes of pain can be many and varied. Most physicians, therefore, feel the term runner's knee can be a catch-all for a number of conditions involving any one of the various tissues and structures which contribute to the joint and its action. For our purposes we will restrict its use to knee pain brought about by faulty gait associated with exaggerated foot pronation. As we have seen, the pronated foot tends to "toe out," with resultant outward rotation of the entire leg, including the hip joint. This puts the knee at a mechanical disadvantage. The hinge has to move obliquely to the body's line of progression instead of parallel with it. There is an abnormal pulling force to the inner side of the joint, resulting in strain and inflammation of the structures in that area. In addition a grating develops between the kneecap and thigh bone, causing its under-surface to become painfully roughened and eroded. This latter condition is known medically as *chondromalacia patellae*. Since the kneecap is attached to the upper end of the shin bone (or tibia) by a tendon (the patellar tendon), the grating can also involve this structure, inflaming it and giving rise to the condition of *patellar tendonitis*.

Satisfactory treatment almost invariably requires correction of the pronation deformity by means of an orthotic device. This doesn't have to be of the rigid custom-made type. Indeed, you should first try a temporary soft support which you can make yourself or, if you wish, buy a semi-rigid one from the drug store. It should lift and support the arch of the foot and also the inner side of the heel bone. If you find after two or three weeks that this is not helping, then you may have to consider the more expensive orthotic. If the hip tends to externally rotate, then stretching exercises for the hamstring and hip rotators should be instituted. Quadriceps strengthening exercises are essential, but because of the undersurface roughening of the patella, they should be of the isometric or static weight-loading type with the knee joint fully extended as described on page 210. If quadriceps exercises are not carried out and a jogger begins to favour the leg by restricting knee movement, noticeable wasting of the thigh muscles will occur within a matter of two or three weeks. An elastic knee support should never be worn; it tends to press the kneecap against the thigh bone. You can modify the support, however, by cutting out a hole through which the kneecap protrudes; this will relieve the pain, and can be used while jogging. In the early acute stages of the condition, ice therapy will help and later heat in the form of hot packs or short-wave diathermy can be tried. Aspirin will also help.

Don't expect a cure in a matter of days; it may take months. That is not to say that you won't be able to jog for months. You can keep going if you slow your pace, avoid hills, stay off roads which are highly cambered, avoid rough surfaces, and maintain a good jogging technique. Don't be afraid to back off your workouts for a day or two if the condition flares up, but start up again as soon as you notice signs of recovery. Don't become discouraged if progress seems to be slow. In some cases it can take as long as a year for the condition to resolve, and even then it has a tendency to recur from time to time.

Shin Splints   This again is an imprecise term which has no medical meaning, although it is very familiar to physicians who make a habit of treating injured track men or joggers. It merely means pain in the shin region. It can occur in two forms, depending on the location of the pain. An *anterior* shin splint refers to pain felt in the muscle of the front of the lower leg and along the outside border of the shin bone. The commonest causes are over-striding, the wearing of shoes which are too heavy, excessive downhill running, pronated foot deformity, and strength imbalance between the muscles of the calf and front of the leg.

In all these situations the front lower leg muscle (the anterior tibial muscle) is being made to work too hard. In the case of over-striding, the toes and forefoot are too high in the air at the moment of heel-strike, and so, in order to prevent uncontrolled foot-slap, the anterior tibial muscle has to work like a stay-rope, gradually paying out the tendons attached to the top of the foot and letting the sole meet the ground with a minimum of shock. Repeat this thousands of times in a run, and you can see why the muscle would start to complain of over-use. Heavy shoes require effort to keep the toes from stubbing against the ground during the swing-through phase of jogging — again, extra work for the anterior tibial muscle. Pronated feet are "loose" feet, and the excessive joint mobility has to be compensated for by additional muscular work. As for the muscle strength imbalance, most joggers have very powerful calf muscles which tend to overpower the anterior tibial muscles. Since the action of the calf muscles is to rotate the foot downward, and the action of the anterior tibial muscle is to pull the foot upward, it can be readily seen that weak anterior tibials are constantly fighting to resist the action of the calf muscles.

There is another symptom sometimes associated with anterior shin splints. Because the anterior tibial muscle shares a rather cramped compartment in the front of the leg with both a nerve and an artery, swelling of the muscle due to over-use sometimes compresses both these structures, particularly the nerve. This results in numbness and tingling in the foot and sometimes stubbing of the toe because of weakness in pulling the toes up during the swing phase.

In the acute stages of anterior shin splints, treatment consists of ice massage. Correction of over-striding, choosing shoes of suitable weight, the fitting of an orthotic device, and strengthening exercises for the anterior tibial muscle are all measures to be used if indicated. Once the cause of the condition has been established, then the treatment becomes obvious.

Posterior shin splints describes pain in the lower leg along the inside border of the shin bone. Again, the culprit is the pronated foot. To understand this, you have to realize that one of the major deep muscles of the calf, the tibialis posterior, is attached at its upper end to the back and inner border of the shin bone and then forms a tendon which hooks around the inside of the ankle to fan out and be attached to most of the bones which form the sole of the foot. The action of the muscle is to pull the foot into the supinated position. Therefore in the pronated foot, the tibialis posterior muscle is working constantly to correct the deformity. The greater degree of pronation during jogging, the greater the likelihood that the muscle will give trouble. First, the workload may be so great that tiny parts of the muscle attachment to the back and side of the shin bone tear away. In a bad case of posterior shin splints, you can feel tiny bumps if you run your finger along the inside border of the shin. These can be very tender and probably represent the areas where fibres of the muscle have pulled away from the bone. This is the commonest presentation of the condition. Another symptom of the overworked tibialis posterior is pain and swelling just behind and beneath the inner ankle bone, where the tendon is constantly sliding back and forth through a tunnel formed by bone and fibrous tissue. If this movement is excessive, then the tendon becomes inflamed, swollen and sore. The way to treat posterior shin splints is to correct the pronation deformity. In the acute stage, once again one can use ice massage to the painful area, and reduce the workouts to a level which do not cause pain.

I have heard it said that shin splints occur most frequently in inexperienced runners whose enthusiasm leads them to change too rapidly from slow running to speed training, or from soft to hard running surfaces. This may be so, but I haven't found that the novice has any monopoly on these errors, and, in fact, some of the most stubborn cases I have ever treated have been in world-class distance runners. In these individuals, excessive mileage may be an additional aggravating factor, but I am satisfied that in the chronic case, relief can only be achieved by successful treatment of the foot deformity.

Stress Fracture   These are fine, almost invisible, cracks in the bones of the foot or lower leg, and are due to excessive mileage, faulty jogging technique, foot or leg deformity, non-resilient shoes or a combination of any or all of these factors. In a way, they resemble the fatigue faults that develop in a metal that has been exposed to excessive stress. The symptom of the stress fracture is pain, usually severe enough to stop your jogging, present at night, and throbbing in character. Occasionally, there will be swelling also. Tapping the bone in the area of the stress fracture will aggravate the pain. X-rays are of little value, since the crack is so fine that it doesn't appear on the x-ray until it has started to heal and lay down a fine line of extra calcium which then shows up on the x-ray plate. The treatment is rest. On no account try to run through a stress fracture; otherwise, you will only delay healing. The healing period is about six weeks, and during that time, you should attempt to maintain your fitness level by switching to some non-weight-bearing exercise like swimming or cycling. There is no need for you to sit around and mope because you are missing your customary daily jog.

Most stress fractures occur in one of the long bones (metatarsals) of the foot, although they can also occur in the two long bones of the lower leg (the tibia and fibula). A stress fracture in the tibia should be treated more seriously than elsewhere because this bone bears a good deal of the body's weight and occasionally even excessive walking may extend the fine hairline crack into an out-and-out break. Otherwise, stress fractures heal very well. Indeed, the bone is a good deal stronger after healing than it was before. If you wish to avoid a recurrence of the condition, you have to be careful not to repeat the cause. Since the supinated foot is more susceptible because of its relative inability to absorb landing shock, insoles and well-padded shoes are a must.

Runner's Heel   The muscles of the sole of the foot are covered by the plantar fascia, a sheet of tough tissue which is attached to the front of the heel bone, passes forward under the longitudinal arch and then fans out to insert into the under-surfaces of the toe bones. Because of its fore and aft attachments, it acts as a sort of tie, joining the two ends of the bony arch of the foot. Since this arch flattens when the foot is taking body weight and resumes its curved shape when the foot is off the ground, the plantar fascia is being stretched and relaxed with every step. Excessive mileage, or unaccustomed sprinting (an action which requires powerful "toe-off") or just the old fault of too much too soon, can result in plantar fasciitis, or inflammation of the structure. Microscopic tearing of fibres occur at the attachment of the heel bone and sometimes further forward, closer to the arch of the foot. The complaint is one of pain under the heel just where the heel pad joins the arch when walking or jogging, and pressure in this region, even when the foot is resting, reproduces the discomfort.

Runner's heel is particularly likely if you start to train too vigorously after a long lay-off. The weeks of inactivity tend to tighten and weaken the plantar fascia. Shoes that have poor arch supports or are too stiff, requiring a vigorous toe-off in order to bend them, will obviously throw an extra strain on the fascia. On occasion, the area where the fibres pull away from the front of the heel bone becomes infiltrated with calcium and forms a so-called spur, which is seen on an x-ray. Some surgeons advocate the removal of this spur, although in my experience this rarely helps. The general treatment is to look for and eliminate the cause; however, in the early, very painful phase, an internal heel raise with a cut-out which coincides with the painful area, together with an arch support, will help. Some physicians advise local cortisone injections, but while this does relieve some of the inflammation and soften the scar tissue, it may cause even more tearing to occur especially if the individual persists with his jogging. Cortisone should only be used as a last resort, and then only if you are prepared to lay off for a period of one week after the injection. Physical therapy treatments consist of ice massage, or application of ultra-sound.

Achilles Tendonitis   This is the inflammation of the heel cord and is a major headache for a significant number of runners. The reason is not hard to find. Even under normal everyday circumstances, the heel cord has to take an incredible strain. If you balance on one foot, and then stand on tip-toe, your heel cord is being subjected to a pulling force equivalent to twice your body weight. For the average jogger, that means some 250 to 300 lbs. on each heel cord with each step. If you start to sprint, which means landing and driving off the toes rather than the heel or flat foot, then the strain is even greater. Actually, the healthy heel cord, or Achilles tendon, is capable of taking the strain of up to 5,000 to 6,000 lbs. per square inch before it snaps, and can bear about one third of this weight with perfect safety. Notice, however, that I said the *healthy* tendon. By the time we get into our mid-thirties, the blood supply to the tendons begins to get less, with the result that the safety level begins to drop. This is why in elderly individuals an apparently minor strain, such as stepping awkwardly off the curb, can result in rupture of the tendon. While a partial or even complete tear can occur in joggers, it is relatively rare. More likely are the repeated microscopic tears in the deep fibres of the tendon, resulting in a generalized inflammation. The commonest causes are tight heel cords (you should make a point of carrying out stretching exercises to alleviate this), a shoe with an inadequate heel lift or one which allows the heel to wobble from side to side, running up hills, excessive speed work, or running on the toes. If you have perfected the short stride, flat-foot landing, then you should rarely be troubled with Achilles tendonitis.

In the early stages of the condition, the jogger notices aching pain in the heel cords both during and after the run. He finds that when he gets up in the morning, he has to hobble across the room for the first few minutes before the tendons loosen up. As the condition develops, swelling and thickening is apparent. The treatment consists of reducing the intensity and duration of the workouts, adding a half-inch heel raise, and correcting any shoe faults. Ice massage can be carried out after each jogging session, and aspirin often helps. In severe cases, the physician may want to apply a plaster cast to prevent the tendon moving too much during ordinary walking. I have rarely found this necessary, and when it is, an attempt should be made to find an alternative form of exercise for the sufferer. Under no circumstances should cortisone injections be given into the tendon. This is only likely to soften the tissue up and lead to an extension of the tear, or even a fully fledged rupture. If the tendon does tear through, then surgical repair will be necessary. Ultra-sound using a technique in which it is given through water may help to reduce chronic inflammation. In the final analysis, however, improvement in jogging technique is the only answer.

Before leaving the subject of Achilles tendonitis, mention should be made of *calcaneal bursitis* or inflammation of the fluid sac which forms an interface between the back of the heel bone and the heel cord at its point of insertion. This is usually caused by ill-fitting shoes which press against the back of the heel and rub up and down with each step. The fluid sac becomes inflamed, reddened and painful. The differentiation between this condition and Achilles tendonitis is largely by location of discomfort. Pain from bursitis is lower down, often over the back of the heel bone itself, and is aggravated by thumb pressure in this area. The cure is removal of the offending pressure from the shoe. In the acute stage, ice, ultra-sound, or even a hydrocortisone injection into the sac itself will bring quick relief.

An occasional cause of foot pain in the jogger is *Morton's metatarsalgia,* named after Dr. T. G. Morton, who first described it in 1876. This is due to the development of a spindle-shaped swelling, or neuroma, about three-quarters of an inch long, on the small nerve which lies between the third and fourth toes. Actually, it is a thickening of the nerve sheath, or covering, which has been irritated by constantly being nipped between the adjoining bones that form the base of the third and fourth toes. It is seen most frequently in an individual with the broad, or splayed, forefoot. It occasionally occurs between the second and third toes, or the fourth and fifth toes. The presenting symptom is sharp or burning pain in the ball of the foot, sometimes shooting into the affected toes. It is not constant, but occurs at varying intervals, and each attack has a sudden onset. Characteristically, relief is not obtained by sitting down and taking weight off the foot, but by taking off the shoe and squeezing or manipulating the forefoot. Diagnosis is usually made on the history, and by the fact that the pain can sometimes be aggravated or brought on by squeezing the bases of the toes together. Very occasionally, it is possible to detect a patch of numbness on the affected toes. X-rays are negative, since nerve tissue doesn't register on an x-ray plate. Treatment consists of altering the alignment of the toe bones by the use of an orthopedic felt insert which raises one of the two offending toe bones so it no longer squeezes the nerve. A shoe with a broad toe box is also advised. In addition, injections of cortisone and local anesthetic between the affected toes can often help. In the last resort, the neuroma can be removed by a relatively simple surgical procedure.

Ever since the New Jersey cardiologist Dr. George Sheehan referred to the subject of Morton's Toe in his *Runner's World* column, joggers have become excessively conscious of the length of their toes. Dr. Dudley J. Morton, in his book, *The Human Foot,* described a congenital abnormality consisting primarily of a shortened big toe or, more precisely, a shortened first metatarsal (the long bone which extends from the base of the big toe to the apex of the longitudinal arch). Because of this shortening, the big toe cannot take its fair share of bearing the body's weight, with the result that the second toe and the corresponding second metatarsal bone have to take an additional load. The result is a painful callous on the ball of the foot under the second toe and discomfort in the forefoot due to the excessive motion of the second metatarsal. X-rays will show the shortened first metatarsal, and also a thickening in width of the shaft of the second metatarsal, due entirely to its extra weight-bearing chores. This is the so-called atavistic foot, or Morton's Toe. How common is it? Not very, in its classical and complete form. Just because your second toe is a smidgeon longer than your big toe doesn't give you the right to blame Dudley Morton for all your foot woes. In short, I suspect the condition is probably grossly over-diagnosed.

The condition can be relieved by fashioning a metatarsal insert which, by providing a platform under the base of the big toe, shifts the maximum point of weight-bearing away from the second toe back to where it belongs. The painful callous under the second toe, if present, is pared down and should not recur.

Hematuria   This is the medical term for the passage of blood-stained urine. It can occur in long distance runners and joggers after a particularly hard workout. Needless to say, it is a frightening symptom, especially since, in a sedentary individual, it usually heralds disease of the kidney or lower urinary tract. However, careful investigation of a large number of marathon runners who were found to have the problem failed to reveal any evidence of the disease. What then is the cause of the bleeding? Until recently, we assumed that it was due to a temporary failure of the kidneys' filtering system, allowing red blood cells to leak into the urine along with other waste products being excreted. Since the filtration failure was temporary, no structural damage ensued, and investigations found nothing. But in 1977, a British surgeon, Dr. N. J. Blacklock, came up with an alternative explanation. By passing an instrument through the penis and into the bladder of runners with "10,000 metre hematuria," he observed that the back wall of the bladder showed considerable bruising and tiny bleeding points. He concluded that this was the origin of the bleeding and that the state of the posterior wall was due to repeated banging against the base of the bladder during running.

The only way that this could happen would be if the bladder were flaccid, or empty. On questioning the runners, it was indeed found that invariably they had not taken any fluid before or during their runs. The moral, then, is never to undertake a long, hard jog without ensuring a partially full bladder by adequate intake of fluids.

Not all red-stained urine contains blood. On occasions, the colour may be due to the breakdown of red cells, releasing the pigment from the blood protein hemoglobin into the urine. Why do the red cells break down? The theory is that as they pass through the fine blood vessels in the sole of the feet, the more fragile ones are literally pounded apart with the impact of each jogging step. Hemoglobin pigment is a harmless substance and its excretion does not damage the kidney. The remedy for the situation is to be found in good-quality jogging shoes which contain well-padded soles.

Another brownish-coloured substance which when present in the urine may mimic hematuria is myoglobin. This is a muscle protein, and its presence in the urine indicates some muscle destruction, the commonest causes of which are severe and exhausting bouts of exercise, or advanced dehydration amounting almost to heat stroke. Neither of these situations should occur, except in the most imprudent or fanatical jogger. Myoglobinuria is a dangerous business. The muscle breakdown substance does not pass easily through the kidney and can, in fact, block its filtration mechanism and lead to renal failure and death.

In general, then, blood-stained urine occurring occasionally in a long distance jogger is a benign condition which can be controlled by ensuring a partially full bladder. However, a sample of the urine should be examined by a physician to confirm that no other substances are present which might indicate true kidney disease. The bleeding usually clears up quite rapidly, within a couple of days. If it lasts longer, however, or recurs frequently, then the physician should assume it is due to some other abnormality until thorough investigations have proved the contrary.

Minor Discomforts and Irritations   It is the little things that get you. You finish your first marathon, you bask in the awe-struck deference of your sedentary fellow species, and that night you drift off to sleep in a mood of jubilant ecstasy — only to get out of bed the next morning, and find that you have developed an exquisitely painful pea-sized bluish swelling at the edge of your anus. Which reduces your triumphant healthy stride into the office into a sort of crab-like shuffle. You have developed a thrombosed *external hemorrhoid*. It is really nothing to do with the internal hemorrhoids that sedentary individuals frequently complain of; this is a clotting of blood in a small subcutaneous vein close to the opening of the anus, and it is caused by friction. Despite the acute pain, it usually settles down of its own accord within a few days. If not, then the out-patient treatment is evacuation of the hardened clot by making a small incision through the wall of the vein after injection of a local anaesthetic. Prevention is easy. Just apply a liberal amount of vaseline between the buttocks before the marathon starts.

Muscle stiffness after a lengthy jog can be avoided. The longer you have been jogging, the less likely you are to be bothered by this problem. However, it can be a nuisance, and in the early stages of your jogging career, you may find that large doses of Vitamin C (500 to 1,000 mg daily) may help. If you can manage to jog just two or three miles the day after a long run, it helps to relieve muscle discomfort. The first few steps may be difficult, but take your time, don't be afraid to walk every so often, and you'll be surprised to find that at the end of the first few miles, you feel a good deal better.

Numbness of the toes, usually the third, fourth and fifth, bothers some joggers. It usually comes on after about five or six miles, and once started, is difficult to relieve except by slowing to a walk. You can avoid the problem by lacing your shoes quite loosely or, better still, not lacing the bottom two or three holes. Again, prevention is better than cure. I find that once the numbness commences on a run, even loosening your laces helps only partially. The high arched foot is particularly susceptible to this condition. When buying jogging shoes, it is better to choose ones in which the lace holes are continued down to the level of the toes; this allows you to ensure looseness at the lower levels.

Some joggers complain of *swollen, tingling fingers* after a lengthy workout. This may be due to two causes. Holding the elbows in the bent position for too long without straightening them restricts blood flow and so gives rise to a puffy swelling which, in turn, causes the nerves of the fingers to tingle. Middle-aged joggers who have wear and tear degenerative changes of their spine and run with hunched shoulders and tight neck muscles may compress the roots of the nerves which emerge between the neck vertebrae and pass down through the arms to the hands. This will also cause tingling and numbness. Learn, then, to run loosely, with relaxed shoulder and neck muscles, occasional straightening of the elbows and clenching and un-clenching of the fingers.

Nipple irritation, soreness, and even frank bleeding will occur during a long jog in hot weather when the running shirt becomes soaked in sweat and rubs against the unprotected nipples. Vaseline is the runner's friend. It should be applied liberally to all potential areas of friction, especially the nipples, in the anal cleft and the insides of the thighs.

Regular joggers expose their skin to the sun for long periods of time. In the sunnier climates, this can lead to bad cases of *sunburn,* especially in light-skinned individuals. The best solution is to apply any one of the commercial sun screens which contain the substance Paba. You can use these in various strengths, depending on the susceptibility of your skin to sunshine. I have had good results with Pre-Sun, and Coppertone's Supershade, both screens containing 5 per cent Paba. (The former stains clothing slightly.) Some individuals are allergic to Paba, and so they should try a small amount first and then check for the development of a skin rash. Heavy sweating will tend to dilute the effect of the screen; reapply it every hour or so. Tanning oils do not give adequate protection and, in fact, in a very hot sun, merely "fry" the skin. Remember to wear a hat with a sufficiently wide brim to protect your face. White clothing tends to reflect the sun, but the light material of a running shirt will often let a high percentage of the sun's rays through. The more porous the material, the more likely this is to happen. Constant over-exposure to sun and wind will dry your skin out, and age it prematurely. Both in winter and summer, then, it makes sense to apply a protective cream or lotion. Skin cancer is on the increase, and is directly related to the number of hours of expo-sure to the sun. It is slow-growing, does not spread to other parts of the body, and can be cured by a simple surgical excision or exposure to radiotherapy, but better to avoid it in the first place. Classically, the skin cancer appears anywhere on the face above the level of the mouth, commences as a small pearl-like tumour with raised edges and dimpled centre, often with a scale-like covering from a slight discharge. If you knock this transparent crust off, it quickly forms again. Anything resembling this should be checked out by your dermatologist.

The Air We Breathe

If you live in a large city, you have to be prepared to pay a price for the vocational and avocational advantages of massive "togetherness." There, in a word, I may have alienated those readers whose whole aim in life is to find some quiet, sparsely populated retreat in which only the sound of the wind or sea or solitary bird call disturbs their contemplative life. So be it. I have always loved cities, and found their fascinating mix of inhabitants both personally and professionally stimulating. I am aware of the dire predictions about the imminent demise of the urban way of life; yet, like the hundreds of millions of city dwellers all over the world, I continue to live where I feel I can best fulfill my mental, emotional and material wants.

There are, of course, drawbacks to this type of living. Among other things, we have to contend with the pollution of our air by the waste products of our automobiles and our industrial plants. Lately, the jogger has had to contend with the charge that all of the benefits which he thought he was getting from his hobby are being neutralized by the increased inhalation of these harmful substances. All that huffing and puffing, say the local Jeremiahs, fill your lungs with so much poison that you would be better off sitting in your living room with all the doors and windows tightly closed, watching television and enjoying a six-pack. I think this argument may be somewhat exaggerated.

What are the common air pollutants? What affect do they have on us? The answer to the first question depends to some extent on the area in which you live. In Los Angeles, for instance, the pollutants are composed largely of compounds that arise from the chemical interaction between sunlight and the various combustible products of automobile fumes. In other cities, we may be dealing predominantly with carbon monoxide, sulphur dioxide, or a number of airborne chemicals in particulate form.

Carbon monoxide is a major component of cigarette smoke, and we have already described its cuckoo-like occupancy of the red cells of the blood, displacing the vital oxygen being carried to the body's cells. Inhaled even in minute quantities by the jogger, in theory, it could reduce the efficiency of his oxygen transport system and turn an easy workout into a relatively tough one. Inhalation of enough carbon monoxide to affect about 20 per cent of hemoglobin, the oxygen-carrying protein in the blood, will lead to headache behind and over the eyes, breathlessness, muscular weakness and dizziness. When about 40 per cent of the available hemoglobin is saturated with carbon monoxide, there is a feeling of nausea together with dimming and blurring of vision; judgment becomes impaired and the individual becomes belligerent.

Since the major source of carbon monoxide is from automobile exhaust fumes, the highest concentration will be along heavily travelled highways. Exhaust smoke disperses slowly, so if your regular jogging route is 40 to 60 feet or more away from the edge of a busy highway, you should be home free.

Ozone is a key component in the smog which results from the action of sunlight on fuel oil hydrocarbons and nitrogen dioxide. It has been found in aircraft cabins at altitudes above 30,000 feet, and also in association with various welding devices. In recent years, a good deal of work has been done on the effect of ozone on the human body, and while much is still to be learned, we do have some indications that in high concentrations (greater than 0.15 parts per million of air), it can have some toxic effects. Its major target is the respiratory organs, where it can cause breathlessness, chest pain and coughing. Experimental animals have been shown to develop edema of the lungs and pulmonary hemorrhage when exposed to very high concentrations of ozone. In addition to the respiratory symptoms, high ozone levels can cause headaches and reduce one's ability to concentrate. The heart rate may drop, and this can give rise to increases in blood carbon dioxide. At ozone levels in excess of 0.2 parts per million there may be a considerable decrease in central visual acuity and ability to see in the dark, together with an increase in peripheral vision. Some coaches have reported that when ozone levels are high, athletic performance is adversely affected.

A few cities now operate an ozone alert when the level reaches more than 0.15 parts per million, which warns susceptible individuals to reduce physical exertion. When the level becomes in excess of 0.2 parts per million, even healthy persons should limit their outdoor exercise. It is possible, however, to defeat the ozone problem if you remember one or two basic principles. In the first place, keep in mind that on a sunny, humid day the maximal ozone levels are between 11 a.m. and 6 p.m., and the lowest levels are in the early morning. Therefore, if you wish to be on the safe side, run early in the morning or late at night. Older individuals (and that means us) are more susceptible to the effects of ozone than young people. Don't forget that the hotter it gets, the more ozone is produced. For instance, a rise of 15°F., from 75°F. to 90°F., doubles the amount of ozone which can be generated. Secondly, if you have a chest infection, you are obviously more susceptible. Interestingly, the ingestion of Vitamin C would appear to substantially reduce the effect of ozone on the lungs. Finally (and this must be a consolation to Los Angeleans), the more exposure you have to ozone, the more likely you are to develop a tolerance toward it. At least you are less likely to be overcome by the more acute and unpleasant symptoms. Whether the long-term effects are worse, only further research and time can tell. Again, a sensible jogger who understands the dangers and is prepared to alter his normal workout times to suit the conditions has little to fear.

There is no doubt that running in the city on a hot, humid, muggy day when the traffic is heavy and the industrial pall is hanging close to the ground can be uncomfortable and sometimes downright unpleasant. Nevertheless, if you follow some of these simple guidelines you should not come to any harm, and the benefits of jogging will far outweigh any minor and transitory discomforts brought about by breathing polluted air.

The Perils of Heat

Whenever I watch an old late-night movie about the exploits of the British army in India or the French Foreign Legion in the Sahara, I make a bet with myself that more soldiers or legionnaires died from dehydration than ever succumbed to a tribesman's bullet. In those days, the way to avoid sunstroke was to protect the head and back of the neck. The most essential article of tropical kit was the pith helmet; it practically became the symbol of Empire, the Raj, Kipling and all that. Unfortunately, picturesque as it may have been, the sun helmet did little to protect from the real killer, fluid lack from excessive sweating — in other words, dehydration. But can we, in our daily jog or our easy-going marathon attempt, become dehydrated? If so, can the results really be that serious? What precautions can we take to avoid them? To answer these questions, we should know how dehydration occurs.

Our body temperature results from heat generated by our working muscles and organs and heat absorbed from the surrounding atmosphere. As you sit reading this book, hopefully relaxed and calm, with easy breathing and slowly beating heart, you are generating about 75 calories of heat every hour. If you were to put the book down (not yet, please), stand up and go for a three-mile walk, you would have generated about 300 calories. Intense brief activity can burn about 800 to 900 calories an hour.

If the body had no means of dissipating its internal heat, then even under resting conditions, your temperature would rise about 2°F. (1°C.) an hour; under moderate working conditions, the rise would be in the order of 9°F. (5°C.) an hour. Like any other machine, the body has a temperature at which all the various parts function most efficiently, 98.6°F. (37°C.). If the inside temperature of the body climbs above 108°F. (42°C.) or falls below 84°F. (29°C.), essential organs such as the heart, kidneys and liver, cease to work, and death is imminent. But since, as we have seen, even staying alive generates enough heat to kill us in a matter of hours, we must have a very efficient mechanism of dissipating this excess heat and holding the body temperature consistently close to the 98.6°F. level. How does this system work?

Exercising requires oxygen, and this results in the shunting of as much as a gallon of blood through the blood vessels of the muscles every minute. Since these muscles are working, their internal temperature is raised, and this heats the blood which passes through them. This heated blood then returns to the heart where it is pumped around the body again. As it flows through the brain, it triggers off the "Benzinger Reflex," a mechanism by which the blood vessels to the skin are reflexly opened up and the sweat glands stimulated to work overtime. Warm blood can now dissipate its heat into the surrounding cooler air by the processes of convection, conduction and radiation. Notice I said *cooler* air — that is, air temperature lower than the skin temperature. What happens when the air temperature is high, approaching that of the skin? Under these circumstances, the body has to depend more and more on the evaporation of sweat to drop the body temperature. The mere act of sweating has no cooling effect per se; it is the vapourization, or evaporation of the sweat from the surface of the body which is all important.

A 1-calorie increase in body heat can be balanced by the evaporation of about 1.5 c.c. of sweat. But there is a limit to the rate at which one can sweat. In the average unconditioned individual, this amounts to about two to three pints per hour; in a trained, heat-acclimatized jogger, this figure may be increased to as much as five pints per hour.

Evaporation of sweat can be influenced by a number of conditions. If the air is humid, it is already saturated with moisture and cannot accept any more. So the sweat will not vapourize; it will merely drip down the face and body like water, in which form it cannot have a cooling effect. In conditions of very high humidity, therefore, sweating becomes less effective as a means of reducing body temperature.

On a windy day, the mechanism of evaporation has an advantage. The air next to the sweating skin, as soon as it becomes heavily laden with sweat moisture, is blown away, and its place is taken by air which is drier and more receptive to further vapourization.

Clothing is an important factor. It should allow free movement of air over the skin. Trapped pockets of air become saturated with vapourized sweat and prevent further evaporation from that area. Air is a very good insulator, and prevents body heat from escaping by conduction or radiation. Perfect examples of clothing which prevent adequate heat loss are the rubberized training suit, or the footballer's uniform, with its plastic helmet and padding, designed to protect against bodily contact injury but not against the ill effects of high heat conditions. Deaths from heat stroke due to the wearing of such apparel are, sad to say, recorded from time to time in the medical literature.

The fourth condition affecting sweat evaporation has to do with blood volume. Why is it that when you go for a long jog on a very hot day (usually the first hot day of the summer, when you are not as yet acclimatized to the heat), you tire so quickly? As we have seen, a portion of your circulating blood volume is shunted into your muscles during exercise; furthermore, because of the heat of the day, you are sweating heavily and losing water from your blood stream at a rate of five pints an hour. Unless you replace the sweat loss by drinking fluids, the net result will be a reduction in blood volume. But as long as you keep jogging, your muscles require oxygen and thus your heart is committed to pumping a steady supply of oxygen-laden blood to the scene of action. With the drop in the amount of blood available, however, there is a concomitant drop in the amount ejected with each heart beat — i.e., the stroke volume. The only way that the heart can now maintain its output of blood is by increasing the number of strokes per minute. In other words, the heart rate must go up if the heart is to maintain an adequate blood supply to the exercising muscles.

But, as we have seen in Chapter Three, each of us has a maximum heart rate; if we continue to jog at the same intensity, this maximum is eventually reached. When that happens, cardiac output cannot keep pace with demand. Actually, we can gain a very slight respite by constricting the blood vessels of the skin, a stratagem which can be detected by the sudden change which occurs in the jogger's complexion, from ruddy and sweating to ashen pale. This constriction of the skin's blood vessels shunts some blood back into the central pool, raising the central blood volume, and making more blood available, again, for the heart to pump. For a short period of time, stroke volume increases and cardiac output is maintained. Unfortunately, the price you have paid for this temporary postponement of the inevitable is a high one. By diverting blood away from the skin, you have deprived yourself of your major mechanism of heat loss. Thus the temperature inside your body rapidly begins to climb and the whole heat control compensatory system begins to break down. Unless you stop exercising, or unless you have been drinking ample quantities of fluid to keep your blood volume up, you have reached the stage of dehydration.

There are three clinical conditions associated with exercising in the hot weather, and although they may merge imperceptibly and insidiously into one another, it leads to a better understanding of the whole mechanism of dehydration if they are dealt with as separate entities.

Heat Cramps   Heat cramps occur in highly trained individuals who have been working out for some time in hot weather. In the case of the jogger, the cramps occur in the legs. They may come on toward the end of a run (the last four or five miles of a marathon) or after the jog, for example, in the shower or walking home. They can be extremely severe and may last for many minutes. Sometimes they involve the muscles of the abdomen and then may simulate a surgical condition, such as an acute appendicitis.

Such cramps are thought to be due to a chronic lack or loss of sodium. As I explained earlier, the highly conditioned athlete has a copious sweat production, much greater than the sedentary individual. While his sweat contains less sodium than normal (the body's attempt to conserve its supply), this can be outbalanced by the speed with which sweating occurs, so that eventually, he tends to lose sodium. He can replace the fluid by drinking water, but this does not replace sodium. Ingestion of a dilute salt solution (1 teaspoonful of salt to 2 pints of water) will relieve his cramps very rapidly.

The average jogger is not likely to be bothered by this. It is much more frequent in the individual who is training for long periods in the heat, such as the competitive marathon runner who is averaging 150 miles a week in a hot climate. Incidentally, your best source of salt is catsup, bran, fish, nuts and meat. Do not use salt tablets; they are far too concentrated.

Heat Exhaustion   This is due to inadequate replacement of the water lost in sweat. The early signs are fatigue and weakness. I cannot emphasize enough that thirst is a very poor indicator that you need fluid. There are several reasons for this. It has been shown that the mere act of putting something in the mouth, a pebble, for instance, reduces the sensation of thirst for about 15 minutes. Also, laboratory experiments have shown that the introduction of a small amount of fluid through a tube directly into the stomach has the same effect — even though the water has not been absorbed through the stomach wall. So a jogger may take just a mouthful of cold water, swallow it, no longer feel thirsty, and carry on for another half an hour before he feels he needs to drink again. Yet the amount of fluid taken is totally inadequate, and dehydration is inevitable.

With water losses of up to 5 per cent of his body weight, the dehydrated jogger develops a flushed, hot skin, his judgment becomes poor, and he may become inco-ordinated and irrational. I recall an athlete in Boston, screaming at his coach and a group of people who were providing fluid, that they had given him "the wrong bottle." In fact, he was given the fluid that had been made up for him, but in his confused state, he didn't recognize it. It didn't taste right to him, and he became extremely belligerent. After the race, he couldn't remember the incident at all!

Other symptoms of heat exhaustion are light-headedness, a very rapid heart rate, and severe frontal headaches. Heat exhaustion can occur in varying degrees of severity, and may become chronic during a long spell of hot weather training, until noticed by a coach, a friend, or the jogger himself who is familiar with the effects of dehydration. Drinking adequate water before, during and after training jogs is just as important as during a marathon race. Heat exhaustion can also develop rapidly during a run and may progress to heat stroke, the third and most dangerous manifestation of dehydration.

Heat Stroke   Heat stroke is the popular term for hyperpyrexia, that is, body temperature in excess of 108°F. (42°C.). Again, the cause is lack of water. Its onset can be insidious and rapid. The victim, after demonstrating evidence of extreme heat exhaustion, collapses into a coma, from which he may never recover. Death is frequently due to renal failure.

The effects of heat stroke on the body are widespread. In the posterior portion of the brain, the cerebellum, there is destruction of specialized cells. This is why survivors may be left with staggering gait, or speech disorders. Bleeding into the cortex of the brain is responsible for various mental disturbances. The kidneys can be irreparably damaged, making renal dialysis necessary. Hemorrhage into the heart muscle, and even heart attacks in spite of perfectly normal coronary arteries have been reported. The liver may be damaged, causing intense jaundice. Clotting of blood in the blood vessels may lead to damage in a whole host of organs. As you can see, an incredible number of deadly pathological changes all stem from simple failure to drink adequately during a hot weather run.

How to Avoid Dehydration   Anyone who exercises on a hot day, old or young, male or female, jogger or runner, is a potential dehydration victim. If you are a fun jogger, never forget that the number of calories burned (and therefore the amount of body heat generated) doesn't depend on the speed you jog, but rather on the distance you cover. For example, whether you jog three miles in 24 minutes or in 36 you will still burn approximately 300 calories. Actually, the slower the pace, the longer you are exposed to the sun, and so the greater the likelihood of dehydration. The heavier you are, the more calories you will burn as you jog and, therefore, the greater your need for fluid. The following rules apply equally to the middle-aged novice jogger and the highly trained athlete:

1. Allow time for heat acclimatization. The body learns to cope with heat if you give it enough time to adjust. The process takes about 7 to 10 days, and during this time, the workouts should be low key to commence with, gradually building up to your usual intensity and duration. When the temperature is above 85°F. (30°C.) and the humidity above 30 per cent, the cardiac jogger should miss out the session altogether. (See page 294 for use of the Heat Safety Index.)

2. Always prehydrate 10 to 20 minutes or so before exercising on a warm day. Drink about half a pint of fluid, then another half a pint every 20 minutes or so while working out. Don't wait to feel thirsty before drinking. You should train yourself to prehydrate and hydrate, otherwise you won't be able to do it in competition. Carried out for the first time under the stressful conditions of an official marathon, your stomach will feel distended, you won't be able to absorb the fluid, and it will swill around inside you at every step.

3. The best fluid to use is water. It should be comfortably cold (best temperature for absorption is 40°F.), and if you require a flavour you may add a little fruit juice according to taste. Minerals such as sodium and potassium aren't really essential; the body can replace them later. However, if you do add sodium, it should be in small amounts of 4 teaspoons of salt to a gallon of water.

What about potassium? During prolonged physical exertion, potassium leaks out of the muscles, resulting in relatively high levels in the blood. Even though some or this excess is excreted in the urine and sweat, it is rarely enough to drop blood potassium levels below normal. Therefore, there is no need to add potassium to the fluid which is taken during the run. It has been our experience that most proprietary hydration fluids contain too much potassium and, therefore, if given consistently during the marathon, result in excessively high potassium levels. After the run, however, potassium passes back into the muscles, dropping the blood concentration. Therefore, potassium should be used in the post-race drinks, in concentrations about half that normally found in sweat. Diluted orange juice is an excellent source.

Chronic potassium loss in sweat and urine can occur from exhaustive hot-weather training day after day, especially before heat acclimatization takes place. This is best prevented by eating a diet high in potassium-containing foods, e.g., whole grains, nuts, fruits such as bananas, oranges and prunes, tomato catsup. In general, the potassium-deficient athlete will have a craving for such foodstuffs, and will not have to be urged to eat them.

Some post-coronary joggers may be taking hydrochlorothiazide medication, a diuretic which is given to treat mild cases of high blood pressure. Diuretics encourage the kidneys to excrete sodium and, therefore, water. Potassium is lost in the urine at the same time, and the prescribing physician often suggests that a patient on such medication increase his consumption of potassium-containing foods or, alternatively, prescribes a potassium pill to take. Obviously, a patient taking diuretics (trade names, Diural, Hydrodiural, Esiberix) is most susceptible to low blood potassium levels in high heat training and should be aware of this. Too much or too little potassium in the blood can give rise to various abnormalities of cardiac rhythm, and in unexplained cases of palpitations or skipped beats appearing in a healthy jogger, analysis of a blood sample for potassium concentrations should be carried out.

Sugar, usually in the form of glucose, is often added to replacement fluid to provide energy. Actually, there is little to recommend this practice. Glucose solutions which exceed 2.5 per cent strength are too concentrated to be absorbed through the gut wall and therefore lie in the stomach, causing nausea and vomiting. Worse still, to dilute the glucose, water is actually drawn out of the blood stream and cells of the body into the intestine, thus aggravating the dehydration! If, on the other hand, you prepare a solution containing less than 2.5 per cent glucose, the amount of energy provided is probably too small to be of any value.

The best replacement fluid, then, is still cold water, plus a mild flavouring agent if desired.

4. Clothing should be light, porous and comfortable. Fishnet

vests are most suitable, allowing easy circulation of air and free evaporation of sweat from the skin.

5. Cold water sponging helps, as will putting ice under your hat. If you sponge your legs, be careful not to wet your shoes and socks, otherwise you will run into problems with blisters.

6. Get into the habit of weighing yourself naked before and after each workout. If you have hydrated adequately, you should have lost no more than 3 per cent of your body weight; more than 5 per cent, and you have definitely dehydrated.

7. Finally, when the air temperature and humidity are both extremely high even copious quantities of water will not hold your body temperature down. Slowing your pace, or even walking, will reduce your body's rate of heat generation, but if you start to develop symptoms of excessive high body temperature (severe muscle and abdomen cramps, dizziness, extreme irritability, a tendency to stumble), then smarten up and drop out of the run. Failure to do so may have very unpleasant consequences.

Cold Weather Jogging

While indoor exercising has its advocates, I believe that walking and jogging out of doors is of most benefit. Apart from the sheer boredom and discomfort of indoor exercising (when did you last sweat your way round four miles of a "26-lap-to-the-mile" track?), the outdoor jogger achieves an exhilaration and sense of satisfaction which can only be obtained by physically coping with the natural elements. The feeling one gets from hacking four miles through the pouring rain or driving snow is no less rewarding than the pleasure of an early morning run through the park in the spring. Even allowing for your reluctance to accept this philosophy, there is another more cogent reason for advocating out-of-door exercising. If you are going to work out five days a week for the rest of your life, surely the most convenient way to do so is by merely stepping through your front door and using your own district as a training ground. You fit your exercising into your lifestyle, and you make it part of your daily living.

I have found that patients who resort to indoor stationary exercycles and the like rarely persist with their programs. Instead of arranging their day's activities around their one hour workout, they attempt to fit the exercise session into their already rather hectic lifestyle. They try to watch television while cycling, or rig up a stand so that they can read a book during the session. They fit the activity in just before supper, and if they arrive home late from work, they find it all too easy to miss out "just this once." Eventually the bicycle, or rowing machine, or other exercise gimmick, is relegated to the basement because it looks so forlorn, untidy and unused in the living room; and that's the end of that. As for the indoor fitness club, this certainly has its place, provided you don't have a half hour's drive each way, and provided its facilities include a jogging track big enough to allow you to cover four miles without injuring your ankles, knees or inner ear balance mechanism from pivoting around a miniscule circle.

The ideal temperature for outdoor exercising is between 40°F. and 60°F. (4°C.-15°C.). Actually, it is possible to enjoy walking and jogging in temperatures as low as 15°F. above zero (-10°C.). My post-coronary patients are taught to train outdoors as long as the temperature remains above this level. However, you should always take the wind chill factor into account. Even though the temperature is 20°F., a 5-mile-an-hour wind will produce an equivalent chill temperature of 15°F. (see chart on page 293). Running in cold weather, even for post-coronary patients, is not the hazard it appears. Provided certain basic principles are understood and the necessary precautions taken, it can be both enjoyable and safe.

Whenever somebody expresses amazement when you venture out in temperatures below zero and still enjoy yourself, you know for sure that you are talking to a sedentary type. Any jogger or cross-country skier realizes that the body heat generated by exercise can keep you quite warm. For instance, even jogging at a 12-minute-mile pace will cause a tenfold increase in heat production over and above that associated with the resting state. Naturally, when the surrounding air is cold, then the body will tend to lose heat in a variety of ways (e.g., evaporation of exhaled breath from the lungs, transfer of heat from the mucous membranes of the nose and mouth to warm the cold inspired air, radiation to colder surrounding objects, and conduction and convection to air currents). Nevertheless, despite this loss, exercise-induced heat is often sufficient to let you operate out of doors in below freezing temperatures with only a minimum amount of additional clothing.

Scientists use the Clo unit as a measurement of the amount of body covering required to maintain body comfort at various temperatures. One Clo unit keeps you comfortable at an indoor temperature of 21 °C. (70°F.). The number of Clo units, or layers of clothing, that you need to protect you when out of doors on a cold day will depend upon the speed of your walk or jog and thus the body heat you develop, and the temperature of the surrounding air. Obviously the ideal to aim at is a balance between heat production and heat loss, so that your body temperature remains constant and you feel comfortable.

At first glance, this seems a simple matter to work out. For instance, you can calculate the heat generated by the speed of your walk or jog and then, taking into account the precise temperature of the outside air, judge the number of layers of clothes required. In theory the whole business becomes a simple matter of using a pocket calculator.

As you might have guessed, there are one or two complications. In the first place, absolute air temperature applies only on those calm, still days when there is a complete absence of wind. We must take the wind chill into account. If we use our chart, however, this is hardly a chore. Look at the prevailing air temperature, listen to the radio for wind strengths, and then determine the "effective" temperature. For instance, assuming an outside temperature of 35°F. (2°C.), and a 10-mile-an-hour wind (16 km/h), we have an effective temperature of 20°F. (-6°C.). If you went out for a walk in these conditions, at 3½ mile an hour pace, then you would have to wear clothing equivalent to two or three Clo units (i.e., two or three layers).

Another point. Is the sun shining or is it overcast? Direct sunshine is worth an additional 12°F. (7°C.). This can be critical. You may start your walk on a calm day, with the sun shining brightly. If you are using an out-and-back course, by the time you head for home you may find yourself battling a 10-mile-an-hour headwind, with the sun long since disappeared behind the clouds. Net result? You are no longer wearing enough layers of clothes to retain your body heat, and things begin to become pretty miserable. You can, of course, pick up your pace to generate more body heat. But this may require a level of exertion beyond your capabilities, in which case, you will fatigue, lose body heat even more rapidly or, if you are a post-coronary patient, develop angina and have to slow down again. So you see, winter jogging requires the ability to allow for sudden shifts in weather.

I have left the most crucial of all variables to the end. If safety and comfort depend upon a nice balance between heat production and heat loss, then the greatest threat to equilibrium is wet clothing. Whether the result of driving rain, melting snow, or drenching perspiration, the effect is the same. Evaporation from the wet material will drop your body temperature at an alarming rate. This is one of the most potent causes of hypothermia. With every degree fall below normal, you go through the successive stages of slurred speech, inco-ordination of hands and feet, unsteadiness, confusion, collapse, and finally coma. Hypothermia is hardly the lot of everyone who goes for a jog on a cold day and gets his clothes wet, but you should take precautions to see that you never put yourself in the position of risking such a tragedy. The trick is to wear suitable layers of clothing so as to trap air, a poor conductor of heat, between each layer and so prevent body heat from "wicking out" into the surrounding air. Pure wool is ideal as the middle and outer layers; its natural oils cause it to shed beads of moisture, and it traps air bubbles between its fibres, making it the perfect heat insulator. Wet cotton, on the other hand, is a poor insulator, and wicks heat from the body at an alarming rate. The current "uniform" of cotton blue jeans and shirt has been incriminated on more than one occasion in the deaths from hypothermia of individuals who have fallen into lakes or rivers and managed to swim to shore, only to die from exposure within the relative short time it has taken rescuers to reach them.

Putting all of this together, we can lay down the following guidelines for cold weather jogging:

1. Clothing should be light, capable of absorbing sweat, and non-restrictive. Warmth should be obtained by adding layers, rather than by utilization of one thick, bulky garment. A cotton vest should be worn next to the skin so that it can absorb sweat. Over this should be a woollen vest and then a track suit top made of a mixture of wool and cotton. If an additional layer is required on the torso, you can add a

wool sweater. Some joggers like to wear a nylon-type wind-breaker over the track suit top, but this aggravates sweating, and so I usually save it for a rainy mild day, and then merely wear it directly on top of the cotton vest. If possible, all of the upper body garments should be zipped or buttoned in such a way that they can be loosened at the neck when you are overheating, but closed up, in polo fashion, if you begin to chill. Obviously the number of layers you use will depend upon how cold it is. Darker coloured outer garments don't reflect the sun too readily, and so tend to conserve body heat. However, at night time, they should be decorated with reflective strip material.

The lower limbs are protected with panty hose (yes, men too!) either on their own or covered with the cotton/wool mixture sweat suit pants. In the winter time, I tend to avoid the all nylon type sweat suits; they don't absorb sweat very well. If you have to wear long-johns, I suggest that you cut them off about the knees; your leg action will feel a good deal freer, and the lower legs rarely need extra covering.

Socks should be of a cotton/wool mixture, the hands (which are poorly muscled, used little in jogging, and become cold quite easily) are best protected by woollen mittens. Twenty per cent or more of body heat is lost through the head and so a woollen cap or hat is mandatory. This should pull down well over the ears to protect them from frostbite. The exposed parts of the face should be heavily vaselined, otherwise the combination of cold and wind will cause lip chapping and cold sores. As for shoes, you might want to consider waffle soles for greater purchase on the ice, and a slightly flared heel to give greater stability in soft snow. Some runners prefer leather uppers in the winter. The leather can be treated with a mixture of musk oil and silicone to make it waterproof.

2. If the effective temperature is below 15°F. (−10°C.) post-coronary joggers should question the wisdom of exercising out of doors. To be honest, over 90 per cent of my patients exercise at below this temperature during the winter time, but only after they have been adequately instructed in all of the safety measures mentioned above. In their case, it is particularly important that they allow for wind, wet conditions, presence or absence of sunshine, etc. But probably the

most important factor is whether or not they enjoy cold weather. I know it's hard to believe in this day and age of science, but the only way to predict whether or not an individual functions better in cold or in the heat is to ask him! There are some people who can happily work out of doors in temperatures down as low as 0°F; there are others who shiver miserably at one degree below freezing. Your body metabolism is your affair, and only you know the type of climatic conditions most suitable to your own machinery.

For those who suffer from angina on exposure to the cold, either a scarf over the mouth, or a simple face mask proves to be beneficial. The mask that we use is a disposable type connected to a corregated tube which is placed under the clothing and permits the walker or jogger to breath from the warm surface layer of air covering the body (see Appendix, page 294).

3. On an out-and-back course, remember to take the wind into account. Two miles on a cold day, with the sun shining and a slight wind at your back, can feel great; but by the time you turn and start to wend your two miles home, you may find that the sun has waned, the light following breeze has turned into a cold headwind, and that pleasant perspiration is now freezing your face and body solid.

4. Frostbite is an unusual occurrence for the jogger, although I recall reading in a medical journal some years back of a physician who, on returning from a cold weather jog, discovered that he had lost all sensation in his penis. Horror of horrors! The thought of frostbite in such a crucial part of his anatomy almost lead to hysterical breakdown. However, his professional training came to his aid and he manfully treated the situation with sufficient competence that all was not lost. To his eternal credit, he was sufficiently civic-minded that he immediately wrote a letter to the *New England Medical Journal* informing the medical profession far and wide to be on the lookout for this catastrophic possibility.

Frostbite occurs when the temperature of the skin drops below freezing. The skin develops a white bloodless appearance, is completely numb, and the condition may only be noticed when it has been present for some time. If you suspect frostbite, get yourself into the emergency department of the nearest hospital post haste. The treatment is immersion of the area in lukewarm water (105° - 108°F.), and when thawing has occurred, measures to preserve the damaged structures. In the worst cases, gangrene occurs and portions of tissue may be lost or have to be amputated. If you want to avoid this condition, then keep the exposed parts of your body well covered, and always be alert to the development of numbness and change of colour in your fingers, toes or ears. Never try to thaw the area with excessive heat, and never rub it with snow.

5. Despite the fact that there are individual variations in the reaction of the body to cold, it is possible to cold acclimatize. Have you noticed that butchers or people who work in cold storage depots have warm hands and never seem to complain of the freezing temperatures? This is because their cardiovascular system has adjusted so as to conserve body heat. Careful physical activity in the early stages of winter can do the same for you. The trouble is, by the time winter has come to an end, you have to start acclimatizing to the heat again. Such is life!

The Other Side of the Coin

Jogging has become one of the most popular participation sports in North America. I am delighted. I enjoy jogging for its own sake, and I am happy to see so many others, young and old, male and female, share my delight. One of the many spinoffs, because of the increased feeling of well-being which accompanies a regular jogging program, is the development of a greater interest in other physical pastimes. At last count, my post-coronary patients were actively engaged in and enjoying any one of a total of sixteen different sports and physical recreations. In addition to jogging and walking, they included cycling, golf, swimming, tennis, squash, curling, bowling, ice skating and roller skating, cross-country and Alpine skiing, ice hockey, ballroom dancing, square dancing, various types of calisthenics, horse riding, sailing, and canoeing. There is no doubt that North America is on the greatest exercise kick in history. Are there any disadvantages to this? Maybe. Whether you call them side effects, drawbacks, or just the inevitable consequences of the latest vogue, depends on your point of view. In any event, a few comments on these various aspects are probably timely at this particular stage in the development of what I hope is now our mutual hobby.

The Cult of Jogging　　　Any mass movement tends to attract the cultist, the individual who by nature is impelled to add a ritualistic and mystic aura to the most mundane of pursuits. I am the last to gainsay the psychological advantages of jogging, but to listen to the cultist, every workout should be akin to a religious experience. This super-charged attitude makes me feel a trifle uncomfortable, and I feel that it should be put in perspective.

A recent book on jogging stated that 78 per cent of all the subjects questioned by the author admitted to experiencing a "high" at least once while jogging. They described the experience in various terms, but in essence it seemed to mean a feeling of increased self-awareness, often associated with a pleasurable heightening of sensory input. The colours of sunsets or sunrises seem more intense. Familiar objects such as buildings, bushes, trees, billboards, assume unfamiliar but intriguing shapes. The very air itself develops a texture, an odour and a dimension which it never had before. Some even describe a state bordering on self-hallucination, in which "the true meaning of life is revealed." All well and good, except that in questioning thousands of joggers on my program and talking to as many or more fun runners in the British Isles, Europe and Australasia, I have never been able to find more than a handful of individuals in whom running induced such bizarre sensations. For most of us, there are days when every step is a drag and the nicest thing about the whole session is the hot shower and the glass of beer that follow it. Running too hard or too fast doesn't "grey out our peripheral vision" as one eloquent cultist put it, it merely makes our heart rate go up, puts us into oxygen debt, gives us a head-ache, and from time to time causes us to throw up at the end of the race.

Believe it or not, but I have even heard one "high priest jogger" describe how, at a certain stage in a marathon race, his ecstasy of superlative fitness reached such heights that he experienced an orgasm! The reaction of my post-coronary marathoners (admittedly more cynical and hard-bitten than most) to this announcement was something to behold! Some wanted to know the exact mile at which it happened (so that they could prepare for the great and eagerly anticipated event should it happen to them); others, with more practical turns of mind, were inclined to implicate an excessively tight jock strap rather than the "ecstasy of fitness." Our erstwhile captain, Harry B., put forward the theory that the 67-year-old marathoner in question was probably confusing ejaculation with micturition.

But surely, I hear you say, the jogging enthusiast who is experiencing the pleasures of exercise and fitness for the first time is bound to see things in a new light and with a different perspective, and cannot this induce a totally new philosophy and outlook on life? I agree entirely. My only point is that one must be constantly on one's guard against exaggerated claims. I have no quarrel with those of poetic bent and eloquent turn of phrase who express the pleasures of jogging in an appealing and attractive manner. My concern is with the zealot, the visionary, who promises Nirvana after a six-mile plod. When the newcomer to the sport fails to experience such spiritual bliss, he naturally blames himself. At which point, he drops the whole thing, and goes back to watching television.

The other problem with cultists, of course, is that they are notoriously fickle. One year it's jogging, the next, dynamic breath-holding. Since they don't stay long enough with anything to obtain all the benefits, and since they often have to rationalize their reason for forsaking the last craze, they tend to bad-mouth it. These are people who are constantly looking for the unattainable; they are rarely, if ever, satisfied. Jogging can do without them. Not only do they add complex, unnecessary and exaggerated dimensions to what is essentially a very simple activity, but they inevitably entice other undesirables. If I may paraphrase Wordsworth, "The huckster is too much with us; late and soon, getting and spending, he lays waste our powers." Hucksters are attracted to cults like flies to a jampot. What better market for their wares? Jogging magazines are full of ads for "jogging aids," which are of questionable value. Self-styled experts lacking any formal training and short on experience, to say the least, promise to advise you by book, correspondence course, seminar, or "running camp" how to achieve your jogging heart's desire — at a substantial price, of course! Pseudo-scientific mumbo-jumbo is used to impress the unwary and confuse the intelligent enquirer in search of genuine help.

The answer to all this? Merely be aware that it's happening. Try to get your advice, whether verbal or written, from individuals who have been running or jogging long before the present craze started. When reading a column or a book on jogging, make it your business to find out the author's qualifications. That's not to say that you need a piece of paper or a string of letters after your name to make you an authority. Some of the greatest track and field coaches in the world never had a formal lecture on the subject. But the knowledgeable layman will never try to infer that he is what he is not. If he speaks of scientific matters, he will invariably give you the source of his basic data, and when he expresses his own interpretation of that data, he will make it equally plain what he is doing. The bottom line for the huckster, naturally enough, is dollars and cents. Bear that in mind, and you shouldn't be too easy a mark!

The Fanatical Jogger   A few weeks ago, I had a phone call from an orthopedic surgeon friend of mine. He was treating a jogger patient who had developed a stress fracture but, against advice, had continued to jog and had now developed a second fracture. My friend, in a desperate attempt to enforce a period of rest, had decided to apply a below-knee plaster cast. To his astonishment, the patient was still reluctant to accept the inevitable six-week layoff and was demanding that "something else" be tried that would allow him to get back to jogging within a few days. "What in God's name," said my friend, "makes a guy like this tick? Are all joggers this crazy?" I assured him that not all of us were this crazy, but I admitted that from time to time there are some who go a trifle overboard.

I have referred earlier in this book to the "beneficial addiction." By that, I mean the development of a reliance on your jogging workout, so that when you miss a few days, you begin to feel the worse for it. You get a little irritable, you feel a little down, you don't sleep quite as well, and you certainly miss the familiar rhythmic movement of your body along the roads and paths of your customary route. I believe there is a chemical reason for these mild, quite bearable, withdrawal symptoms. The trouble is, we have not as yet identified the chemical. This makes me wonder if the fanatical jogger, the individual who cannot bear to stop running for even a day, becomes a great deal more dependent upon that chemical than the rest of us. Could it be that he is deficient in it even before he starts jogging?

The jogger who cannot stop is often the one who attains the greatest degree of mental satisfaction and contentment from the workout. Our own studies have shown that the most depressed post-coronary patient is the one who obtains the greatest alleviation of that depression as a result of the jogging program. The individual with the normal psychological profile shows little change as a result of jogging. He feels better, he enjoys life more, and he uses jogging just as much as a relief from the tensions and anxieties of his everyday life as his depressed counterpart, but scientific analysis does not reflect this. In short, if you have a normal outlook on life, jogging is not going to do anything other than reinforce it. If, on the other hand, you have deep-seated psychological problems, then they may respond very gratifyingly to a regular jogging regime. Not only that, but the improvement may be readily measured by the clinical psychologist or psychiatrist. Drs. Glasser, Hackett, Greist and Kostrubala are all psychiatrists who confirm that jogging therapy can be effective in the treatment of chronic depression, phobias, anxiety neuroses, schizophrenia, and anorexia nervosa. In the hands of such experts, jogging is a welcome alternative to, for instance, the excessive use of various psychotropic medications.

But what if a runner, all unwittingly, is practising running self-medication — in other words, treating himself for any of the above conditions without realizing it? All he knows is that until he started running, life was miserable; since he began to jog, he is happy and functioning at a level of contentment that he has never experienced before. If he stops running, the old feelings of insecurity and despair begin to return. Under these circumstances, is he not likely to minimize any symptoms, be they musculoskeletal or cardiovascular, which might prevent him from running? Herein may lie the explanation for my orthopedic friend's patient who continues to work out with two broken bones in his foot. Or the marathoner described by cardiologist Dr. Tim Noakes of Cape Town who, against medical orders, ran five marathons in the 28-month period between his first heart attack and his second fatal one, and whose training log book recorded numerous episodes of pain in the chest, jaws or arms during training runs, for none of which he sought medical advice. Or the American congressman jogger who had two exercise stress tests which indicated severe disease of the coronary arteries but who, spurning all warnings, continued to run vigorously — until he dropped dead some months later at the end of a fifteen-mile training run! The examples are frequent enough, I think, to make my point. Certainly the theory could explain the unaccountable behaviour of some apparently intelligent joggers.

There is a fine line between enthusiasm and fanaticism, between dedication and a death wish. I have nothing but congratulations for the individual who so successfully organizes his work schedule and his spare time that he can fit in his jogging session as part of his life. I have the greatest admiration for those who overcome the vagaries of weather and the inevitable daily unexpected crises of life and still maintain their regular exercise schedule. But there is a difference between reorganizing your social life and totally demolishing it. What of the jogger who, because of his early morning workout, must get to bed between 9 and 10 o'clock every night, weekends included? As far as his wife, family and friends are concerned, he is strictly a party pooper. Not only that, but evening theatre, movies or late-night dinner engagements become a thing of the past. If this is the way it is, then something has to be wrong. Life does not consist only of working, sleeping and jogging.

Like everything else, moderation is the key to success. While not gainsaying the mental and physical benefits of jogging, these benefits must be put in perspective. As goals, they must never be lost sight of, but to become compulsive about the method of attaining them is, paradoxically, to destroy their value. The compulsive jogger is an uptight, strung-out individual who is worrying about his work schedule when he is jogging and about his jogging when he is working. He is the antithesis of the relaxed, loping, easy-breathing image that he is aiming for. The compulsive jogger is sick and a complete pain in the buttocks to all the normal people who have to share his life.

If, on reading this, you begin to see the beginnings of a self-portrait, then do me a favour — stop running for two weeks, and then, at the end of the second week, make a list of the reasons which started you jogging in the first place. Do you still consider these reasons worthwhile? If so, how many of them have you realized? Finally — and be honest here — has there been any deterioration in your mental equanimity, your home life, your relationships with the members of your family or your oldest and dearest friends, your social and cultural life, or your job? If the answer to this last question is yes, then is it due to your new life-style? In a nutshell, have the gains outweighed the losses? If not, then the chances are that you have become a compulsive jogger. The remedy lies in your own hands. The fact is that if you don't change, you'll wind up without any of the health advantages, and maybe even minus your wife and friends. The choice is yours.

The Media   The recent explosion of interest in jogging has intrigued those whose job it is to report and comment on the opinions, habits and daily activities of the rest of us. The result has been considerable media coverage of mass marathon runs, as well as features about the jogger, the jogger's wife, the jogger's shoes, and almost every conceivable aspect of jogging that you can mention. The high incidence of heart disease, and its association with the sedentary lifestyle, has given added impetus to this trend. I find that a goodly number of media workers are themselves joggers. They are often highly intelligent individuals who are quick to perceive the validity of the pro-exercise arguments. As a group, they have traditionally tended to smoke too much, eat irregularly and unwisely, take little if any exercise, drink too much, put on too much weight, and to add insult to injury, live notoriously hectic and stress-filled lives. They are, in short, prime candidates for heart attacks, and they know it. Small wonder that some of the most enthusiastic joggers are now to be found in their ranks.

This is all to the good. Not only have the media done a great job in fostering public interest in a more healthy lifestyle, but both the style and substance of the message has usually been both mature and well-informed. There is so much information available today on exercise, training, fitness, and the like that one is hard put to keep abreast of it all. It is no exaggeration to say that the intelligent layman who merely touches base from time to time with the larger circulation jogging magazines, news-paper fitness columns, and occasional radio and television programs knows more about the topic than most coaches of ten years back — and certainly than the vast majority of present-day physicians. The North American jogger is now thoroughly familiar with such terms as HDL cholesterol, fast-twitch fibres, carbohydrate loading, and similar jargon.

A word of caution. All honeymoons must come to an end. The business of the media is to present the news. The time is approaching when stories about joggers will have become about as interesting as the contents of the obituary column. Before leaving the topic of jogging, however, the media can still extract some interest by panning it. The time will come when a freelance writer is much more likely to get an article accepted if it decries jogging as a highly dangerous activity than if it merely repeats all of its advantages. Ten years ago, my post-coronary joggers had to endure the ridicule and warnings of their neighbours and friends as they plodded through the streets. They showed admirable singleness of purpose, faith in the program, and imperviousness to public opinion. Patients who join the program today find things a good deal easier. The streets are full of joggers, old and young, ridicule is stilled, and the media are with them every step of the way. I hope that when the brickbats come, they will not be intimidated back into their old way of life. I don't think they will, because I feel we have taught them to do all the right things for the right reasons. But I suspect that there are a group of latter-day joggers who enjoy swimming with the stream, but who, at the first appearance of the anti-jogging articles, will quickly put away their sweat suit and jogging shoes, and paddle about waiting for the next wave to ride.

Jogging Deaths

Sudden, unexpected death is not a recent phenomenon; it has been with us since antiquity. The commonest cause in recent times is a malfunction of the heart. Interestingly, while 50 to 60 per cent of heart attack victims die within a few hours, it should not be assumed that all cases of sudden death are caused by a heart attack. Actually, on autopsy only about one-third exhibit classical evidence of blocked coronary vessels and death of heart tissue. The other two-thirds, while frequently showing atherosclerosis of their coronary blood vessels, have no evidence of a myocardial infarction. Why is this?

The prevailing theory is that death has occurred too quickly (within a matter of minutes) for the classical, pathological changes to take place. But this doesn't explain why the coronary arteries should show no signs of a recent blood clot. Another explanation is that the heart has "fibrillated" or developed a defect in its rhythm-conducting system which interrupts its continuous pumping action and leaves it quivering ineffectually, thus starving the vital organs of oxygen. Sounds reasonable enough, but what caused the electrical failure in the first place? At present we don't know for certain; all we have are a good many clues.

We may be close to a breakthrough, however. In the first place, we have begun to accept that while cardiac atherosclerosis is probably at the root of 90 per cent of sudden deaths (the rest have non-cardiovascular causes), a frank myocardial infarction is not the only, or even the major mechanism responsible. It has been noted that in a number of cases of sudden death, tiny vital microscopic blood vessels supplying oxygen to the leashes of rhythm-conducting nerves of the heart are blocked by what are called platelet microemboli. Platelets are tiny round cells, about half the size of a red blood cell, which circulate in the blood in large quantities and prevent bleeding from cut or broken blood vessels by clumping together, plugging the break, and initiating the formation of a blood clot. The trouble is that they can be fooled into mistaking an atherosclerotic plaque inside the blood vessel for a break in its wall, or a slowing down of blood flow in a fat narrowed vessel for a compensatory slowing due to excessive bleeding; in which case, with true sense of duty, they clump together and block off the blood flow through the blood vessel in question entirely. Deprivation of oxygen supply to the heart's rhythm pace-maker (the sino-atrial node — see p. 72), or any of its message-conducting systems, can be fatal in a matter of minutes.

But whether sudden death is due to a large clot in a major coronary artery which leads to destruction of heart tissue, or a microscopic clot in a microscopic artery which leads to fatal cardiac rhythm disturbances, what's the difference? Well, reduction in the incidence of sudden death depends upon our concept of its cause. If we assume that practically all cases are due to classical heart attacks, then prevention becomes strictly a matter of eliminating coronary atherosclerosis. But if disturbance in platelet cell function, superimposed upon coronary atherosclerosis, is the major risk factor, then actions and drugs which reduce platelet clumping may be critical in reducing the incidence of sudden death.

This theory of the cause of some sudden deaths does explain some hitherto paradoxical and puzzling scientific findings. For instance, a four-year follow-up in Seattle of 234 patients who were successfully resuscitated after "dying" suddenly showed that the subsequent "sudden death" rate was more than three times higher in those who, after their first episode, failed to go on to a full-blown heart attack. It would seem, then, from this study, that risk from sudden death can be a characteristic separate from myocardial infarction risk. There have also been a number of drug trials which have shown that certain medications have been woefully deficient in preventing heart attacks, both primary and recurrent but, apparently coincidentally, have been associated with the reduction in sudden deaths. Could it be that such therapeutic agents, while not affecting atherosclerosis per se, have been acting as anti-platelet aggregation substances? Or, looked at another way, since we know that smoking accelerates platelet clumping, would this explain why sudden death is apparently much higher in smokers than non-smokers?

The precise cause of sudden death in all cases is still a matter of conjecture, which makes it difficult to evaluate the effect of any one of a number of activities which the unfortunate victim is carrying out at the time of his demise. If a jogger drops dead, was jogging the cause? Unless an autopsy has been carried out, not even the immediate mechanism of death is certain, never mind the reason. And even if a post-mortem uncovers the immediate cause as being myocardial infarction or "electrical failure," can we incriminate exercise, or is it merely a coincidental association? In other words, would the episode have occurred anyway, irrespective of the activity? For instance, a study by Yater et al on young U.S. army men showed that while sudden death was twice as frequent during strenuous activity, autopsy demonstrated the presence of recent coronary thrombosis, i.e. silent heart attacks. In other words, the exercise had not caused the heart attack. The coronary artery clot had already developed, prior to the strenuous event.

But what about the newspaper reports which confront you from time to time? "Congressman Drops Dead While Jogging." "American Medical Association Journal Reports 18 Cases of Sudden Death in Joggers." "Two South African Physicians Report Death from Heart Attacks in Four Marathon Runners." Well, you must realize that deaths occurring during exercise are news, especially if the victims are well known; they occur in full view of onlookers. How often do you read of surgical deaths? Yet if it made headlines in the press every time a patient failed to survive a coronary by-pass procedure or died while undergoing a coronary arteriogram (x-ray of coronary arteries using injection of radio opaque dye), it would give a totally false impression. Both coronary arteriography and coronary by-pass surgery are now extremely safe procedures. That's not to say that from time to time a death doesn't occur on the operating table, but when you consider the complex and intricate procedures being carried out, and the critically severe nature of the disease in those who are being treated, this is not surprising.

Medical science uses statistical methods to assess the odds for success. The bottom line is the same as in any other endeavour: the greatest good for the greatest number. In the long run, it all comes down to a mathematical assessment of benefit achieved balanced against harm done. Does that sound callous? If so, I don't mean it to. I, like many physicians and surgeons before me, have watched one of my patients die. It's something you never quite accept, never quite get used to. You analyse the circumstances for a cause. You ask yourself if you could have prevented it.

Jogging and exercise deaths are no exception. It's no good merely noting their presence. The cause of death must be identified wherever possible. Not only that, but because of the relative rarity of exercise deaths, they must be estimated mathematically in terms of their occurrence relative to other activities. For instance, do more sudden deaths occur during sleep, or sexual intercourse, or at work, or watching a football game, or in the sauna, or in the doctor's waiting room, etc.? In order to discover this, we must look at a large number of sudden death cases, and examine the circumstances under which they occurred. Not only that, but we must ascertain the time spent by the group under study in various activities. For instance, if one-third of their day was spent on work, one-third in sleep, and one-third in recreation, then, statistically at least, you would expect the same relationship to apply to the incidence of sudden death. A disturbance in this distribution might incriminate any one of these three activities. For instance, if you were to postulate that jogging or exercise was associated with a high incidence of sudden death, then you have to ascertain the amount of time spent by the group under study in exercising, and calculate the anticipated incidence of death accordingly.

Actually, it has already been estimated that in the United States, given the current incidence of death from heart and blood vessel disease, for every 250,000 joggers as many as 6.5 deaths could occur during or within two hours of the workout by chance alone — and that assumes an average jogging session of only 20 minutes, three times weekly. Given the most recent Gallup poll estimate that there are now some 20 million Americans jogging, as many as 520 of them can be expected to die by chance while jogging — just as some will die while eating, sleeping, watching television, or carrying out some other activity of daily living. I think this sheds some statistical perspective on the relationship between jogging and sudden death.

In 1971 Jokl and McClellan reviewed sudden death and exercise in a monograph and noted that "Not one instance was encountered in which death could be regarded as due to the effects of extreme exertion in a previously healthy heart. It is significant that there is no case in our list." In 1978, Dr. Ilkka M. Vuori, of the University of Turku, Finland, published one of the classical reports on sudden death in the *Journal of Cardiology*. He examined the circumstances surrounding 2,606 sudden deaths, with the specific purpose of ascertaining whether or not they were associated with physical activity. He concluded that sudden deaths connected with sporting activities were rare. Ten sudden deaths occurred in connection with day-long ski-hikes, and strenuous physical exercise seemed to have played an important role in these cases. However, most of the subjects had serious cardiovascular risk factors which were known in advance or which could have been identified by medical examination. Daily physical activities or sports could not be incriminated as an important contributory factor in sudden death in the general population. However, he suggested that there was a risk of cardiac complications in connection with strenuous physical exercise in subjects who had cardiac disease.

Our own studies and investigations in Toronto have corroborated these findings. The immediate factor triggering a heart attack in about one-third of the patients referred to us for post-coronary rehabilitation seemed to have been intense and unaccustomed exercise, sometimes associated with emotional excitement. This is hardly surprising. The majority of epidemiological studies support the conclusion that prolonged inactivity increases the overall risk of myocardial infarction. Unaccustomed exercise, then, when it acts as a precipitant for a heart attack, does no more than reveal a previously damaged coronary system which is highly susceptible to both physical and emotional stress.

Are we saying, then, that exercise can be dangerous in individuals who have severe coronary artery disease? Of course. Otherwise there would be no need for the medically supervised type of post-coronary exercise program offered at the Toronto Rehabilitation Centre. For those males over 35 in the general population who have latent heart disease but are not aware of it, there must surely be a danger in ill-advised, excessive, and non-medically prescribed competitive jogging. The cardiac contra-indications to exercise are dealt with fully in Chapter 5 and, in the interests of space, will not be repeated here. However, they are obviously of paramount importance in this particular context and will bear reading again.

There are a number of circumstances surrounding exercise which, either alone or in combination, may precipitate irregularities of cardiac rhythm or maybe sudden death. First and foremost is *exercising when one has a fever*. This has been stressed previously, but one cannot over-accentuate the dangers of forcing the heart to work when it may well be suffering from an infection. Flu-like illnesses may often be harmless, but from time to time they will give rise to a myocarditis, or inflammation of the heart muscle cells, in which case any additional strain placed on the heart may be fatal. In order to prevent the unnecessary risk of exercise-related sudden death in association with myocarditis, we apply the absolutely strict ruling that anyone suffering from a flu-like illness must not exercise until a full seven days have elapsed since his temperature has returned to normal. An unexplained persistent rapid or irregular heart rate following or accompanying a flu-like illness is strongly suggestive of active myocarditis.

The problems of *exercise in the heat* have been discussed in detail already, but one cannot over-emphasize the dangers. When one exercises in high temperature, there is a progressive fall in the ability of the heart to pump blood. In these circumstances, output of blood from the heart can only be maintained by an increase of the heart rate. All of this is due to the fact that a significant proportion of circulating blood volume has to be shunted to the skin in order to dissipate heat. The entire detrimental consequences of this major hemodynamic fluctuation is not as yet fully understood, but on first principles it seems advisable to pay particular attention to adequate fluid intake, and cold sponging during prolonged exercise in the heat. Deaths during long distance runs in high temperature have been ascribed to heart attacks, and yet on more than one occasion autopsies have failed to reveal any evidence of coronary atherosclerosis. It is not unreasonable to assume that such deaths have been due to dehydration and consequent alteration in blood electrolytes. No one is immune to all of the terrible consequences of dehydration, but middle-aged males with latent coronary artery disease are more susceptible.

A less tangible, but nonetheless important, factor in the equation balancing the benefits and hazards of exercise is that of *personality*. The driving, ambitious, individual, who tends to take on too many projects and may have some concealed hostility, once introduced to an exercise program is usually over-eager to excel. Such individuals must be rigorously controlled from misapplying their natural aggression and competitiveness. Not infrequently they become compulsive, and when business pressures mount will try to complete their workout in less and less time. Even worse, they may deny cardiac symptoms so that they can continue both their exercise program and still keep up their heavy business and social commitments. In effect, they ignore symptoms, attributing them to non-cardiac ailments, or else they dismiss them as being of no consequence.

The inherent danger in this attitude is that it always causes a delay before these symptoms are brought to the attention of the doctor. For this reason I take warning signs such as excessive fatigue, tiredness and especially anginal-type pain on exercise extremely seriously. They are an indication that the training must be immediately reduced, pending a detailed re-examination of the exerciser's cardiovascular status.

We have evolved five exercise rules as applied particularly to these deadline fighters:

- train regularly without excessive peaks of activity;
- avoid intensive competitions;
- adhere to the prescribed limits;
- reduce the exercise load when either physical symptoms, mental tension or depression develops;
- report all "cardiac type" symptoms such as exercise-related chest pain, arm pain, excessive palpitations, dizziness, "black-outs", or undue breathlessness—even if they appear for the first time after years of steady symptom-free training.

The recent tragic death in the United States of an outstanding young female tennis star while warming-down after a competitive tennis match illustrates another potential presage to sudden death. Although the post-mortem failed to establish a cause of death, a detailed inquiry revealed that prior to her death, she had suffered episodic black-outs. It was, therefore, assumed that these black-outs and her death were both due to a cardiac arrhythmia which on this occasion failed to reverse spontaneously — so-called "electrical death."

The lesson here is that all episodes of *loss of consciousness*, however brief, occurring during or immediately after exercise, should be assumed to be cardiac in origin. The patient should be subjected to a thorough physical and cardiovascular examination including an exercise test, and his cardiac rhythm should be monitored for prolonged periods until either a treatable abnormality is found, or until it can safely be concluded that the likelihood or further dysrhythmic episodes is remote.

To sum up, exercise-induced deaths are rare, but inevitably they do occur. Despite suggestions to the contrary, those physicians who are involved on a day-to-day basis in training individuals with latent and overt coronary artery disease can often recognize and prevent potential hazards. Needless to say, it is impossible to prove that anticipatory action in the form of anti-dysrhythmic medications, or advice regarding reduction of exercise intensity has been successful in preventing an exercise death. However, results of successful post-coronary exercise programs are revealing. The Toronto program, in the period between 1968 and 1979, has accumulated a total of almost one million hours of exercise. This has been associated with only five jogging deaths, not one of which could be directly ascribed to the effects of physical exertion per se. This reflects the findings of William Haskell who summarized the experience of 103 different post-coronary exercise programs, involving a total of 1,629,634 patient hours of supervised exercise. The average complication rate for all programs was one non-fatal and one fatal event for every 34,673, and 116,402 patient hours of participation respectively.

In the final analysis, surely the fact that the recent worldwide explosion in the number of joggers has not been accompanied by an immediate and proportionate increase in sudden jogging deaths attests in the most dramatic and eloquent way possible to jogging's inherent safety.

CHAPTER TEN

The Marathon

SINCE the first edition of this book appeared in 1976, marathon running has become the North American national participation sport. In 1979, there were over 300 official marathon races held in the United States; the most prestigious of all, the Boston Marathon, had well over 5,000 official entrants, as well as 2,000 unofficial starters! A far cry from the mere handful of runners who customarily started out from Hopkinton, Massachusetts in the 1930s and 1940s. The upstart New York Marathon, with a route which winds through all five boroughs of the "Big Apple," had to cope with some 14,000 entrants in 1979. And so it goes, with larger and larger numbers of people wanting to finish the gruelling 26¼ miles.

Who are these masochists? Are they the new wave of hippies and weirdos? Anything but. Many of them are business executives and professionals. Yet the number of honest-to-God hardcore competitive marathon runners has not increased significantly. Undoubtedly, there are more sub-2½ hour marathoners than there were ten years ago, but one swallow doesn't make a summer. No, the bulk of this new wave of joggers is made up of people who enter for the same reason that my post-coronary joggers did when they took part in their first Boston Marathon back in 1973. It is a goal, a target to aim for. In a world where regretfully (but all too frequently), the winner is not just the smartest on the job but also the one who happens to know the right people (and in the right order), one cannot deny the appeal of making it on your own. One of my post-coronary marathoning patients put it to me like this, "When you train for a marathon, you know that no-one can do your homework for you."

Certainly anyone who takes up marathon jogging for his health can expect it to provide the physiological and psychological advantages of long distance running in general. But there is no magic in the marathon distance. Actually, in recent years, the original Bassler theory (that the completion of the marathon distance in $4^{1}/_{2}$ hours or less confers an immunity from a fatal heart attack for two to three years), has become magnified out of all proportion.

The story of the "marathon controversy" is worth the telling if only to demonstrate how, from time to time, even the most clear-thinking scientists can get themselves sidetracked. The stage was set when Dr. Tom Bassler, a Californian pathologist, stated that he had never performed an autopsy on a non-smoking marathoner and found the cause of death to be coronary atherosclerosis. Neither, he said, did he expect to. He then propounded his contentious theory maintaining that the marathoner's lifestyle was incompatible with fatal coronary atherosclerosis. Further, he challenged physicians to produce autopsy evidence that would contradict his statement.

The outcome was predictable. Most physicians, as well as the lay media, accepted the claim for what it was worth. After all, our own Toronto post-coronary program had already demonstrated in the most dramatic way that individuals with indisputable evidence of coronary atherosclerosis, including angiography, can train for and complete marathons. A few responded more vigorously, producing case after case which purported to destroy the Bassler hypothesis. But that wasn't as easy as it looked. Electrocardiographic evidence of heart disease was not acceptable, nor were classical symptoms of a heart attack. Nothing more than an autopsy would suffice! Not only that, but the findings at autopsy had to show that death was due to a heart attack brought about by recent blockage of a coronary artery, and Bassler demanded proof that the deceased had *completed* a marathon within a specified period of time. When subjected to these criteria, the counter-arguments failed. Meanwhile, as the increasing hordes of joggers went quietly about their daily training programs, the hard-core protagonists on both sides continued the debate as if it were of apocalyptic magnitude. For myself, I always saw Bassler's theory as a novel and provocative philosophy, something to discuss over a friendly beer or even during a fun marathon jog. Besides, even if I cannot accept Bassler's argument in total, I share his belief in the health value of jogging.

The recent blows against the Bassler bastion have come from Cape Town, South Africa, where Dr. Tim Noakes reports four cases of autopsy-proved coronary atherosclerosis in marathon runners. One runner with severe coronary atherosclerosis died during a 15-mile race; another had a heart attack and died in hospital while awaiting coronary bypass surgery. Two others killed in an automobile accident were found to have coronary atherosclerosis on post-mortem examination. (Interestingly, one of the two runners who actually died as the result of a heart attack was a smoker. The other had only been running long-distance events for 14 months; in this period, he entered and finished eight standard marathons, a 35-mile race and a 56-mile race.) Thus it would now seem, at least on the face of it, that the Bassler imperative can be laid to rest. If so (and we have to see Bassler's rebuttal yet), then we can all take pleasure in the fact that the coup was delivered by a likeable young physician who is a keen marathoner himself and who, gracious in victory, is quick to comment: "We cannot prove that marathon running did not reduce the rate of progression of coronary atherosclerosis in these or other athletes. Nor can we prove that if these men had not been marathon runners, they would not have died sooner."

This attitude is in sharp contrast to the Jeremiahs who, startled by Bassler's approach, have attacked the whole concept of long distance running on the basis that it is too dangerous. I am all for caution; recklessness can never be the hallmark of a successful exercise program. But I think we should be very careful that we don't frighten people away from healthy, strenuous endeavour. After all, what is left for the individual to challenge in today's world? Politics, business, interpersonal relationships are all so complex that effort is synonymous with stress. In the sixties, the young turned left from all this; they dropped out, refused to play, made failure a fetish. The seventies generation has, I believe, developed a much healthier approach. Like the Greeks (and even the much despised Victorians), they sense the harmony that must exist between a healthy mind and a healthy body. They seem to be discovering that discord in this interrelationship can have disastrous consequences. Oh, I admit that the symbolism is obvious. We are all running away from something. But in a way, that is a perfectly healthy reaction. Nature intended that we only stand and fight if we have a good chance of winning. If we can't win, then we were meant to run. Standing still in the face of imminent danger or, to put it another way, leading a sedentary life of constant anxiety, is an inappropriate action which ultimately leads to health breakdown. Movement placates the primitive brain, keeps it happy and ensures the efficient operation of all those intricate bodily mechanisms which are totally independent of the brain.

All of the foregoing may help you decide whether or not you want to prepare for a fun marathon. In the final analysis, you have to make your own decision. But maybe it will help if we look at the practical pros and cons.

Pros

Despite the introduction of such unofficial distances as 50 miles and 100 miles, the marathon 26 miles, 385 yards (or, in metric, 42 kilometres) still remains the longest official foot-race held under the auspices of the International Amateur Athletic Federation, the world's governing body of track and field. Thus, all official marathon races have to receive approval of that body or its local representative. This means that the course must be over a road surface, must be very accurately measured, must be kept clear of vehicular traffic during the competition and, while being challenging, should not be "impossible." The officials, including the timers, must be certified as competent, and the timekeeping apparatus must be checked for accuracy. The official nature of the contest endows it with a considerable air of status. Make no mistake about it, there is a great feeling of achievement in finishing. You walk ten feet tall for weeks afterwards.

Even the start of a marathon race is exciting. The atmosphere is almost carnival-like. Gathered together behind the starting line are thousands of individuals with similar interests, but from all walks of life. You are all there for the same purpose — to test your body's capacity to finish the same course under the same climatic conditions and in accordance with the same rules. Favouritism is impossible. In such circumstances, one can appreciate the deep sense of camaraderie which exists among fun marathoners.

For them, it is a paramount ingredient of the whole proceedings. In this regard, you have to pity the serious competitor who can only allow himself the luxury of empathizing with his fellow runner after the race is over. The occasion, then, is a great motivator. Wherever it takes place, be it New York, Boston, Detroit, Toronto or Honolulu, its anticipation sustains you through those days when cheerless circumstances all combine to make those first few steps of your workout a supreme triumph of will over won't!

As a benchmark of your cardiovascular fitness, you probably couldn't choose better than a marathon, for more than fitness is required. You also require self-discipline not only in training, but also on the day of the race when you must keep a pace that is well within your capacity. There is nothing like a marathon to expose the foolhardy, those who consistently over-estimate their own capabilities.

Finally, when all the shouting has died down, most of us have to agree that marathoners seem to have the sort of metabolic and biochemical programming that scientists have consistently associated with a low incidence of coronary heart disease: slim, almost skinny, with minimal body fat, non-smokers, possessing a slowly beating, powerfully stroking heart and with high levels of so-called protective (or HDL) cholesterol. It would be suprising if such types didn't have noticeably less incidence of heart attacks.

Cons

If you don't like crowds, then you'd better pick your marathons carefully. Since becoming a national craze, the number of entrants in most of the major events can be counted in the thousands rather than the hundreds. So you are now faced with the hassle of finding suitable accommodation before the race. The last time I brought thirteen of my patients to take part in the New York Marathon, we had to book our rooms six months ahead of time! On the plus side, the New York Marathon is a model of efficiency. The same cannot be said for many other less well-organized races. What worked beautifully for 300 or 400 competitors becomes a disaster area when applied to 5,000 or 6,000 runners. On balance, the increased numbers tend to bring out more cheering onlookers and enhance the carnival atmosphere, and so can't be entirely condemned. Nevertheless, the mass marathons are not for the fastidious!

Another side effect of mass participation is the arrival of the pseudo-scientific gimmickery, the exhibitions which are now associated with the run and in which one must endure the spectacle of stall after stall displaying running shoes, sweat suits, stop watches, socks, pedometers, vitamins, food supplements, insoles, arch supports, shoe repair outfits, heart rate monitors, energy drinks, T-shirts, I.D. bracelets, treadmills, wrist radios, head band radios, reflective tape, anti-chafe cream, anti-sunburn cream, books on running, magazines on running, audio cassettes on running, etc., etc., etc. Some of the products currently on the market are of great help to runners. But for those who relish the simplicity of jogging, today's commercialism comes as a bit of a jolt.

The decision to enter a marathon requires, as you will see later in this chapter, a considerable commitment on your part. If you are to do yourself justice, avoid injury or accident, then you must be prepared to invest roughly the equivalent of a day a week in training time. If you are compulsive, competitive or careless of the signals given out by a tired or strained body, then you should think twice before you take up marathoning. Remember that all athletic injuries are self-inflicted wounds invariably caused by 1) exceeding your current level of competence either in terms of speed, duration or frequency of workout session; 2) not allowing for the effect of external conditions such as hills, head wind or rough ground; or 3) ignoring the signs of fatigue, lack of sleep, infections, etc. You can only draw on your body's reserve of energy for so long; sooner or later, the debt must be repaid. The marathon is the day of reckoning. It tests your personality as much as your physical endurance. If you suspect that either is likely to be found wanting, then better give it a miss — at least until you come to terms with yourself.

Having read all of the above, let's assume you decide to have a go. What's the next step? You must prepare yourself. That means a training program. It is not my intention to compete with the avalanche of running books which have appeared on the market over the past ten years or so. My advice will be strictly limited to the middle-aged jogger who is planning to enter his or her first marathon, whose sole aim is to finish — not necessarily in good time, but certainly in good shape. Furthermore, it is assumed that you are already at the stage of being able to jog six miles in one hour (10-minute mile pace) five times weekly; that is, you are jogging 30 miles a week. If you are not yet at this stage, then you have to work up to it before following the marathon training plan. I do have some patients who have successfully completed a marathon and cannot jog faster than a 12-minute mile pace, but they are exceptions, and I invariably like to train them on a personal basis, running with them myself.

Preparation

First, pick your initial marathon carefully. Avoid a very hilly course or one that has a reputation for strong head winds. Try to stay away from the hot part of the year; if the temperature is likely to be high, make sure the organizers of the race have a good track record for supplying plenty of ice and fluid along the route. Most important of all, make sure that the race is one which welcomes joggers. A serious, competitive marathon attracts top-class runners whose sole purpose in being there is to win or make a good time. In such company, joggers will invariably get under the feet of runners and officials alike. Not only that, but it is expected that no one will be out on the course longer than 3 hours, or $3^1/_2$ at the most. So when you cross the finish line in $4^1/_2$ or 5 hours, you may be shattered to find that there is no line; it has been erased, the timekeepers have gone home, and the changing rooms are probably locked. A large marathon nowadays often caters to both top-flight runners and fun joggers (the overwhelming numbers of joggers providing a most welcome bonanza in entry fees). In this case, the rule at the start is runners in the front rank, joggers behind. These days it is not unusual for joggers like myself to discover it takes five or six minutes from the time the gun goes off to reach the starting line! Incidentally, your best source of information for all of the above points is a good journal such as *Runners World* or, better still, another jogger. You will be surprised to find how anxious other joggers are to help.

Well, you've picked your first marathon. How do you train for it? Before getting into that, I would like to make one point which I suppose should be self-evident. If there were such a thing as the perfect training method, then every coach and every athlete would be using it. In reality, there are as many training schedules as there are athletes using them. The more one studies the training methods of world-class athletes, the more variations you see. Why is that? Again, I think the answer is obvious. When one is striving for excellence, every strength must be exploited, every weakness must be minimized. The game plan, if it is to be successful, must be custom-designed, not an off-the-shelf item. Your needs are not so critical. Nevertheless, you should take a lesson from your betters. The smart thing to do is to learn the accepted basic training principles for your chosen event, and then use them to modify the program you are following. Tables printed in a book, no matter how good that book is (and that includes this one), should never be adhered to slavishly. Look at it like this: the more successful the book is, the more copies it will sell and, therefore, the more individuals will read it. Do you honestly think that a training schedule drawn up for a million aspiring athletes is going to suit all of them? I would be surprised if it worked for 50 per cent.

Basic Principles of a Long Distance Training Program

In order to jog 26 miles, 385 yards non-stop, you have to cover a considerable number of miles in training. Furthermore, the mileage must consist of both medium and long distance runs. In addition to increasing your ability to utilize oxygen, long runs teach the body to become more efficient in utilizing fat as a working fuel. The primary source of energy used by muscle is carbohydrate, in the form of glycogen (see Chapter 2). When the muscle burns up all its available supply of glycogen, it is no longer able to function. This is what happens when your legs give out on a long run — "hitting the wall," they call it. But the muscles can also burn fat and don't hesitate to do so when their glycogen store starts to run low. Fat-burning becomes a significant factor in muscle metabolism on any run in excess of 6 miles, which is why that distance has been chosen as the basic training unit in the marathon training tables that follow on page 271. It is only by running six miles and up that you accustom your system to using fat as a fuel, thus eking out the precious supply of energy-rich glycogen.

Given that mileage is a prerequisite, the next obvious question to be answered is, how much? There is a theory that if you want to be sure of finishing a certain distance in a race, your average weekly mileage (seven days a week) for eight weeks before the race should be one-third of the race distance; that is, for the marathon you would have to jog $8^3/_4$ miles a day or $61^1/_4$ miles a week for eight weeks prior to the day of the race. This rule of thumb works quite well and has stood the test of time. However, I have found that for the fun jogger who is maintaining a year-round average of about 30 miles a week and who is not concerned with finishing times, this order of mileage may be a little on the high side and can be reduced by about 10 per cent. Is there a total mileage which you should have completed before entering your first marathon? Empirically and based on experience with post-coronary middle-aged patients, I have established the "1,000-mile rule." Simply put, it states that the beginning marathoner must have jogged a minimum of 1,000 miles in training before being allowed to enter. In addition, for the reasons stated above, the mileage should be calculated in units of six miles in other words, anything less than six miles d sn't count — only six miles and over. In the final three months before the marathon, the requirement is for 48 to 60 miles a week (eight to ten six-mile units), using a judicious blend of six (one unit), twelve (two units) and eighteen (three units) jogs.

Build-up versus Breakdown   You can define training as the repeated application of measured doses of stress to the body to stimulate the development of beneficial chemical and biological changes. The net result is greater resistance to the stress applied. Strength through adversity, as it were. However, it is not too difficult to imagine a situation in which the amount or duration of stress is so great that it overwhelms the body's defences completely before it has had time to become stronger. In some ways, excessive training is worse than no training at all. This may seem obvious, but this is probably the most difficult point to put across to any athlete. It seems we always get back to the old business of "if one pill is good for you, then two pills are twice as good for you, and four pills are four times as good for you!"

It may help to look at it like this. Training is a two-stage process. The first stage consists of the application of the stimulus or, in our terms, the workout. The second stage consists of the body's responses to that stimulus. This latter stage is just as important as the first and, as a matter of fact, requires a greater period of time. Thus, if you are to get benefit from your workout, you must allow time for the body to complete the job. If you apply the stimulus again and again, not allowing for any response, a training effect can never occur. Worse, the whole system begins to break down, the athlete's performances rapidly deteriorate, resistance to disease drops, and illness occurs.

How can we avoid this? Firstly, by adopting a training schedule which alternates periods of heavy work with periods of light work, long runs with middle-distance runs, faster runs with slower runs. We can also be constantly on the lookout for signs of over-training. The main ones are:

- fall in body weight below the usual training level;
- irritability and insomnia;
- muscle ache in the legs at night in bed;
- running nose, often lasting only for a day or two and frequently attributed to a cold or allergy;
- tendency to minor gastro-intestinal upsets (e.g., nausea, diarrhea);
- vague aching pain in the joints, not accompanied by redness or swelling;
- sore throat; enlarged glands in the neck, under the arms, or in the groins; and
- tendency to inco-ordination (e.g., tripping, becoming "accident-prone").

If you suspect over-training, then obviously the first thing to do is check your average mileage over the previous few months. Remember to take into account the speed of the jogs, the presence of adverse physical conditions such as high humidity, hills, poor running surface. And finally, make sure you're not burning the candle at both ends. You can't expect to keep up a heavy training schedule if you are working twice as hard at your job.

Natural Endowment   Never forget that all the training in the world is not going to turn a cart-horse into a Kentucky Derby contender. As a fun jogger, that shouldn't worry you. But if you start to become too ambitious, you might bear it in mind. There are such things as born marathoners just as there are born sprinters. These days, exercise physiologists are prone to carry out what they call muscle biopsies and talk knowingly about fast-twitch and slow-twitch fibres. The procedure consists of removing a minute piece of muscle tissue from deep within the muscle by means of a small needle-like instrument. Examined under a microscope, the muscle is seen to contain two types of fibres, slow and fast twitch. The higher the percentage of slow-twitch fibres present, the more the individual is suited to endurance type running. Conversely, the greater the percentage of fast-twitch fibres, the greater the propensity for speed. While training is thought to be able to improve the metabolic efficiency of both types of fibres, it seems unlikely that it can effect any marked change in their relative proportion. So don't expect training to achieve miracles. You are in it for your health, not just to beat that scraggy guy with the thin legs who always seems to run farther and faster than you, no matter how hard you try to catch him.

The training tables that follow are designed for the fun jogger, post-coronary or otherwise, who has achieved Level 6 of Phase 3 of the general training tables: i.e., six miles at the 10 or 12-minute mile pace, five times weekly, and who has been carrying this out easily and without symptoms or discomfort for a period of at least three months. The aim is to enable you to finish a marathon safely in a time of between $4^1/2$ and $6^1/2$ hours, depending on your initial level of fitness. They incorporate the following principles:

1) There are five stages, each of three weeks, between the basic 30 miles a week level and the start of a three-month preparation period for the marathon itself. When you are "coasting" between marathons, depending upon the weekly mileage you wish to maintain, you can choose any one of the five stages as a "holding pattern."

2) Since endurance, not speed, is our goal, no training jog is shorter than six miles.

3) Distances in excess of six miles are at proportionately slower pace (see Table 3). The purpose of training is to build up, not tear down. I am well aware that you are capable of running these longer distances quicker than the times specified, just as I am also aware that a 60-minute six-miler can run one single mile in 8 minutes or less. The fact is that many world-class marathoners do the bulk of their training at speeds 30 to 40 per cent slower than their best competition times. If it is good enough for them, why not us? Try, therefore, not to exceed the prescribed speeds.

4) Included in the workouts are a number of "speed-play" sessions where only the actual duration of the training session is given; the distance covered is ignored. For instance, a 4-hour speed-play session means that you walk and jog, comfortably and easily, for that period of time. I enjoy these sessions. They make a pleasant break, boost your morale, and help to prepare you mentally for being out on the marathon course for that period of time. The trick is to start slowly, and introduce the walk/jog sessions (say 5 minutes walk followed by 10 minutes jog) right from the outset. Don't jog until you are too tired to go any further, and then have to start walking.

5) Because the body needs rest as part of its building-up program, long, hard workouts are alternated with shorter jogs or rest days, both on a daily and weekly basis.

6) Our customary five days a week training shedule has been retained, and the highest weekly mileage has been held to between 45 and 53 miles. Admittedly, running six or even seven times a week will "up" the mileage considerably and produce faster racing times. But we are not racing, and 30 minutes or even 60 minutes saved in a marathon is scant compensation for the fun jogger whose hitherto enjoyable workout has become a relentless, deadly grind. So, if you want to race, or feel that you are too good for the 60-minute six-mile class, then skip these tables, and look elsewhere for advice.

Table 1
You are already jogging 30 miles a week, comfortably

		Stage 1			Stage 2			Stage 3			Stage 4			Stage 5		
Week	1	2	3	1	2	3	1	2	3	1	2	3	1	2	3
Day															
1	R	R	R	R	R	R	R	R	R	R	R	R	R	R	R
2	6	6	6	6	6	6	9	8	9	8	9	8	6	9	6
3	6	6	6	6	6	6	7	8	7	8	9	8	9	9	9
4	6	6	6	9	9	9	7	8	7	8	9	8	9	9	9
5	6	6	6	6	6	6	7	8	7	9	9	9	9	9	9
6	R	R	R	R	R	R	R	R	R	R	R	R	R	R	R
7	9	9	9	9	9	9	10	8	10	12	9	12	15	SP	15
Total														(4 hr)	
Mileage	33	33	33	36	36	36	40	40	40	45	45	45	48		48

Key: R = Rest   SP = Speed Play   M = Marathon

Table 2
Three-month preparation leading to marathon

		Month 1				Month 2				Month 3			Marathon
Week	1	2	3	4	1	2	3	4	1	2	3	4	Week
Day													
1	R	R	R	R	R	R	R	R	R	R	R	R	R
2	8	9	8	10	10	6	6	8	R	8	9	9	10
3	9	12	9	10	6	10	10	10	12	6	9	9	R
4	9	10	9	6	10	10	9	8	10	12	9	9	R
5	9	10	7	12	9	12	10	6	12	10	9	7	R
6	R	R	R	R	R	R	R	R	R	R	R	R	R
7	18	12	20	SP	18	SP	18	SP	12	12	10	10	M
Total				(4 hr)		(4 hr)		(5 hr)					26¼
Mileage	53	53	53		53		53		46	48	46	44	36¼

Table 3
Pacing table

	Time	
Miles	Min. per mile	Total (hours)
6	10	1:00:00
7	10	1:10:00
8	10	1:20:00
9	10½	1:34:30
10	10½	1:45:00
12	11	2:12:00
15	11	2:45:00
18	12	3:36:00
20	12	4:00:00

The Big Day

Finally, the moment of truth has arrived. Your training has gone to plan, you have by luck as much as by good management avoided injury, and in a matter of hours you will be embarking on one of the most interesting if not most exciting experiences of your life. If you are smart, you will have checked out all your final preparations with an experienced marathoner. If you are lucky, you will be in the company of such an individual who will inevitably save you from the classic beginner's mistakes. Failing both, you will just have to read this section carefully. If you find it a little trite, then I assure you you are the very person who needs it. Admitted, these are the sort of obvious comments which you won't find in the high-powered training manuals — but I'll bet the majority of marathoners would have welcomed them in the early stages of their careers.

The Week Before   To deal with the question of carbohydrate loading, we have to go back to the week before the big event. Even if you don't follow this procedure, you should know something about it. Carbohydrates, sugars and starches are the body's major sources of energy. After digestion, they are broken down into glucose, a substance easily burned up by working muscle. Glucose, however, is an immediate source of energy and so when we eat more carbohydrate than we need for the time being, the body changes it into glycogen and stores it in both muscle and liver. This store can be called upon in times of need (e.g., running a marathon) and converted back into the easily utilized glucose. Obviously the greater the store of glycogen in your muscles, the more muscular work you will be able to do. Carrying the argument further, the way to increase the glycogen stores is to increase the intake of carbohydrate foods while at the same time limiting muscular action to a minimum.

This is the basic theory of carbohydrate loading. There are one or two refinements. If you drain the muscle of its glycogen content first, then you can stuff more glycogen in during the high carbohydrate ingestion. How do you drain the muscle of glycogen? Once glycogen is stored in muscle, the only way to get it out is for the muscle to burn it. This means going for a run which is long enough and fast enough to make your legs ache and become a little wobbly — and then plod on for about another mile! Obviously the distance will vary with individuals, but for the fun jogger it is probably around six to ten miles. On the three succeeding days following this workout the muscle glycogen level is kept at extremely low levels by adhering to a diet which contains only minimal amounts of carbohydrates (about 60 grams a day), and is very high in fat and protein. During this "depletion" stage, you may jog three miles or so daily but don't be surprised if your legs feel like lead and you find yourself becoming increasingly ill-tempered and depressed. The three days of high-fat, high-protein diet finishes with another leg-aching depletion run of about five miles (if you really restricted the carbohydrates you may be labouring as early as two miles). Finally, you reward yourself by switching to very high carbohydrate foods for the final three days before the marathon. Since you are trying to conserve every gram of the extra muscle glycogen you have managed to store, you do not do any exercising or running at all during this stage. Eat little and often, use natural carbohydrates such as fruits, cereals and whole-wheat bread, rather than cakes and candies, which are loaded with refined sugar. If all works to plan, then you can expect to have a good deal more spring in your legs over the last four to six miles of the marathon run.

Are there any provisos? The first thing to note is that for every molecule of glycogen stored by the muscle, three molecules of water are stored at the same time. It is for this reason that you should drink plentiful supplies of water during the three-day carbohydrate loading phase. But this additional stored water means an increase in body weight, and all that much more to carry over the 26 miles, 385 yards; which is why some world-class marathoners who are strong on endurance but slow on speed do not carbohydrate-load before an important race. The additional weight slows them up in the initial stages of the race, the period in which they are most vulnerable. This increase in weight, as a matter of interest, provides a method of checking the effectiveness of your carbohydrate-loading program during the high carbohydrate stage. You should weigh yourself every morning; when maximum glycogen storage has been achieved, your weight will increase by about two or three pounds. So you must balance the advantages of the extra glycogen against the disadvantages of the additional weight. There is one set of circumstances in which the stored water, extra weight or no extra weight, can come to your help. When you know that the run is going to be held in conditions of high temperature or high humidity and that dehydration is an ever-present threat, then maximal glycogen loading means that you start the run with a water storage of about $2^{1/2}$ pints. This represents a reserve within the muscle cells which can afford to be lost in heavy sweating.

I have one other reservation to make on the subject of carbohydrate loading. A preliminary high-fat, high-protein diet is the least important aspect of the process — in fact, some authorities feel that it has no value at all. But, more important from the point of view of the middle-aged male, it may result in a precipitate rise in blood fat levels, with all its attendant dangers to the cardio-vascular system. For those of us in that age group, then, I suggest you miss out this stage.

The Day Before the Day   This can be a critical period. Your diet should be light, easily digested. You will receive all sorts of advice from faddists, ranging from fruit juices for 24 hours to steaks for breakfast, and I suppose there will be the odd individual who performs well on these regimes. In general, you will do best to stay with small amounts of what you fancy. I never cease to be amazed by the unerring accuracy by which the long distance jogger's appetite chooses that which his body needs the most!

But diet isn't everything. You should try and get an early night; even if excitement keeps you awake until the early hours, console yourself with the thought that insomnia will not take its toll on your physical performance until the day *after* the race. Of course, you will have checked all the practicalities. You will have packed your shoes (in which you have run at least 200 miles) and also packed a spare pair of laces. There is nothing more frustrating than breaking a lace just before the start and not having a spare. I hate to admit it, but I have arrived in Reno the night before the Silver City Marathon and been devastated to find that I had forgotten to pack my running shoes. If it were not for the incredible tolerance and kindness of the race organizer who persuaded the proprietor of the local Athlete's Foot Store (another jogger) to open his establishment and help get me fitted with a pair of Etonics, I would have had to pad the entire distance in bare feet! I have even been known to pack two left shoes. Fortunately, my jogging patients are now familiar with this weakness and invariably check my running gear before I leave Toronto.

Another invaluable item is a jar of vaseline. There is nothing worse than trying to run the last three or four miles of a marathon with agonizingly chafing thighs. Never mind that flies, road dirt and assorted airborne items stick to your person, you should be sure to apply vaseline liberally to your inner thighs, nipples, armpits and anal area.

The Morning of the Race   No matter how early the race starts, you are obliged to get out of bed about four hours beforehand. Otherwise, you won't have left enough time to digest your breakfast. Many competitors are happy to go to the starting line with just a slice of toast and a glass of orange juice. Others require something more substantial. Whatever you do, try not to eat within three hours of the starting time; that will leave enough time for digestion. Breakfast should be light enough to have passed the stomach within a three-hour period which means that protein (bacon, sausage, steak) and fatty foods are prohibited.

Immediate pre-race nutritional needs are minimal. I advise my joggers to pre-hydrate, and so 20 minutes before the start, they drink half a pint of water. Don't worry about having to urinate during the run; marathon joggers, both male and female, never suffer from false modesty and always manage to find convenient bushes or stone walls along the route. Some runners have the false impression that high sugar content drinks or glucose tablets taken within 30 to 60 minutes of the start will provide extra energy. Nothing could be further from the truth! The intake of sugar just before physical exercise results in a compensatory drop in blood glucose; this leads to a premature breakdown of the glycogen store in the muscle in order to bring the blood glucose back to normal levels. Thus, the muscle glycogen is used at an earlier stage in the race than normal and, consequently, is used up all the more quickly.

During the Race   Try to drink fluid, about 8 to 10 ounces, every 20 to 30 minutes. Water is probably best, although a slight fruit flavouring may be more appealing to the taste.

The more efficiently your muscles burn fat, the more sparing you are of your glycogen store. Recently there has been some evidence to suggest that the ingestion of caffeine about an hour before a long run will stimulate the breakdown of fat. So you might try a strong cup of coffee or tea 60 minutes before the start; but remember that caffeine also has a diuretic effect (i.e. it makes you pass urine more frequently). This may be a nuisance under normal conditions, but in the hot weather, it could aggravate the risk of dehydration.

You are now ready to make your way to the starting line. Unless it is very warm, you should keep your sweat suit on until a few minutes before the one-minute warning gun. You have applied your vaseline, adjusted your sweat headband, double-tied your shoe laces, pinned your number to the front of your running vest, made the last of what seems to have been innumerable visits to the toilet over the past few hours, put a dime in your sock in order to make a telephone call in case you get stranded along the way, and handed your carefully wrapped belongings to your long-suffering wife or the appropriate race official. You are ready to go.

For those who merely want to finish, the die is cast in the first two miles. This is especially true for the novice marathoner. It's not until you enter your first race that you have any conception of the excitement at the start. You need a will of iron not to go charging off with the other thousands, elbow to elbow and shoulder to shoulder, caught up in a human cavalry charge that will take you to the five-mile point at a speed you never thought you were capable of. By then, it's too late. You've blown it. By the tenth mile, you are uncomfortable; by the fourteenth, you are praying you can finish; and by the twentieth, you have accepted the inevitability of having to drop out.

The answer is obvious. *Start slowly!* I can't emphasize that enough. Don't worry about letting people get ahead of you. I can assure you that if you have trained properly, and if your only aim is to finish, you will invariably experience the ecstasy of passing people one by one in the last two to three miles. If you feel embarrassed at being so far behind in the initial stages of the run, console yourself with the thought that the onlookers reserve their cheers for the first 50 and the last 200 finishers. If it's crowd adulation you want, then you can always double the cheering by putting on a teeth-gritting, true blue, stiff upper lip expression over the final 100 yards.

Two other points. If you fall into a conversation with a fellow jogger along the way, make sure you don't unintentionally fall into running at his pace — unless you know him well and are sure that he plans to finish in the same time as you. It's easy to get carried along and find you've run two or three miles at a minute or more faster per mile than you had planned. Secondly, don't experiment with new drinks along the way. If you trained using water, then don't try some other type of drink. I can recall Jerome Drayton experimenting with a proprietary electrolyte drink in the Fukuoka Marathon in Japan and having to drop out with severe cramps. There was nothing wrong with the drink, it was just that he wasn't used to it. If a runner of Jerome's stature and experience can fall into that trap, how much easier for you as a novice.

From time to time in the first 20 miles, remind yourself that the marathon really only starts at 20 miles! That will keep you from squandering your energy too early in the game. Let's face it, many people can complete a 20-mile jog. It's the last six that separates the men from the boys. If your legs begin to feel very tired before the finish, there is no shame in walking for a few hundred yards and then picking up the jog again. In fact, I believe that it is better to slow to a walk from time to time when you still have some strength left, rather than grimly plodding along in a pathetic semblance of the jog only to slow to a walk out of complete necessity. When that happens, it is extremely unlikely that you will be able to get back into jogging tempo again.

Above all, don't race! Leave that to the talented young guys — or the dumb old ones. I realize it may require will power, but it really isn't going to make that much difference whether you finish in 4 hours, 30 minutes or 4 hours, 20 minutes. If you have a problem with your ego, don't let your nearest and dearest watch you. They won't be impressed by the sight of their hero, slack-jawed and blue in the face, trying to grunt his way past a sweet, smiling old lady or a rotund, middle-aged executive with a "Joggers Make Better Lovers" message on his T-shirt. Actually, it is probably better not to have your nearest and dearest anywhere near the finish at all. You probably look so haggard by then that you might be delivered an ultimatum to stop all this mara-thoning nonsense immediately — or else!

You've finished! I won't attempt to describe the feeling. Any words of mine would be superfluous. Now it's time for that beer (after a light sandwich), a shower, change, and start to put together the step-by-step, mile-by-mile narrative with which you are going to bore the office staff for the next few months — or until the next marathon!

Epilogue

This book started with the story of a rehabilitation success. Eight men ran along a road in Boston, and proved a point. There was nothing miraculous in what they did. In a way, the whole purpose of the exercise was to prove that very point; namely, it does not require a miracle for men or women who have had a heart attack to perform feats of physical endurance with safety. What it does require is motivation on their part and some informed medical guidance. Given these two ingredients, any post-coronary patient can learn to function maximally.

The results of the Toronto Rehabilitation Centre's post-coronary exercise program have been most encouraging. Acceptance of the program by the community, family physicians and cardiologists has been high, with some 2,500 patients joining the program over the past eleven years. Currently the referral rate is running at 10 to 15 new patients a week, with the result that an additional wing to the Centre has been built which will be devoted entirely to the rehabilitation of cardiac patients.

The exercise compliance rate has been excellent. A careful follow-up of our first consecutively referred 610 patients showed that 82.8 per cent continued to exercise at least three times weekly, and that only 2.8 per cent have ceased to exercise altogether. Considering that the compliance rate in most programs is less than 50 per cent after two years, it is apparent that these results are exceptional and indicate that in virtually all patients the program effects a sustained alteration in their exercise pattern. These facts also give the lie to the repeated charge that jogging is boring and that few individuals will ever stick with a regular exercise regime that emphasizes only jogging.

To date, some 38 of our patients have taken part in a total of over 148 official marathon runs. These cardiac marathoners have not differed greatly in terms of their clinical history and running experience from the general post-coronary population. On admission to the program their cardiovascular fitness level was similar to that of the other patients, but in response to long and careful training they showed as much as a 55 per cent increase in their maximum oxygen consumption. These post-coronary marathoners have been generous in sharing their experiences with other patients and have continued to provide a constant source of encouragement for everyone else involved in the program.

How have our patients fared in terms of a second heart attack? In following the history of our first 610 patients for a period of ten years, there has been an annual fatal recurrence rate of 1.1 per cent and a non-fatal recurrence rate of 1.0 per cent. Fatal and non-fatal recurrence rates were particularly low among patients who had exercised on the program for more than two years. In this group the recurrence rate was only 0.85 per cent per annum. These rates are considerably lower than the usual annual mortality of between 4 per cent and 6 per cent per year in the first five years after a heart attack; they are also consistent with the reports of others who have found that recurrence rates are lower in exercising than in non-exercising post-heart attack patients.

However, while detailed statistical analysis is not appropriate for a book of this type, some interpretation of these results is necessary. It should be recognized that while they are highly suggestive of the efficacy of exercise in reducing recurrence, they cannot be accepted entirely as proof positive. Too many factors must be taken into account. For instance, like most other studies, we did not have an adequate control group of heart attack patients who were not exercised and who therefore could be compared with our patients. Then again, were the patients referred to the program the ones with the lowest recurrence risk? Were they, in other words, pre-selected or self-selected? My impression is that this is not so, but without assessing every other patient in Toronto who had a heart attack during the same period of time, one cannot be absolutely certain. Even if the referred patients are truly representative of all the other post-coronary patients, is it the exercise per se which is exerting this specific beneficial effect, or is it some other as yet unsuspected factor in the program's format? Again, one cannot be sure. All we can say is that the results indicate that our patients do well, and that the carefully prescribed vigorous exercise which they undertake does not increase their risk of dying suddenly or of suffering a further heart attack. In fact, our data and the data of William Haskell indicate that the risk of a heart attack occurring *during exercise* in a medically controlled rehabilitation program is no greater than that for the non-exercising post-coronary individual by chance alone.

At the same time, we must never lose sight of our goal: to successfully rehabilitate. Academic righteousness and statistical propriety should not be allowed to deny patients a method of therapy which cannot harm, and is to all intents and purposes, most effective in improving the quality even if not the quantity of life. After all, in the final analysis, it is the quality of life which matters most.

I daresay 43-year-old Al V. would be happy to think he had another thirty years to live, but right now he is delighted to be able to work full-time, look after his young family, and go jogging five mornings a week — especially when you consider that just after his heart attack five years ago, he was referred to the Centre with the label "suitable for modified sedentary work only." At that time, he was well on his way to becoming a complete neurotic, imagined every ache and pain was the sign of another heart attack, and was reluctant to try anything but the lightest type of work. An immigrant from Europe, his comprehension of the English language was not as good as it might have been, and he responded poorly to the usual rehabilitation techniques involving psychotherapy and work assessment. After attending the Centre daily for almost a year, he was still no closer to going back to work. Finally, he was discharged to the evening exercise program where the only form of therapy was supervised jogging. Almost immediately his mood began to improve. With each increase in his prescription came renewed confidence until by the time he was able to jog three miles comfortably in 30 minutes, he had enthusiastically started to look for a job again. Right now, his greatest problem is low back trouble resulting from the heavy lifting required in his trade!

For some, the attraction of the program lies entirely in its ability to make life more enjoyable. This type of individual will usually continue to enjoy his cigarettes, his double martini before dinner, and his late-night weekend party, despite the possibility that all of these things, especially the smoking, may increase the risk of a recurrence. One advertising executive put it like this, "I'm not jogging to live longer. I'm jogging because it's made me fit, and I can now enjoy certain pleasures in life which have always been important to me. I no longer have angina when I stay up late at night, I can play longer and harder than ever before, and for me that's what living is all about." Obviously this man is interested in something more than marking off the days on a calendar, and mortality statistics mean nothing to him.

While we have talked much of the healthy, simple life associated with recreational running, we shouldn't become cult-like in our approach. I do have two patients who have given up their jobs to become mailmen. One had his own business, and the other was a salesman. In both their cases, the combination of heart attack and the running program made them realize that they preferred an active, open-air job. It's fair to say, however, that the vast majority of patients have returned to their previous employment, and a significant number have obtained better positions than they held before the heart attack. An analysis of their economic situations showed that less than 1 per cent had suffered a drop in living standards since their heart attack and as a result of the illness. This is a far cry from the state of affairs which existed before the era of rehabilitation, when many state and provincial authorities reported sadly that as much as 50 per cent and higher of heart attack survivors never returned to work.

Even in the more advanced countries, the position isn't as bright as it might be. The following is an excerpt from a British Joint Working Party Report on Rehabilitation after Cardiac Illness, published in 1975.

Among previously employed survivors of myocardial infarction, 80 per cent returned to work eventually, but unnecessary delay is common. This encourages invalidism and causes unnecessary economic loss to the individual and the community. The reason for the delay may be summarized as physical (heart failure and angina), psychological (chiefly anxiety and depression), and social (redundancy, a job now considered unsuitable, or the discouraging advice and habits of family, friends and employers). Only a few patients have persisting disability from heart failure, crippling angina or mental breakdown. Most can return to the level of physical and intellectual activity which preceded the attack.

That the fit post-coronary patient is also successful at his job is hardly surprising. The old dictum "a healthy mind in a healthy body" may have some justification after all, since numerous reports have verified that fitness is frequently associated with a superior self-image, better emotional control, increased self-confidence, and improved mental activity.

With increased self-confidence may come both welcome and sometimes unexpected bonuses. An example of the first is the heavy drinker or borderline alcoholic who now finds that he doesn't need liquor to bolster his self-esteem. An example of the second is the bachelor who had open-heart surgery, went on to complete two marathon runs and, if that weren't enough, proceeded at the age of 48 to get married. The week this chapter was written, his wife presented him with an 8 lb. baby girl.

Or, in a lighter vein, there is the patient who came to us with a cholesterol phobia so big that he wouldn't eat in a restaurant until he had inspected the kitchens and satisfied himself that the cook was using unsaturated cooking oil; he weakened once, ate a shrimp cocktail, and didn't sleep for weeks. He can now dare to contemplate eating an egg, and has almost ceased driving his wife and family physician crazy.

But, I can hear you say, what of the failures? Surely every case history is not a success story. You are right. Life isn't a fairy tale, and there is no medical treatment or rehabilitation program which promises immortality. I have already referred to the men who have suffered a fatal recurrence. A small group, admittedly, but none the less important for all that. That is why their histories are continuously reviewed in order to see if they contain a clue as to what went wrong. In most cases, one can only surmise the answer. Wherever there is a lesson to be learned, it is quickly introduced into the program format for the benefit of the other patients.

And then there are the dropouts. These are the individuals who couldn't accommodate to the new lifestyle required of them. Again, they are small in number, but there is less comfort in that, for these are often the very people who need the most help. It might have been easier to retain them by asking for an easier commitment, by making less demands, by bending the truth so as to make it more palatable; but that wouldn't be doing them any favours, and it would hardly be fair to the vast majority who have been prepared to go the whole course, both uphill and downhill.

On balance, I would say that the failures are so heavily outweighed by the successes that their main value is not to deter but rather to help formulate a better program. This is not meant to sound callous. It is the customary approach taken with any form of medical treatment, and is both rational and humane. The problem for those who use exercise in the treatment of heart disease is that they are allowed very little, if any, margin for failure.

It is this which, in my opinion, has been largely responsible for the medical profession's reluctance to mobilize the post-coronary patient. Consider for a moment what happens if a heart patient undergoing rehabilitation drops dead in your local Y. Chances are that the incident will be fully reported in the morning paper, will probably receive mention on the town radio station, and might just make the tail-end of the late night T.V. news round-up. What if that patient were to die during heart surgery? It would likely receive no mention whatsoever in the media, unless he or she were someone of great importance. I realize that the exercise death may seem to be a more dramatic occurrence, taking place as it does in full view of the lay public. On the other hand, in some areas, post-coronary exercise rehabilitation is more common than by-pass surgery, has been around for a longer period of time, and has a far lower mortality rate. Which may put things a little more in perspective.

Yet, every achievement has its failure, and every success story has its sad note. On February 15, 1975, "Big John," one of the original eight who ran the Boston Marathon in 1973, died in his sleep. An autopsy, while revealing the scars from his previous two heart attacks, failed to show any recent thrombosis of the coronary vessels or, indeed, any acute myocardial damage. It must be assumed that he died from a cardiac arrest, possibly due to some form of electrical failure. A regular distance jogger, he had been faithful to his program, although remaining a fairly heavy cigarette smoker, and there is some indication that his cigarette consumption increased in the months before his death.

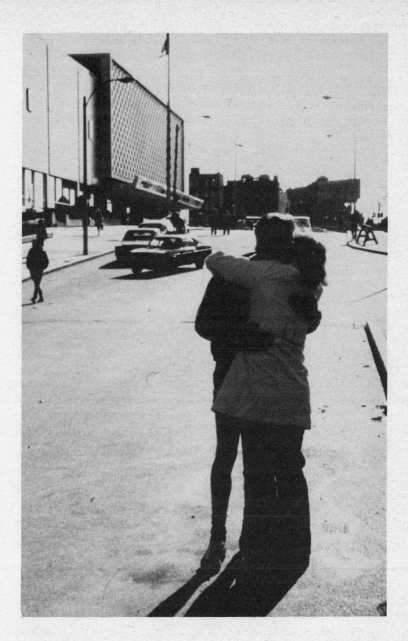

No medals, no crowds — but he made it! A T.R.C. *jogger in Prudential Square, Boston, 1975.*

He had not run a marathon since 1973, largely because of business and social commitments, but was planning to take part again in 1975. Of the men who ran with him in 1973, some returned to Boston again in 1976, and their elation at doing so well was tinged by sorrow at the loss of a good friend. The mood was not entirely melancholy, however, for at the post-race dinner we all recalled again the letter from his wife which expresses better than I can, the sum and substance of these pages. I can think of no better way to end than with an appropriate excerpt:

> "Knowing John's temperament, no one could have wished him a lingering end. I feel the program gave him seven vigorous and enjoyable years, living life the way he wanted to — to the hilt.
>
> "He was a fine man — so have a brandy or a martini for him and we'll all be with you in spirit at the 'Boston'."

Figure 14

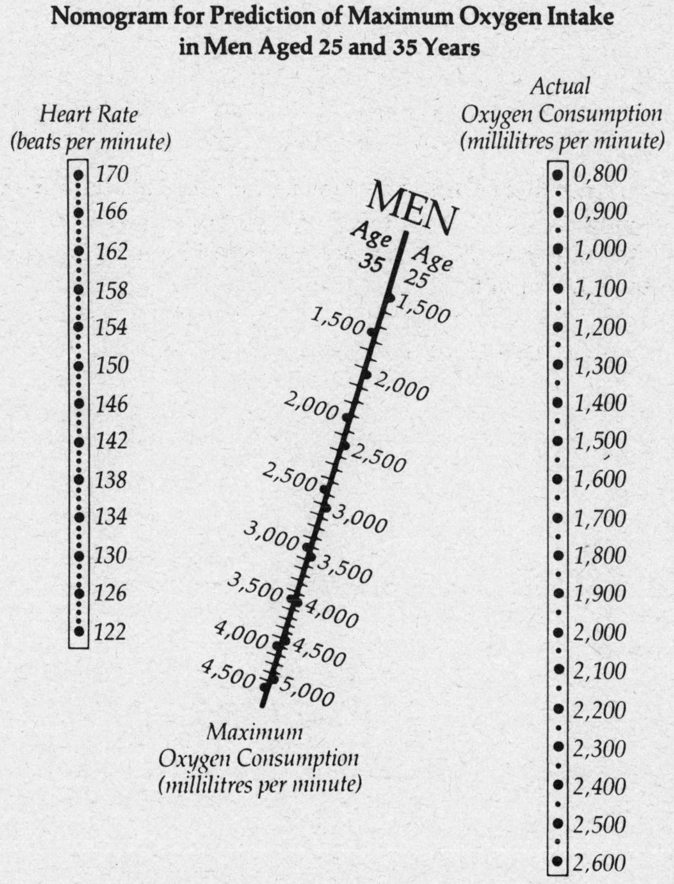

Nomogram for Prediction of Maximum Oxygen Intake in Men Aged 25 and 35 Years

Heart Rate
(beats per minute)

Actual
Oxygen Consumption
(millilitres per minute)

MEN

Age 35   Age 25

Maximum
Oxygen Consumption
(millilitres per minute)

*A line joining your heart rate and actual oxygen
consumption will intersect the centre line at
your maximum oxygen consumption.*

Figure 15

Nomogram for Prediction of Maximum Oxygen Intake
in Women Aged 25 and 35 Years

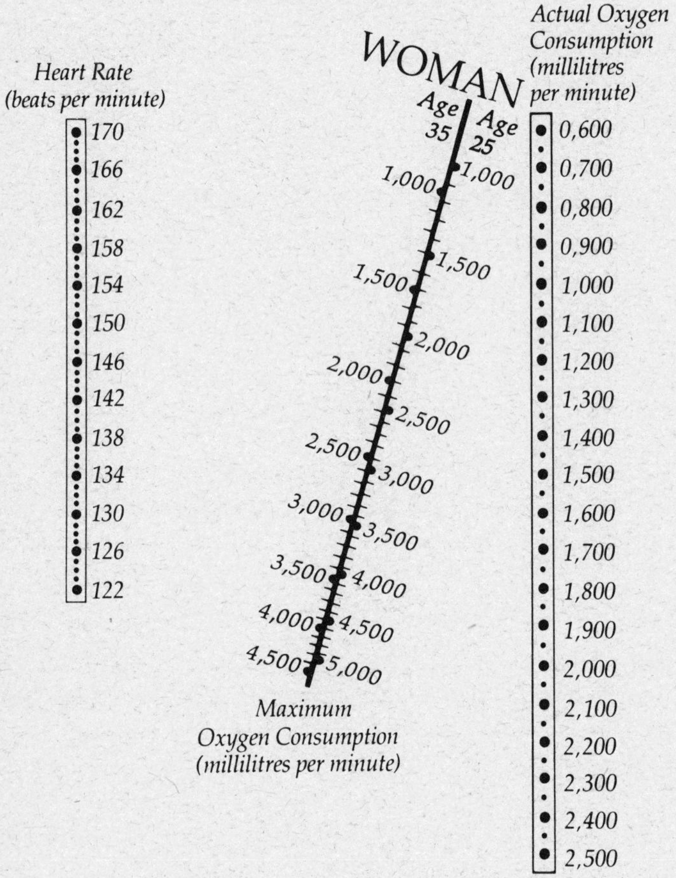

Heart Rate
(beats per minute)

WOMAN
Age 35   Age 25

Actual Oxygen
Consumption
(millilitres
per minute)

Heart Rate		Actual Oxygen Consumption
170	1,000 / 1,000	0,600
166		0,700
162		0,800
158	1,500 / 1,500	0,900
154		1,000
150	2,000	1,100
146	2,000	1,200
142	2,500	1,300
138	2,500 / 3,000	1,400
134		1,500
130	3,000 / 3,500	1,600
126	3,500 / 4,000	1,700
122	4,000 / 4,500	1,800
	4,500 / 5,000	1,900
		2,000
		2,100
		2,200
		2,300
		2,400
		2,500

Maximum
Oxygen Consumption
(millilitres per minute)

*A line joining your heart rate and actual oxygen
consumption will intersect the centre line at
your maximum oxygen consumption.*

Figure 16

Nomogram for Prediction of Maximum Oxygen Intake in Men Aged 45 and 55 Years

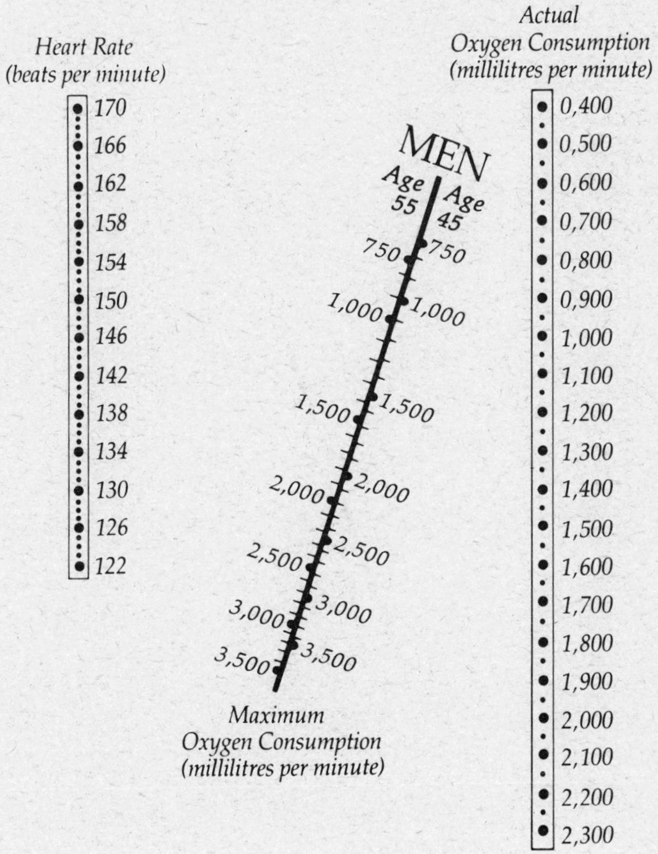

*Heart Rate
(beats per minute)*

170
166
162
158
154
150
146
142
138
134
130
126
122

MEN
Age 55   Age 45

750   750
1,000   1,000
1,500   1,500
2,000   2,000
2,500   2,500
3,000   3,000
3,500   3,500

*Maximum
Oxygen Consumption
(millilitres per minute)*

*Actual
Oxygen Consumption
(millilitres per minute)*

0,400
0,500
0,600
0,700
0,800
0,900
1,000
1,100
1,200
1,300
1,400
1,500
1,600
1,700
1,800
1,900
2,000
2,100
2,200
2,300

*A line joining your heart rate and actual oxygen
consumption will intersect the centre line at
your maximum oxygen consumption.*

Figure 17

Nomogram for Prediction of Maximum Oxygen Intake in Women Aged 45 and 55 Years

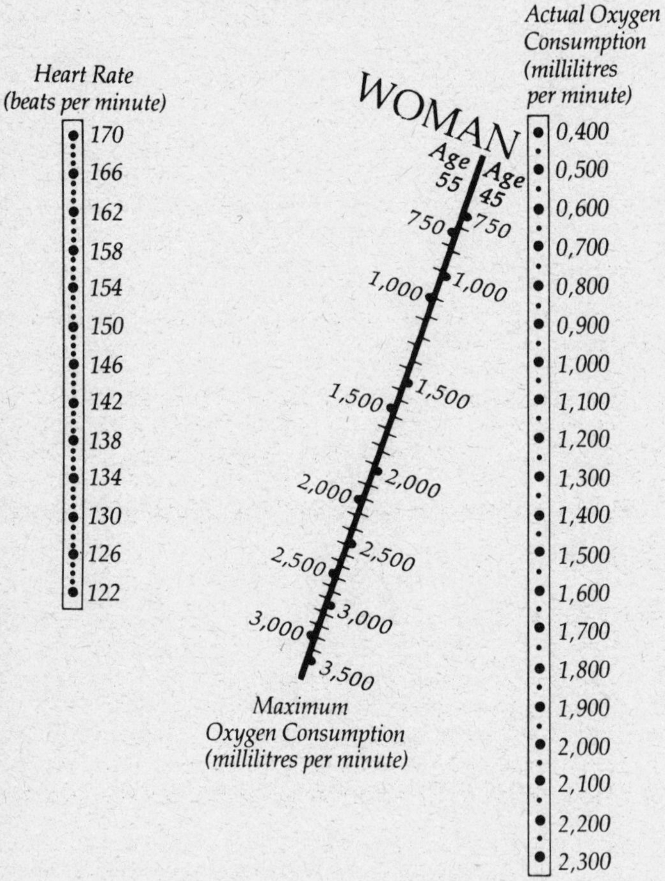

Heart Rate
(beats per minute)

- 170
- 166
- 162
- 158
- 154
- 150
- 146
- 142
- 138
- 134
- 130
- 126
- 122

WOMAN
Age 55   Age 45

750   750
1,000   1,000
1,500   1,500
2,000   2,000
2,500   2,500
3,000   3,000
3,500

Maximum
Oxygen Consumption
(millilitres per minute)

Actual Oxygen
Consumption
(millilitres
per minute)

- 0,400
- 0,500
- 0,600
- 0,700
- 0,800
- 0,900
- 1,000
- 1,100
- 1,200
- 1,300
- 1,400
- 1,500
- 1,600
- 1,700
- 1,800
- 1,900
- 2,000
- 2,100
- 2,200
- 2,300

A line joining your heart rate and actual oxygen consumption will intersect the centre line at your maximum oxygen consumption.

Appendix

Training Tables

To be used for determining your exercise prescription, *but* only after careful reading of the text.

If your predicted maximum oxygen consumption (VO_2 max.) is below 16 millilitres per kilogram per minute, or if you do not actually know what it is, begin at the Preliminary Phase, Level 1. If your maximum oxygen consumption is more than 16 millilitres per kilogram per minute, begin at the appropriate level in Phase 1 (see pages 124-25).

Ideally, in all Phases you should plan to exercise 5 times weekly.

Preliminary Phase

Levels to be taken in sequence.

Level 1   For 2 weeks walk 1 mile in 30 minutes
Level 2   For 2 weeks walk $1^1/_2$ miles in 42 minutes
Level 3   For 2 weeks walk 2 miles in 50 minutes
Level 4   For 2 weeks walk $2^1/_2$ miles in $57^1/_2$ minutes

When you have completed the Preliminary Phase progress to Phase 1, Level 1.

Phase 1

For instructions on progressing through the levels of Phase 1, see pages 121-22.

If you begin your exercise program at one of the levels in Phase 1 (see pages 124-25), do not attempt at first the full prescription for your starting level. Instead, start with one third the starting prescription (eg. at Level 1, walk 1 mile in 20 minutes if you are under age 45). After two weeks progress to two thirds the starting prescription (eg. 2 miles in 40 minutes, if under age 45 and at Level 1) for a further two weeks. Then, provided there are no adverse symptoms, proceed to the full three miles in the time prescribed for your starting level.

Level	Predicted maximum oxygen consumption (millilitres per kilogram per minute)	Distance (miles)	Time (minutes)	
			Under age 45	Over age 45
1	16.1 to 17.5 ml/kg/min	3	60	63
2	17.6 to 18.4 ml/kg/min	3	57	60
3	18.5 to 21.3 ml/kg/min	3	54	57
4	21.4 to 22.7 ml/kg/min	3	51	54
5	22.8 to 25.6 ml/kg/min	3	48	51
6	25.7 to 28.5 ml/kg/min	3	45	48
7	28.6 + ml/kg/min	3	42	45

When you have completed Phase 1, Level 7, progress to Phase 2, Level 1.

Phase 2

For instructions on progressing through the levels of Phase 2, see pages 122-23.

Level	Under age 45			Over age 45		
	Distance (miles)	Time (minutes)	Approx. Pace (mins/ mile)	Distance (miles)	Time (minutes)	Approx. Pace (mins/ mile)
1	$2^3/_4$	$36^1/_2$	$13^1/_4$	$2^3/_4$	41	$14^3/_4$
2	$2^3/_4$	35	$12^3/_4$	$2^3/_4$	39	$14^1/_4$
3	$2^3/_4$	34	$12^1/_4$	$2^3/_4$	$37^1/_2$	$13^1/_2$
4	$2^3/_4$	33	12	$2^3/_4$	$36^1/_2$	$13^1/_4$
5	$2^3/_4$	31	$11^1/_2$	$2^3/_4$	35	$12^3/_4$
6	$2^1/_2$	27	$10^3/_4$	$2^1/_2$	31	$12^1/_2$
7	$2^1/_2$	26	$10^1/_2$	$2^1/_2$	30	12
8	$2^1/_2$	25	10	$2^3/_4$	33	12
9	$2^3/_4$	$27^1/_2$	10	3	36	12
10	3	30	10	3	36	12
11	$3^1/_4$	$32^1/_2$	10	$3^1/_4$	39	12
12	$3^1/_2$	35	10	$3^1/_2$	42	12
13	$3^3/_4$	$37^1/_2$	10	$3^3/_4$	45	12
14	4	40	10	4	48	12

If you have completed Phase 2, Level 11, and are now an enthusiastic jogger, you may progress to Phase 3.

Phase 3

For instructions on progressing through the levels of Phase 3, see pages 123-24.

Level	Under age 45		Over age 45	
	Distance (miles)	Time (minutes)	Distance (miles)	Time (minutes)
1	$4^1/_4$	$42^1/_2$	$4^1/_4$	51
2	$4^1/_2$	45	$4^1/_2$	54
3	$4^3/_4$	$47^1/_2$	$4^3/_4$	57
4	5	50	5	60
5	$5^1/_2$	55	$5^1/_2$	66
6	6	60	6	72

The predicted maximum oxygen consumption figures used in the Training Tables are based on values obtained from routine use of a sub-maximum, 9-minute, bicycle ergometer stress test.

Wind Chill Factors

Wind Speed
mph (km/h)*   Temperature °F (°C)*

Calm	40 (5)	35 (2)	30 (−1)	25 (−3)	20 (−6)
5 (8)	35	30	25	20	15
10 (16)	30	20	15		
15 (24)	25	15			
20 (32)	20				
25 (40)	15				

Do not exercise out of doors
when the wind chill factor
is below the level indicated
to the left of the heavy line.

*Metric equivalents are approximate

SOURCE: Adapted from a chart by Dr. Charles Egan,
Colorado State University.

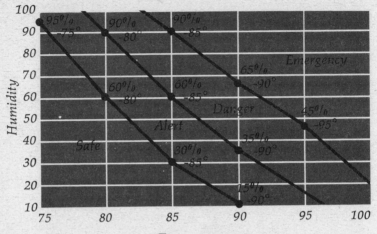

Heat Safety Index

(Chart: Humidity vs. Temperature)

- 95% −75°
- 90% −80°
- 90% −85°
- 60% −80°
- 60% −85°
- 65% −90°
- 45% −95°
- 30% −85°
- 35% −90°
- 15% −90°

Regions: Emergency, Danger, Alert, Safe

Y-axis: Humidity (10–100)
X-axis: Temperature (75–100)

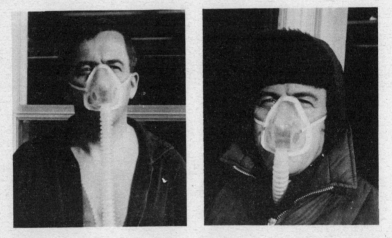

Cold Weather Jogging Mask

The mask is made by attaching a simple plastic disposable oxygen mask to twelve inches of flexible plastic tubing. (Hudson No. 7 aerosal mask and Bennet No. 0848 flexible tube, $3/4''$ x 12"). A moleskin strip glued to the inner margin of the mask helps to prevent freezing around the edges. The mask fits over the nose and mouth and is held firmly in place by an elastic headband. The tubing extends beneath the subject's T-shirt to about the lower part of the chest. With this device angina patients can continue their outdoor exercise throughout the year.

IDEAL WEIGHT

Height (no shoes) (in.)	MALE Weight (indoor clothing) (lbs.)	(kg.)	FEMALE Weight (indoor clothing) (lbs.)	(kg.)
60	—	—	110	50
61	124	56.2	113	51.3
62	127	57.6	116	52.6
63	130	59.0	120	54.4
64	133	60.3	123	55.8
64.5	135	61.2	125.5	56.9
65.0	137	62.1	128	58.1
65.5	139	63.1	130	59.0
66.0	141	64.0	132	59.9
66.5	143	64.9	134	60.8
67.0	145	65.8	136	61.7
67.5	147	66.7	138	62.6
68.0	149	67.6	140	63.5
68.5	151	68.5	142	64.4
69.0	153	69.4	144	65.3
69.5	155	70.3	146	66.2
70.0	157	71.2	148	67.1
70.5	159.6	72.4	150	68.0
71.0	162	73.5	152	68.9
71.5	164.7	74.7	—	—
72.0	167	75.8	—	—
72.5	169	76.7	—	—
73.0	171	77.6	—	—
73.5	173.5	78.7	—	—
74	176	79.8	—	—
75	181	82.1	—	—
76	186	84.5	—	—

Average "Ideal" Weights in Relation to Height and Sex for Persons of Medium Build

(Based on Data of Society of Actuaries, 1959, as modified by Shephard, 1972)

Recreational Activity and Fitness Levels

When you can comfortably carry out:		You can:
Under Age 45	*Over Age 45*	
Phase 1, Level 2	Phase 1, Level 3	play golf using an electric cart bowl play shuffleboard swim gently horseback ride (walk)
Phase 1, Level 5	Phase 1, Level 6	play golf, pulling club bag play horseshoes cycle leisurely play badminton; doubles and let the hard ones go horseback ride (trot) play ping pong (easy table-tennis!)
Phase 2, Level 2	Phase 2, Level 6	play golf (carry clubs) play badminton; singles, social play tennis; doubles, social play table tennis cycle (don't be in a hurry) ice skate canoe (leisurely)
Phase 2, Level 6	Phase 2, Level 10	downhill ski (leisurely) cycle (moderately) play singles tennis, socially play badminton, briskly
Phase 2, Level 8	Phase 2, Level 12	basketball (easy) horseback ride (gallop) cycle fast downhill ski (vigorous) canoe (5 mph)
Phase 2, Level 12	Phase 2, Level 14	play squash (social) fence basketball (vigorous)
Phase 2, Level 14		probably more than you ever tried before your heart attack!

Adapted from A.H.A. tables.

CATEGORY — *Please check your group*

Service ☐   C.S. ☐   8 week ☐

Day exercise ☐   Home ☐

Used at the Toronto Rehabilitation Centre

EXERCISE DIARY

NAME _____

Present Prescription _____

Resting pulse (average of 3 mornings) _____

Day	Date (mo./day)	Type of exercise	Distance (miles)	Duration (min./sec.)	10 sec. pulse count		Observations of any symptoms during exercise	Remarks
					Just before exercise	After exercise *within 10 sec*		

CATEGORY — *Please check your group*

Service ☐ C.S. ☑ 8 week ☐

Day exercise ☐ Home ☐

Used at the Toronto Rehabilitation Centre

EXERCISE DIARY

NAME _J. Doe_

Present Prescription _3-42_

Resting pulse (average of 3 mornings) _60_

Day	Date (mo./day)	Type of exercise	Distance (miles)	Duration (min./sec.)	10 sec. pulse count Just before exercise	10 sec. pulse count After exercise within 10 sec	Observations of any symptoms during exercise	Remarks
Sun	Feb 8	walk/Jog	3	42.15	11	19		
Mon	9	"	3	42.20	10	19		
Tues	10	"	3	42.0	11	18		
Wed	11	"	3	42.0	12	18	felt good	
Thur	12	"	R	E	S	T		
Fri	13	"	3	42.10	11	19		
Sat	14	"	R	E	S	T		
Sun	15	"	3	42.0	12	21	Slight tightness in chest	
Mon	16	"	3	41.50	11	21	no problems	
Tues	17	"	3	42.15	11	20	"	
Wed	18	"	3	42.15	11	20	"	
Thur	19	"	3	42.15	11	19		
Fri	20	"	R	E	S	T		
Sat	21	"	R	E	S	T		

The Sub-Maximal Exercise Test Customarily Used on the Toronto Program

Patients are exercised on a bicycle ergometer (Quinton Electric or Monark Mechanical). Testing commences at a moderate work intensity and, in the absence of contra-indications, proceeds through three stages, each of three minutes duration, to a final loading of 75% of estimated maximum oxygen consumption (as gauged from age-related maximum heart-rate tables).

Oxygen consumption is measured by a standard open circuit method with collection of expired gas in the final minute of each intensity of exercise. The maximum oxygen consumption is predicted from the work load and the oxygen scales of the Astrand nomogram. Comparison of this scale with direct treadmill measurement has shown this procedure to work well on patients familiar with the Centre staff and equipment.

Blood pressure is measured at rest, at the end of each work stage, at one minute and at four minutes of the recovery phase. The exercise E.C.G. is recorded prior to, during, and following exercise, using CM_5 leads. A resting twelve lead E.C.G. always precedes the test.

Predicted maximum oxygen consumption values obtained from the use of the above protocol forms the basis for the training table system used in the Toronto program. Ideally, therefore, the same testing procedure should be used to ensure accurate interpretation, and physicians who wish to apply the tables in their own cardiac exercise programs are reminded of this. However since this book is written primarily from the patient's viewpoint, as well as those medical personnel who have neither the time nor the equipment for gas analysis, the tables as outlined here are based on heart-rate/work load estimates of vo_2 max; in addition, for safety's sake the various levels of activity have been modified slightly in order to allow for consequent over-estimation of aerobic power.

References

1. Asmussen, E., and Molbech, S. V.: *Methods and Standards for Evaluation of Physiological Working Capacity of Patients.* Comm. Test. Obs. Inst., Hellerup, Denmark, No. 4. October 11, 1959.

2. Shephard, R. J.; Allen, C.; Benade, A. J. S.; Davies, C. T. M.; Di Prampero, P. E.; Hedman, R.; Merriman, J. E.; Myhre, K., and Simmons, R.: *Standardization of Submaximal Exercise Tests. Bull.* World Health Organization 38:765-775, 1968.

3. Astrand, I.: Aerobic Work Capacity in Men and Women with Special Reference to Age. *Acta Physiol. Scand.,* 49 (Suppl. 169), 1960.

4. Blackburn, H., Taylor, H. L., Okamoto, N., Rautaharju, P., Mitchell, P. L., and Kerkhof, A.: "Standardization of the exercise electrocardiogram: A systematic comparison of chest lead configuration employed for monitoring during exercise." In: *Physical Activity and the Heart* (Karvonen, M. J., Barry, A. J., ed) Thomas, Springfield, Illinois, 1967.

5. Kavanagh, T., and Shephard, R. J.: "Maximum Exercise Tests on 'Post-coronary' Patients." In: *Journal of Applied Physiology;* Vol. 40, Number 4: 611-618; April, 1976.

Constitution and Bylaws of the T.R.C. Joggers

The name of the Club shall be the T.R.C. Joggers.

The President shall be T. Kavanagh, M.D.; the Honorary Secretary Johanna Kennedy; the Captain shall be elected annually at or around the time of the Boston Marathon.

Active membership shall not exceed twenty, and is to be drawn from the ranks of the T.R.C. cardiac class.

The purpose of the Club is to maintain interest and provide motivation for long-distance jogging by regular meetings, training sessions, and entry in various road runs and races.

In view of the unique membership, the following rules are mandatory:

1. No member shall exceed his usual training level, enter or participate in any race, competition or road run, involve himself in any form of publicity venture, without the prior permission of the President. Anyone not adhering to the letter and spirit of these rules shall be automatically removed from Club membership. The President's decision shall be final in all matters to do with a member's entry or attempted level of performance in any event.

2. 'Second choice' club running is customarily not acceptable and in general will not be allowed where there is an element of risk involved because of the intensity of the competition, or where the nature of the performance would take rightful credit from the T.R.C. Joggers; judgment in these cases will be made by the Captain, Honorary Secretary, and President.

3. Persistent non-attendance at training sessions shall result in removal from Club membership.

4. Post-training refreshments, liquid and solid, shall be provided by equal contributions from all involved.

5. There shall be no fees for membership except those required by the Canadian Track & Field Association.

6. The Club First Crest shall be the Centre Phoenix, with the words 'T.R.C. Joggers' on a black vest with black shorts, red trim; the Second Crest shall be the Superman on a white vest, with green shorts, white trim. Track suits shall be green or black. The First Crest and uniform will be worn by all who have completed an official marathon run.

References

Prologue

Issekutz, B., Jr., Blizzard, J. J., Birkhead, N. C., and Rodahl, K.: Effect of prolonged bed rest on urinary calcium output. *Journal of Applied Physiology*, 21, 1013 – 1020, 1966.

Kavanagh, T., Shephard, R. J., Pandit, V. "Marathon running after myocardial infarction." *Journal of American Medical Association*, 229:1602, 1974.

Taylor, H. L., Henschel, J. B., and Keys, A.: Effects of bed rest on cardiovascular function and work performance. *Journal of Applied Physiology*, Volume II, No. 5., 223 – 239, November 1949.

Chapter one

Adelstein, A. M. "Some aspects of cardiovascular mortality in South Africa." *British Journal of Preventive Medicine*, 17:29 – 40, 1963.

Auerbach, O., Hammond, E. C., and Garfinkel, L. "Smoking in relation to atherosclerosis of the coronary arteries." *New England Journal of Medicine*, 273:775, 1965.

Clawson, B. J., and Bell, E. T. "Incidence of fatal coronary disease in non-diabetic and diabetic persons." *Archives of Pathology* (Chicago), 48:105, 1949.

The Coronary Drug Project Research Group: *Journal of the American Medical Association*, 231:360, 1975.

Cowie, J., Willett, R. W., Ball, K. P.: Carbon monoxide absorption by cigarette smokers who change to smoking cigars. *Lancet* 1:1033 – 1035, 1973.

Dawber, T. R., Kannel, W. B., Revotskie, N., and Kagan, A. *Proceedings of the Royal Society of Medicine*. 55:265, 1962.

Doll, R., and Hill, A. B. "Mortality in relation to smoking: Ten years observations of British doctors." *British Medical Journal*, 1:1399, 1460, 1964.

Enos, W. F., Beyer, J. C., Holmes, R. H. "Pathogenesis of coronary disease in American soldiers killed in Korea." *Journal of American Medical Association*, 158:912, 1955.

Fodor, J., Lamm, G., et al. "A co-operative trial in the primary prevention of ischaemic heart disease using clofibrate." *British Heart Journal*, 40:1069, 1978.

Gertler, M. M., and White, P. D. *Coronary heart disease in young adults. A multidisciplinary study.* Cambridge, Mass.: Harvard University Press, 1954.

Groom, D., McKee, E. E., Adkins, W., Pean, V., Hudicourt, E. "Developmental patterns of coronary and aortic atherosclerosis in young Negroes of Haiti and the United States." *Annals of Internal Medicine*, 61:900 – 913, 1964.

Hammond, E. C. "Smoking in relation to the death rates of one million men and women," in Haenszel, W. ed., *Epidemiological approaches to the study of cancer and other diseases.* Bethesda, Md.: U.S.

Public Health Service National Cancer Institute, Monograph No. 19, 127 – 204. January, 1966.

Hinkle, L. E., Jr., Whitney, L. H., Lehman, E. W., Dunn, J., Benjamin, B., King, R., Plakun, A., and Flehinger, B. "Occupation, education, and coronary heart disease." *Science,* 161:238, 1968.

Jenkins, C. D., Rosenman, R. H., and Friedman, M. "Development of an objective psychological test for the determination of the coronary-prone behaviour pattern in employed men." *Journal of Chronic Diseases* 20:371 – 79, 1967.

Kannel, W. B., Dawber, T. R., and McNamara, P. M. "Detection of the coronary-prone adult: The Framingham Study." *Journal of the Iowa Medical Society,* 56(1):26, 1966.

Kavanagh, T., Shephard, R. J. "The immediate antecedents of myocardial infarction in active men." *Canadian Medical Association Journal,* 109:19, July 1973.

Kavanagh, T., Shephard, R. J., Tuck, J. A. "Depression after myocardial infarction." *Canadian Medical Association Journal,* 113:23, July 1975.

Kershbaum, A., Bellet, S., Jimenez, J., and Feinberg, L. J. "Differences in effects of cigar and cigarette smoking on free fatty acid mobilization and catecholamine excretion." *Journal of American Medical Association,* 195:1095, 1966.

Keys, A. "Coronary heart disease in seven countries." *Circulation,* Supplement 1:41 – 42, 1970.

Lopez, A., Vial, R., Balart, L., Arroyave, G. "Effect of exercise and physical fitness on serum lipids and lipoproteins." *Atherosclerosis,* 20:1, 1974.

Marble, A. "Coronary artery disease in the diabetic." *Diabetes* 4:290, 1955.

McNamara, J., Molot, M., Stremple, J., *et al.* "Coronary artery disease in combat casualties in Vietnam." *Journal of American Medical Association,* 216:1185, 1971.

Mason, J. K. "Asymptomatic disease of coronary arteries in young men." *British Medical Journal,* 2:1234, 1963.

Medical News: *Journal of American Medical Association,* 232:1319 – 1320, June 30, 1975. Inhaled cigar smoke can be particularly hazardous.

Mitrani, Y., Karplus, H., and Brunner, D. *Coronary atherosclerosis in cases of sudden death; the influence of physical occupational activity on the development of coronary narrowing." Medicine and Sport,* 4: "Physical Activity and Ageing," 241 – 248. Basel/New York: Kargel, 1970.

Morris, J. N. "Towards Prevention – and Health." *Acta Medica Scandinavica Supplement,* 576:13 – 17, 1974.

Neufeld, H. N., Vlodaver, Z. "Structural changes in the coronary arteries of infants." *Proceedings of the Association of European Pediatric Cardiologists,* 4:35 – 39, 1968.

Nixon, P. G. F. "The human function curve." *Practitioner,* 217:765 and 935, 1976.

Osborn, G. R. *The incubation period of coronary thrombosis.* London: Butterworths. 1963.

Rose, G. "Cardiovascular mortality among American Negroes." *Archives of Environmental Health* (Chicago), 5:412 – 414, 1962.

Russek, H. I. "Emotional stress in the etiology of coronary heart disease." *Geriatrics* 22:84, 1967.

Stamler, J. "Atherosclerotic coronary heart disease – The major challenge to contemporary public health and preventive medicine." *Connecticutt Medicine,* 28:675, 1964.

Theorell, T., and Rahe, R. H. "Behavior and life satisfactions characteristics of Swedish subjects with myocardial infarction." *Journal of Chronic Diseases,* 25:139, 1972.

Wolf, S. *Stress and disease in society,* ed. L. Leui. London: Oxford University Press, 1971

Wood, P., Haskell, W., Klein, H., Lewis, S., *et al.* "The distribution of plasma lipoproteins in middle-aged male runners." *Metabolism,* 25(11) 1249 – 1257, 1976.

Chapter two

Birren, J. E., Butler, R. N., Greenhouse, S. W., Sokoloff, L., and Garrow, M. R. *Human ageing.* U.S. Dept. of Health, Education and Welfare. Public Health Services, Publication No. 986, 1963.

Bjorntorp, P., De Jounge, K., Sjostrom, L., and Sullivan, L. "The effect of physical training on insulin production in obesity." *Metabolism* 19: 631 – 638, 1970.

Boyer, J. L., Kasch, F. W. "Exercise therapy in hypertensive men." *Journal of American Medical Association,* 211:1668, 1970.

Brunner, D., and Manelis, G. "Myocardial infarction among members of communal settlements in Israel." *Lancet* 2:1049, 1960.

Brunner, D., Manelis, G., and Altman, S. "Physical activity lipoproteins and ischemic heart disease." *Pathologia microbiologia,* 30:648 – 652, (1967).

Carlson, L. A., and Mossfeldt, F. "Acute effects of prolonged, heavy exercise on the concentration of plasma lipids and lipoproteins in man." *Acta Physiologica Scandinavica,* 62:51 – 59, 1964.

Cash, J. D. "A new approach to studies of the fibrinolytic system in man." *American Heart Journal,* 75:424, 1968.

Cassel, J. C. "Summary of major findings of the Evans County cardiovascular studies." *Archives of Internal Medicine,* 128:887 – 889, 1971.

Chapman, J. M., Georke, L. S., Dixon, W., Loveland, D. B., and Phillips, E. "The clinical status of a population group in Los Angeles under observation for two to three years." *American Journal of Public Health* 47:33 – 42, 1957.

Choquett, G., Ferguson, R. J. "Blood pressure reduction in 'borderline' hypertensives following physical training." *Canadian Medical Association Journal,* 108:699, March 1973.

Cohen, M., and Goldberg, C. "Effect of physical exercise on alimentary lipaemia." *British Medical Journal*, 2:509 – 511, 1960.

Dill, D. B. "Marathoner DeMar: Physiological Studies." *Journal of the National Cancer Institute*, 35:185 – 191, 1965.

Fox, S. M., and Haskell, W. L. "Physical activity and health maintenance." *Journal of Rehabilitation* 32:89, 1966.

Frick, M. H. "Coronary implications of hemodynamic changes caused by physical training." *American Journal of Cardiology*, 22:417, 1968.

Frick, M. H. "Significance of bradycardia in relation to physical training," in *Physical activity and the heart*. Thomas: Springfield, 1967, 33 – 39.

Hall, V. E. "The relation of heart rate to exercise fitness; an attempt at physiological interpretation of the bradycardia of training." *Pediatrics*, 32. (Suppl):723, 1963.

Hames, C. G. "Evans County cardiovascular and cerebrovascular epidemiologic study: Introduction." *Archives of Internal Medicine*, 128:883 – 886, 1971.

Holmgren, A., Strandell, T. "The relationship between heart volume, total hemoglobin and physical working capacity in former athletes." *Acta. Med. Scandanavica* 163:149, 1959.

Iatridis, S. G., Ferguson, J. H. "Effect of physical exercise on blood clotting and fibrinolysis." *Journal of Applied Physiology*, 18:337, 1963.

Joslin, E. P., Root, M., White, P., and Marble, A. *Treatment of Diabetes Mellitus*. Philadelphia: Lea and Febiger, 1959.

Kahn, H. A. "The relationship of reported coronary heart disease mortality to physical activity of work." *American Journal of Public Health*, 53:1058, 1963.

Kavanagh, T. "A conditioning programme for the elderly." *Canadian Family Physician*, July 1971.

Kraus, H., Raab, W. *Hypokinetic Disease*. Springfield, 1961.

Larsson, Y., Sterky, G., Ekengren, K., and Moller, T. "Physical fitness and the influence of training in diabetic adolescent girls." *Diabetes*. 11:No. 2, 109, 1962.

Leaf, A. "Every day is a gift when you are over 100." *National Geographic*, 143: No. 1. 93 – 118. January 1973.

Mann, G. V., Shaffer, R. D., Anderson, R. S., and Sandstead, H. H. "Cardiovascular disease in the Masai." *Journal of Atherosclerosis Research* 4:289 – 312, 1964.

McDonough, J. R., Hames, C. G., Stulb, S. C., Garrison, G. E. "Coronary heart disease among negroes and whites in Evans County, Georgia." *Journal of Chronic Diseases*, 18:443 – 468, 1965.

Mellerowicz, H. "The effects of training on the heart and circulation," in *The Scientific View of Sport*. Berlin: Springer Verlag, 1972. 250 – 261.

Menon, I. S., Burke, F., and Dewar, H. A. "Effect of strenuous and graded exercise on fibrinolytic activity." *Lancet*, 1:700, 1967.

Morganroth, J., Maron, B. J., Henry, W. L., Epstein, S. E. "Comparative left ventricular dimensions in trained athletes." *Annals of Internal Medicine,* 82:4, April 1975.

Morris, J. N., Adam, C., Chave, S. P. W., Sirey, C., Epstein, L., Sheehan, D. J. "Vigorous exercise in leisure-time and the incidence of coronary heart disease." *Lancet,* 333-339, February 1973.

Morris, J. N., Heady, J. A., Raffle, P. A. B. "Physique of London busmen: Epidemiology of uniforms." *Lancet* 2:569 – 570, 1956.

Morris, J. N., Heady, J. A., Raffle, P. A. B., Roberts, C. G., and Parks, J. W. "Coronary heart disease and physical activity of work," *Lancet* 2:1053, 1953.

Nikkila, E. A., and Konttinen, A. "Effects of physical activity on postprandial levels of fats in serum." *Lancet* 1, 1151 – 1154, 1962.

Paffenbarger, R. S., Jr., Hale, W. E., Brand, R. J., *et al.* "Work-energy level, personal characteristics, and fatal heart attack: A birth-cohort effect." *American Journal of Epidemiology,* 105:200 – 213, 1977.

Paffenbarger, R. S., Wing, A. L. and Hyde, R. T. "Physical activity as an index of heart attack risk in college alumni." *American Journal of Epidemiology,* 108:161, 1978.

Raab, W. "Training, physical inactivity and the cardiac dynamic cycle. *Journal of Sports Medicine and Physical Fitness,* 6:38, 1966.

Saltin, B., and Astrand, P. O. "Maximal Oxygen Uptake in Athletes." *Journal of Applied Physiology* 23:353, 1967.

Siegel, W., Blomquist, G., and Mitchell, J. H. "Effects of a quantitated physical training programme on middle-aged sedentary men." *Circulation,* 41:19 – 29, 1970.

Snow, C. C. "Anthropologic and Physiologic observation – Tarahumara endurance runners," in *Symposium on Sports Medicine* (American Academy of Orthopaedic Surgeons, St. Louis: C. V. Mosby Co., 1969, 111 – 117.

Taylor, M. L., Klepetar, E., Keys, A., Parlin, W., Blackburn, H., and Puchner, T. "Death rates among physically active and sedentary employees of the railroad industry." *American Journal of Public Health,* 52:1967, 1962

Weinblatt, E., Shapiro, S., Frank, C. W. and Sager R. V. "Prognosis of men after first myocardial infarction: Mortality and first recurrence in relation to selected parameters." *American Journal of Public Health,* 58:1329, 1968.

Zukel, W. J., Lewis, R. H., Enterline, P. E., Painter, R. C., Ralston, L. S., Fawcett, R. M., Meredith, A. P., and Peterson, B. "A short-term community study of the epidemiology of coronary heart disease." *American Journal of Public Health* 49:1630, 1959.

Chapter three

Astrand, I., Astrand, P. O., and Rodahl, K. "Maximal heart rate during work in older men." *Journal of Applied Physiology,* 14:562, 1959.

Bengt., Saltin., and Per-Olog Astrand. "Maximal oxygen uptake in athletes." *Journal of Applied Physiology,* 23:No. 3. 353 – 358, September 1967.

Blackburn, H., Taylor, H. L., Okamoto, N., Rautaharju, P., Mitchell, P. L., Kerkhof, A. C. "Standardization of the exercise electrocardiogram: A systematic comparison of chest lead configurations employed for monitoring during exercise," in *Physical activity and the heart.* Springfield: Thomas, 1967, 101.

Carlsten, A., Grimby, G. *The Circulatory Response to Muscular Exercise in Man.* Springfield: Thomas, 1966.

Costill, D. L. "Physiology of Marathon Running." *Journal of the American Medical Association,* 221:No. 9, August 1972.

Doan, A. E., Peterson, D. R., Blackmon, J. R., Bruce, R. A. "Myocardial ischemia after maximal exercise in healthy men: A method for detecting potential coronary heart disease?" *American Heart Journal,* 69:11 – 21, 1965.

Eckstein, R. W. "Effect of exercise and coronary artery narrowing on coronary collateral circulation." *Circulation Research,* 5:230, 1957.

Ellestad, M. H., Wan, M. K. C. "Predictive implications of stress testing: Follow-up of 2700 subjects after maximum treadmill stress testing." *Circulation,* 51:363, February 1975.

Frick, M. H., Katila, M. "Hemodynamic consequences of physical training after myocardial infarction." *Circulation,* 37: February 1968.

Frick, M. H., Katila, M., Sjogren, A. L. "Cardiac function and physical training after myocardial infarction," in *Coronary heart disease and physical fitness.* Malmborg: Larsen, 1971, 43 – 47.

Harger, B. S., Miller, J. B., Thomas, J. C. "The caloric cost of running." *Journal of the American Medical Association,* 228:No. 4. 482 – 483. April 22, 1974.

Hinkle, L. E., Jr. Carver, S. T., Plakun, A. "Slow heart rates and increased risk of cardiac death in middle-aged men." *Archives of Internal Medicine,* 129:732, May 1972.

Kavanagh, T., Shephard, R. J. "The immediate antecedents of myocardial infarction in active men." *Canadian Medical Association Journal,* 109: July 7, 1973.

Kavanagh, T., Shephard, R. J., Doney, H., Pandit, V. "Intensive exercise in coronary rehabilitation." *Medicine and Science in Sports,* 5:No. 1, 34 – 39, 1973.

McDonough, J. R., Kusumi, F., Bruce, R. A. "Variations in maximal oxygen intake with physical activity in middle-aged men." *Circulation,* XLI:743, May 1970.

Paffenbarger, R. S., Jr. "Work activity and coronary heart mortality." *New England Journal of Medicine,* 292:11, 545 – 550, 1975.

Paffenbarger, R. S., Jr. Laughlin, M. E., Gima, A. S., and Black, R. A. "Work activity of longshoremen as related to death from coronary heart disease and stroke." *New England Journal of Medicine,* 282:1109, 1970.

Redwood, D. R., Rosing, D. R., Epstein, S. E. "Circulatory and symptomatic effects of physical training in patients with coronary artery disease and angina pectoris." *New England Journal of Medicine,* 286:959, May 1972.

Robb, G. P., Marks, H. H. "Latent coronary artery disease: Determination of its presence and severity by the exercise electrocardiogram." *The American Journal of Cardiology* 603 – 618, May 1964.

Sarnoff, S. J., Braunwald, E., Welch, G. H., Jr. Case, R. B., Stainsby, W. N., and Macruz, R. "Hemodynamic determinants of oxygen consumption of the heart with special reference to the tension-time index." *American Journal of Physiology.* 192:148, 1958.

Shephard, R. J. "Standard Tests of Aerobic Power," in *Frontiers of fitness.* Springfield: Thomas, 1971, 233 – 264.

Siegel, W., Blomquist, G., Mitchell, J. H. "Effects of a quantitated physical training programme on middle-aged sedentary men." *Circulation*, 41:19, 1970.

Sonnenblick, E. H., Ross, J., Jr. and Braunwald, E. "Oxygen consumption of the heart: Newer concepts of its multifactoral determination." *The American Journal of Cardiology*, 22:328, 1968.

Sonnenblick, E. H., Ross, J. Jr., Covell, J. W., Kaiser, G. A. and Braunwald, E. "Velocity of contraction as a determinant of myocardial oxygen consumption." *American Journal of Physiology*, 209:919, 1965.

Chapter four

Brunner, D., and Meshulam N. "Prevention of recurrent myocardial infarction by physical exercise." *Israel Journal of Medical Sciences*, 5:No. 4, 783 – 785, 1969.

Gottheiner, V. "Long range strenuous sports training for cardiac reconditioning and rehabilitation." *American Journal of Cardiology*, 22:426 – 435, 1968.

Hellerstein, H. K. "The effects of physical activity: Patients and normal coronary prone subjects." *Minnesota Medicine.* 52:1335 – 1341, 1969.

Hellerstein, H. K., Hornsten, T. R., Goldbarg, A., Burlando, A. G., Friedman, E. H., Hirsch, E. Z., Marik, S. "The influence of active conditioning upon subjects with coronary artery disease." *Canadian Medical Association Journal*, 96:March 25, 1967.

Kavanagh, T., Shephard, R. J. "Importance of physical activity in post-coronary rehabilitation." *American Journal of Physical Medicine*, 52:No. 6, 1973.

Kavanagh, T., and Shephard, R. J. "Physical exercise and post-coronary rehabilitation." *The Canadian Family Physician*, September 1975.

Kavanagh, T., Shephard, R. J., Doney, H., and Pandit, V. "Intensive exercise in coronary rehabilitation." *Medicine and Science in Sports*, 5:34 – 39, 1973.

Rechnitzer, P. A., Pickard, H. A., Paivio, A. U., Yuhasz, M. S., Cunningham, D. "Long term follow-up study of survival and recurrence rates following myocardial infarction in exercising and control subjects." *Circulation*, 45:853, April 1972.

Weinblatt, E., Shapiro, S., Frank, C. W., and Sager, R. U. "Prognosis of men after first myocardial infarction: mortality and first recurrence in relation to selected parameters." *American Journal of Public Health,* 58:1329 – 1347, 1968.

Chapter five

Astrand, Per-Olof Kaare Rodahl. "Nutrition and Physical Performance," in *Textbook of Work Physiology,* New York: McGraw-Hill, 1970.

Balke, B. "Biodynamics," Glasser, ed., *Medical Physics.* Chicago: Yearbook Publishers, 1960, 50 – 52.

Blankenhorn, D. "Evidence for regression-progression of atherosclerosis." Presented at the Ontario Heart Foundation International Symposium on Atherosclerosis, September 1, 1975.

Cooper, K. H. *The New Aerobics.* New York: Bantam Books, 1970.

Costill, D. L. "Metabolic responses during distance running." *Journal of Applied Physiology,* 28:No. 3, March 1970.

Costill, D. L., Bowers, R., Kammer, W. F. "Skinfold estimates of body fat among marathon runners." *Medicine and Science in Sports,* 2:No. 2, 93 – 95, Summer 1970.

Karvonen, M. J., Kentala, E., Mustala, O. "The effects of training on heart rate: A 'longitudinal' study." *Annales Medecine Experamentalis et Biological Fenniae.* 35:307 – 315, 1957.

Katila, M., and Frick, M. H. "A two-year circulatory follow-up of physical training after myocardial infarction." *Acta Medica Scandinavica,* 187:95 – 100, 1970.

Physical Fitness Research Digest. Series 4, No. 3, July 1974. *Circulatory-Respiratory Endurance Improvement.* Published by President's Council on Physical Fitness and Sports.

Pollock, M. L. "The quantification of endurance training programmes." Jack H. Wilmore, ed, *Exercise and Sports Sciences Reviews,* New York Academic Press, 1973.

Pollock, M. L., Broida, J., Kendrick, Z., Miller, H. S., Jr. Janeway, R., Linnerud, A. C. "Effects of training two days per week at different intensities on middle-aged men." *Medicine and Science in Sports,* 4:192 – 197, 1972.

Puranen, J., Ala-Ketola, L., Peltokallio, P., Saarela, J. "Running and primary osteoarthritis of the hip." *British Medical Journal,* 424 – 425, 24 May, 1975.

Rapaport, E. "Exercise responses in patients with heart failure or valvular or congenital heart disease." *Journal of the South Carolina Medical Association,* p. 61. Supplement, 1969.

Selvester, Ronald H. "Exercise and/or coronary by-pass surgery." Presented at the International Symposium on Exercise and Coronary Artery Disease, Toronto, October 17 and 18, 1975.

Shephard, R. J. "Exercise test methodology," in *Coronary Disease,* Denver, Col.: Dept. of Professional Education International Medical Corporation.

Shephard, R. J. "Intensity, duration, and frequency of exercise as determinants of the response to a training regime." *Internationale Zeitschrift für Angewandte Physiologie Einschliesslich Arbeitsphysiologie,* 32:1973.

Wright, V., Dowson, D., Unsworth, A. "The lubrication and stiffness of joints," in *Modern Trends in Rheumatology* No. 2. London: Butterworths, 1971, 30.

Chapter six

Abelmann, W. H. "Virus and the heart." *Circulation*, 44:950 – 955, November, 1971.

"Alcoholic Cardiomyopathy." *British Medical Journal*, 731, December 28, 1974.

Barnard, R. J., et al. "Cardiovascular response to sudden strenuous exercise-heart rate, blood pressure and electrocardiogram." *Journal of Applied Physiology*, 34:p. 833, 1973.

Bowerman, W. J., Harris, W. E. *Jogging*. New York: Grosset and Dunlap, 1967.

Bruce, R. A. "Prevention and control of cardiovascular complications," in *Exercise testing and exercise training in coronary heart disease*. Naughton and Hellerstein, 1973. 355 – 363.

Bruce, R. A., Hornsten, T. R., Blackmon, J. R. "Myocardial infarction after normal responses to maximal exercise." *Circulation*, 38:552 – 558, September 1968.

Bruce, R. A., Lind, A. R., Franklin, D., Muir, A. L., Macdonald, H. R., McNicol, G. W., and Donald, K. W. "The effects of digoxin on fatiguing static and dynamic exercise in man." *Clinical Science*, 34:29 – 42, 1968.

Cooper, K. H. "Effects of cigarette smoking on endurance performance." *Journal of American Medical Association*, 203:p. 189, 1968.

Cooper, K. H. *The New Aerobics*. New York: Bantam Books, 1970.

Costill, D. L., Kamer, W. F., Fisher, A. "Fluid ingestion during distance running." *Archives of Environmental Health*, 21:October 1970.

Dill, D. B. "Oxygen used in horizontal and grade walking and running on the treadmill." *Journal of Applied Physiology*, 20: No. 1. 19 – 22, 1965.

Elisberg, E. I. "Heart rate response to the valsalva maneuver as a test of circulatory integrity," *Journal of the American Medical Association*, 186:200, 1963.

Hattenhauer, M., Neill, W. A. "The effect of cold air inhalation on angina pectoris and myocardial oxygen supply." *Circulation*, 51:1053 – 1058. June 1975.

Hill, A. V. "The air resistance to a runner," in *Proceedings of the Royal Society*, London, Series B, 102:380 – 385, 1928.

Horwitz, L. D. "Alcohol and heart disease." *Journal of American Medical Association*, 232:No. 9, June 2, 1975.

Kavanagh, T. "A cold weather 'jogging mask' for angina patients." *Canadian Medical Association Journal*, 103:December 5, 1970.

Kavanagh, T., Shephard, R. J. "Conditioning of post-coronary patients: Comparison of continuous and interval training." *Archives of Physical Medicine and Rehabilitation*, 56:No. 2. February 1975.

Kavanagh, T., Shephard, R. J. "Physical exercise and post coronary rehabilitation." *Canadian Family Physician*, September 1975.

Kavanagh, T., Shephard, R. J. "Maintenance of hydration in 'post-coronary' marathon runners." *British Journal of Sports Medicine*, 9:No. 3. October 1975.

Kavanagh, T., Shephard, R. H., Pandit, V., "Marathon running after myocardial infarction." *Journal of the American Medical Association*, 229:No. 12, September 16, 1974.

Knochel, J. P. "Environmental heat illness: An eclectic review." *Archives of Internal Medicine*, 133:May 1974.

Kozlowski, S., Saltin, B. "Effect of sweat loss on body fluids." *Journal of Applied Physiology*, 19:1119 – 1124, 1964.

Lord Moran. *Winston Churchill*. London: Constable, 1966.

Nies, A. S., Shand, D. G. "Clinical Pharmacology of Propranolol." *Circulation*, 52:No. 1. p. 6., July 1975.

Pugh, L. G. C. E. "Oxygen intake in track and treadmill running with observations on the effect of air resistance." *Journal of Physiology*, 207:823 – 835, 1970.

Pugh, L. G. C., Corbett, J. L., Johnson, R. H." Rectal temperatures, weight losses, and sweat rates in marathon running." *Journal of Applied Physiology*, 23:No. 3, September 1967.

Saltin, B. "Circulatory response to submaximal and maximal exercise after thermal dehydration." *Journal of Applied Physiology*, 19:1125 – 1132, 1964.

Selye, H. *The Stress of Life*. New York: McGraw-Hill, 1956.

Society of Actuaries. *Build and Blood Pressure Study*. Chicago, Ill., 1959.

Taggart, P., Parkinson, P., Carruthers, M. "Cardiac responses to thermal, physical, and emotional stress. *British Medical Journal*, July 8, 1972.

Timmis, G. C., Ramos, R. C., Gordon, S., Gangadharan, V. "The basis for differences in ethanol-induced myocardial depression in normal subjects." *Circulation*, 51:No. 6, 1144 – 1148, June 1975.

Tuttle, W. W., Horvath, S. M. "Comparison of effects of static and dynamic work on blood pressure and heart rate." *Journal of Applied Physiology*, 10:p. 294, 1957.

"Viruses and the Heart." *British Medical Journal*, No. 5958, 589, March 15, 1975.

Wyndham, C. H., Strydom, N. B. "The danger of an inadequate water intake during marathon running." *South African Medical Journal*, July 1969, 893.

Chapter seven

Anderson, T. W. "Serum electrolytes and skeletal mineralization in hard-and-soft-water areas." *Canadian Medical Journal*, 107:34 – 37, July 8, 1972.

Anderson, T. W., Beaton, G. H., Corey, P. N., Spero, L. "Winter illness and Vitamin C: the effect of relatively low doses." *Canadian Medical Journal*, 112:823 – 826, April 5, 1975.

Anderson, T. W., and Le Riche, W. H. "Sudden death from ischemic heart disease in Ontario and its correlation with water hardness and other factors." *Canadian Medical Association Journal,* 105:155 – 160, July 24, 1971.

Anderson, T. W., LeRiche, W. H., Mackay, J. S. "Sudden death and ischemic heart disease: correlation with hardness of local water supply." *New England Journal of Medicine,* 805 – 807, April 10, 1969.

Anderson, T. W., Neri, L. C., Schreiber, G. B., Talbot, F. D. F., Zdrojewski, A. "Ischemic heart disease, water hardness and myocardial magnesium." *Canadian Medical Journal,* 113:199 – 203, August 9, 1975.

Asmussen, E. "Some physiological aspects of fitness for sport and work," in *Proceedings of the Royal Society of Medicine,* Symposium No. 11: "The Meaning of Physical Fitness," 62:November 1969.

Bartlett, R. G., Jr. "Physiologic responses during coitus." *Journal of Applied Physiology,* 9:469 – 472, 1956.

Bruche, Hilde. "Energy expenditure of obese children," *American Journal of Diseases of Children,* 60:No. 5, 1082, November 1940.

Burkitt, D. P. "Some diseases characteristic of modern western civilization." *British Medical Journal,* 1:274 – 278, February 3, 1973.

Carruthers, M., Taggart, P. "Paleocardiology and neocardiology." *American Heart Journal,* 48:1 – 6, 1974.

Corrigan, J. J. Jr., Marcus, F. I. "Coagulopathy associated with vitamin E ingestion." *Journal of the American Medical Association,* 230:No. 9, 1300 – 1303, December 1974.

Costill, D. L., Fox, E. "Energetics of marathon running." *Medicine and Science in Sports,* 1:No. 2, 81 – 86, June, 1969.

Hellerstein, H. K., Friedman, E. H. "Sexual activity and the postcoronary patient." *Archives of Internal Medicine,* 125:June, 1970.

Herbert, V. H., Jacob, E. "Destruction of Vitamin B_{12} by ascorbic acid." *Journal of the American Medical Association,* 230:No. 2, October 14, 1974.

Karpannen, H., Neuvonen, P. J. "Ischaemic heart-disease and soil magnesium in Finland." *Lancet,* December 15, 1973.

Kavanagh, T., Shephard, R. J. "Depression after myocardial infarction." *Canadian Medical Association Journal,* 113:23, July 12, 1975.

Keys, A. "Sucrose in the diet and coronary heart disease." *Atherosclerosis,* 14:193, 1971.

Knox, E. G. "Ischaemic-heart-disease mortality and dietary intake of calcium." *Lancet,* June 30, 1973.

Kostrubala, T. "Slow long distance running as a form of psychotherapy." Paper delivered at the Third Annual Honolulu Symposium on the Athletic Heart. American Medical Joggers Association, December 12, 1975.

Mayer, J. *Overweight: Causes, cost, and control.* Englewood Cliffs, N.J.: Prentice-Hall, Inc., 1968.

O'Leary, A. N. "An assessment of patients activity, knowledge and anxiety, after aortic-valve replacement." Paper presented at the annual meeting of the Canadian Cardiovascular Association, Winnipeg, October 1974.

Pauling, Linus. *Vitamin C and the common cold.* San Francisco: W. H. Freeman, 1970.

Shaper, A. G. "Soft water, heart attacks and stroke." *Journal of the American Medical Association,* October 7, 1974.

Taggart, P., Carruthers, M., Somerville, W. "Electrocardiograph, plasma catecholamines and lipids and their modification by oxyprenolol when speaking before an audience." *Lancet* II, 341 – 346, 1973.

Tooshi, Ali. "Effects of Three Different Durations of Endurance Training on Serum Cholesterol, Body Composition, and Other Fitness Measures," Doctoral Dissertation, University of Illinois, 1970.

Yudkin, J. *Sweet and Dangerous.* New York: Bantam Books, 1973.

Chapter eight

Engel, H. J., Page, H. L. Jr., Campbell, W. B. "Coronary artery disease in young women." *Journal of American Medical Association,* 230:No. 11, December 16, 1974.

Kavanagh, T., Shephard, R. J. "The immediate antecedents of myocardial infarction in active men." *Canadian Medical Association Journal,* 109: July 7, 1973.

Mann, J. I., et al. "Myocardial infarction in young women with special reference to oral contraceptive practice." *British Medical Journal,* Vol. 2, No. 5965, 241 – 245, 1975.

Mann, J. I., Thorogood, M., Waters, W. E., Powell, C. "Oral contraceptives and myocardial infarction in young women: a further report." *British Medical Journal,* 3:No. 5984, 605 – 660, 1975.

Chapter nine

Cobb, L. A., Baum, R. S., Alvarez, H., *et al.* "Resuscitation from out of the hospital ventricular fibrillation: four years follow-up." *Circulation,* 52(Suppl. III):223 – 228, 1975.

Haskell, W. "Cardiovascular complications during exercise training of cardiac patients." *Circulation,* 57(5):920 – 924, 1978.

Jokl, E., Melzer, L. "Acute fatal non-traumatic collapse during work and sport," in *Exercise and cardiac death,* ed: E. Jokl, J. T. McLellan. *Medicine and Sport,* Vol. 5. Baltimore, London, Tokyo; University Park Press, 1971, p. 12.

Levy, R. I., "Progress towards prevention of cardiovascular disease: A thirty year retrospective." *Circulation,* 60(7):1555 – 1558, 1979.

Vuori, I., Makarainen, M. and Jaaskelainen, A. "Sudden death and physical activity." *Cardiology,* 63:287-304, 1978.

Yater, W. M., Traum, A. H., Brown, W. G., *et al.* "Coronary artery disease in men 18-39 years of age. *American Heart Journal,* 36:334, 1948.

Chapter ten

Kavanagh, T. and Shephard, R. J. "Fluid and mineral needs of post-coronary distance runners," in *Sports Medicine*, ed. F. Landry and W. A. R. Orban. Miami: Symposia Specialists, 1978, pp. 143 – 151.

Kavanagh, R., Shephard R. J. and Kennedy, J. "Characteristics of Postcoronary Marathon Runners." *Annals of the New York Academy of Science*, 301:455 – 465, 1977.

Noakes, T. D., Obie, L. H., Rose, A. G., et al. "Autopsy-proved coronary atherosclerosis in marathon runners." *New England Journal of Medicine*, 301(2):86 – 89, 1979.

Epilogue

Biddulph, L. G. "Athletic achievement and the personal and social adjustment of high school boys." *Research Quarterly* 25 (1):1, 1954.

Booth, E. G. "Personality traits of athletes as measured by the MMPI." *Research Quarterly* 29(1):27, 1958.

Bucher, C. A. "Health, physical education, and academic achievement." *National Education Association Journal* 54:38 – 40, 1965.

Kavanagh, T., Shephard, R. J., Chisholm, A., et al. "Prognostic indexes for patients with ischemic heart disease enrolled in an exercise-centered rehabilitation program." *American Journal of Cardiology*, 44(7):1230 – 1240, 1979.

"Report of the joint working party of the Royal College of Physicians of London and the British Cardiac Society on rehabilitation after cardiac illness." *Journal of the Royal College of Physicians of London*, 9:281, 1975.

Index

actin, *55-56*
adenosine triposphate (ATP), *56*,
57, 58
adrenaline, *44, 47*
air pollution, *228-30;*
  carbon monoxide, *155-56, 228-29*
  ozone, *229-30*
alcohol, *166, 171*
American Medical Joggers
  Association, *53, 184-85*
Anderson, Dr. Terry, *177, 180-81*
anemia, *61, 116*
aneurysm, *25, 111-13*
angina pectoris, *23-24, 73, 75-76,*
  113, 154, 171;
  and overtraining, *149*
  and training, *136-38, 152-53*
anti-angina mask, *7, 154, 215, 243*
  See also Jogging
arteriovenous oxygen difference
  (avO₂), *61*
ascorbic acid, *177-78*
asynergy (of cardiac muscle), *74*
atherosclerosis, *22-23, 174-75;*
  and acute exercise, *72-74*
  and cholesterol, *31-40*
  development of, *28*
  and diabetes, *43*
  and sympathetic activity, *63*
  See also Coronary artery disease

Balke, Dr. Bruno, *124-25*
Bannister, Dr. Roger, *69*
Bassler, Dr. Thomas, *184-85,*
  261-62
Beta-blockers, *156-57*
Bigelow, Dr. William, *186*
blood fats levels, *35-37, 40-42,*
  67, 75
blood pressure, *63, 66, 71;*
  during acute exercise, *72-73*
  and heart disease, *31, 50, 75, 189*
  inappropriate response to
  exercise, *88-89*
Boston Marathon, *1, 2, 3, 5-12, 28,*
  198, 260, 284-85
  training for (1973), *6-8*
Bowerman, William, *143, 161*
bradycardia, *62-63, 65, 75, 114,*
  131, 150, 157
Bruce, Dr. Robert, *89, 158*
Brunner, Dr. Daniel, *47, 48, 99, 101*

"bulk" diets, *178-79*
Burkitt, Dr. Dennis, *178-79*

carbohydrate loading, *273-75*
cardiac arrest, *24-25*
Chisholm, Dr. A. W., *102*
cholesterol, *31-42, 50, 66, 67,*
  162, 177, 179
  See also lipoprotein, triglyceride
collaterals, *75-76*
contra-indications to exercise,
  111-17;
  acute heart failure, *112*
  anemia, *116*
  aneurysm, *112*
  anginal pain, *113*
  arthritis, *116*
  blood clots, *114*
  congenital heart disease, *115*
  diabetes, *115*
  epilepsy, *115*
  fever, *113, 114*
  heart block, *114*
  high blood pressure, *115*
  irregular heart action, *113-14*
  low back trouble, *116*
  myocarditis, *113*
  pneumothorax, *115*
  valvular heart disease, *114*
Cooper, Dr. Kenneth, *125, 143*
coronary arteries, *22-23, 65*
coronary artery disease, *17, 22-23*
  and chronic exercise, *75-77*
  epidemiology of, *25-27, 29-31*
  latent, diagnosis of, *90-91*
  medication for, *156-57*
  in post-menopausal women, *190*
  and physical activity, *47-51,*
  62-66
  risk factors, *27-45*
  See also Atherosclerosis
coronary by-pass surgery, *186-87,*
  284

dehydration, *230-38, 276;*
  heat cramps, *233-34*
  heat exhaustion, *234-35*
  heat stroke, *235-36*
  and jogging deaths, *257*
denial, of heart attack, *20, 21, 108*
depression, *20, 21, 101, 139, 172-73,*
  193-94, 195, 248